Exploitation and Developing Countries

Exploitation and Developing Countries

The Ethics of Clinical Research

*Edited by Jennifer S. Hawkins
and Ezekiel J. Emanuel*

Princeton University Press   *Princeton & Oxford*

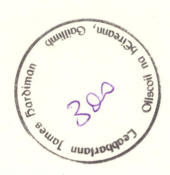

Copyright © 2008 by Princeton University Press

Published by Princeton University Press, 41 William Street,
Princeton, New Jersey 08540
In the United Kingdom: Princeton University Press, 6 Oxford Street,
Woodstock, Oxfordshire OX20 1TW

All Rights Reserved

ISBN: 978-0-691-12675-3
ISBN (pbk.): 978-0-691-12676-0

Library of Congress Control Number: 2008928581

British Library Cataloging-in-Publication Data is available

This book has been composed in Adobe Caslon

Printed on acid-free paper ∞

press.princeton.edu

Printed in the United States of America

1 3 5 7 9 10 8 6 4 2

*To our wonderful colleagues who have helped educate us by pondering
and wrestling with the complex ethical issues
related to research in developing countries*

CHRISTINE GRADY
REIDAR LIE
FRANKLIN MILLER
HENRY RICHARDSON
GOPAL SREENIVASAN
DAVID WENDLER
ALAN WERTHEIMER

Introduction: Why Exploitation?

JENNIFER S. HAWKINS AND EZEKIEL J. EMANUEL

Introduction

The first effective intervention that could dramatically reduce the risk that an HIV-infected woman would pass the virus to her baby was discovered in 1994.[1] The intervention was tested in the AIDS Clinical Trial Group (ACTG) Study 076 and came to be known in the medical community as "the 076 regimen." This regimen was both costly and complicated, involving large quantities of AZT (the trade name for the drug zidovudine) administered in an elaborate schedule. A pregnant HIV-infected woman receiving the 076 regimen was required to begin treatment in the second trimester of pregnancy, so that she would receive the drug for a minimum of twelve weeks. During this time, she took oral AZT five times a day. During labor the woman received intravenous AZT; and for six weeks after delivery the woman's newborn received oral AZT four times a day. A woman following the regimen was not allowed to breast-feed.[2] In 1994, the average cost for the full regimen was $1,000 (U.S.) per woman.[3]

Despite the regimen's cost and complexity, the discovery was a huge breakthrough. The 076 regimen reduced the rate of maternal-fetal HIV transmission by 70 percent, from a baseline rate of 25 percent to a rate of 8 percent.[4] Within a few months of these findings, the U.S. Public Health Service recommended that the 076 regimen be recognized as the new standard of care for HIV-infected pregnant women.[5]

This discovery meant little, however, to most HIV-infected pregnant women, since the vast majority of these women live in developing countries.[6] The annual health budget of these countries is approximately $10 per person.[7] In some cases, available funding is even lower. For example,

in Uganda, the annual health expenditure in the mid-1990s was estimated to be under $3 per person per year.[8] So a treatment regimen that
cost $1,000 per person was not—and still is not—even on the list of re-
mote possibilities. Beyond cost, delivery of the 076 regimen was not
practically feasible in many developing countries—or regions of countries. Most women in such areas do not present for prenatal care until
much further along in pregnancy than required by the twelve weeks of
the original regimen. In many places, there are no facilities for giving intravenous AZT. Most births occur at home. Finally, most women have
no choice but to breast-feed their newborns, since they are unable to
afford baby formula and/or unable to obtain safe drinking water to mix
with the formula.[9]

Nevertheless, the urgent need for some solution to the problem of
maternal-fetal HIV transmission in developing countries, particularly
in Africa, was widely recognized. In the mid-1990s, approximately 1,000
HIV-infected babies were being born each day.[10] And to this day, women
in the developing world "infected through heterosexual sex, are the
fastest growing group with HIV infection, and infected women are the
principle source of infected children."[11]

In June 1994, the World Health Organization held a meeting to discuss strategies for discovering an effective and affordable approach to
the problem of maternal-fetal HIV transmission in developing countries. At that meeting, it was concluded that the best approach was to do
randomized controlled trials (RCTs) of shorter and simpler regimens of
AZT versus placebo controls.[12] Consequently, sixteen trials were designed and approved to be conducted in eleven countries: Burkina Faso,
the Dominican Republic, Ethiopia, Ivory Coast, Kenya, Malawi, South
Africa, Tanzania, Thailand, Uganda, and Zimbabwe.[13] Of these sixteen trials, fifteen used placebo controls, of which nine were funded by
the National Institutes of Health (NIH) and the Centers for Disease
Control (CDC), with five funded by governments other than the United
States and one by the Joint United Nations Programme on HIV/AIDS
(UNAIDS).

It was the fact that fifteen of these trials utilized a placebo control
that first spurred ethical criticism. Controversy erupted into public awareness in 1997, when two researchers from the Public Citizen's Health
Research Group, Peter Lurie and Sidney Wolfe, wrote a letter to the

U.S. secretary of health and human services, Donna Shalala, and followed up with a commentary in the *New England Journal of Medicine*.[14] In both the letter and the commentary, they condemned the NIH- and CDC-sponsored trials as unethical. Simultaneously, Marcia Angell, the executive editor of the *New England Journal of Medicine*, published an editorial strongly supporting Lurie and Wolfe's position and comparing the AZT trials to the infamous Tuskegee studies of untreated syphilis in poor African American men in rural Alabama.[15] These articles sparked an intense and often heated public discussion of the ethical status of placebo-controlled trials in developing countries.

From the very beginning, opinions were deeply divided over these trials. Two members of the *New England Journal of Medicine* editorial board, both of whom were experts on HIV and HIV research, resigned over Marcia Angell's editorial.[16] Harold Varmus, then director of NIH, and David Satcher, then director of CDC, wrote a reply defending the trials as ethical and arguing that the use of placebos was justified by the complexities of the situations in the countries under study and by the urgent needs of these countries.[17] Two prominent bioethics journals—*Bioethics* and the *Hastings Center Report*—devoted whole issues to the debate, with prominent bioethicists writing articles on both sides of the case.[18] From then right up until now, the medical and bioethical literature has been inundated with discussion of the case.

When controversy first erupted, discussion of the ethical problems was confused. Many different arguments were conflated, without clear distinctions being made. With the passage of time and deeper reflection, however, the concerns of ethicists have resolved themselves into three major categories—all of which have relevance far beyond the original maternal-fetal transmission studies that sparked the debate.

Standard of Care and the Ethics of Study Design

Critics of the original AZT trials argued that these trials revealed the application of a morally insidious double standard, since they used placebo controls despite the fact that researchers would not have been allowed *for ethical reasons* to run a placebo trial of AZT in the developed world.[19] After 1994 the 076 regimen was the standard of care in developed countries. This meant that using placebo controls in further transmission studies in (for example) the United States would be unethical, since one significant norm of developed world research ethics requires that in most cases placebo controls not be used once some form of effective therapy exists for the illness or condition being studied. The critics argued that if placebo controls were unethical in developed countries such as the United States, Canada, or the countries of Western Europe, then they must also be unethical in developing countries such as Zimbabwe and Uganda. The criticism was that the choice of placebo controls revealed a lowering of ethical standards, which in turn reflected a lack of equal concern for the welfare of these subjects.

The critics were correct to point out that developed world researchers generally do not use placebo controls once some form of effective treatment exists for the condition or illness being studied.[20] There are, however, recognized exceptions to this rule as, for example, when participants are unlikely to suffer any long-term ill effects from receiving placebo. Still, at the time, critics felt that none of the standard exceptions applied to the AZT perinatal transmission trials.

In addition, some critics cited a provision in the Declaration of Helsinki to justify their objections. This provision, while supporting their favored conclusion in the AZT case, is also very strong. It does not, for example, recognize even the standard exceptions to the rule against placebo use mentioned above. This provision states: "In any medical study, every patient, including those of a control group, if any, should be assured of the best proven diagnostic and therapeutic method."[21] Those critics (such as Lurie, Wolfe, and Angell) who relied most heavily on this provision of Helsinki, felt that once the 076 regimen was proven effective in 1994, every patient in a subsequent research trial should be assured of receiving 076 or a better treatment.

On the other side, defenders of the trials emphasized that placebo controls offered the best way of answering a question that was itself largely dictated by the poor economic circumstances of those being studied. Thus for them, the ethical question was: Could features of the economic and health delivery situation in developing countries justify departure from the norm? Economic constraints were clearly perceived as irrelevant by the critics. But defenders felt that this view was too rigid. They felt that, in this case at least, the answer to the above question was yes.

Defenders pointed out that different trial designs are used to answer different types of questions. The economic constraints such countries face mean that their governments need answers to questions that people in developed countries, with access to the 076 regimen, do not. Only by using placebo controls, it was argued, could information that would actually be useful to the populations being studied be generated. Hence, defenders argued that talk of "double standards" was out of place in discussions of the perinatal trials. It is precisely because all is *not equal* between developing countries and developed countries—because 076 is not affordable there, because women in these settings arrive for care only at the point of delivery, and because intravenous methods of delivery are not feasible in these settings—that it was deemed necessary to find a regimen both cheaper and simpler to administer.

Perhaps most significantly, researchers were open from the beginning to the idea that what they were searching for *was a less effective, but still somewhat effective regimen*.[22] If indeed shorter courses of AZT were likely to be less effective than the 076 regimen, then only a placebo trial could answer the question of *how much more effective than nothing* the alternative regimen was. And this information would, in turn, be key to health policy decision making posttrial.

It is important to emphasize that the defenders of this trial did not think that the importance of a particular research question could justify *just any* treatment of subjects.[23] Rather, they felt that it could justify the use of placebo in these particular settings, given that these people *would otherwise receive no treatment at all*. They clearly recognized that, with these designs, some participants would not benefit as much as they might have, had they been in an active-controlled trial. But they felt that this was morally acceptable as long as (1) using placebo controls was necessary in order to gain the knowledge sought, and (2) no participant was made worse off by participating in the trial than she otherwise would have been.

Controversy over study design also led to controversy over the Declaration of Helsinki. Defenders of the AZT trial noted that requiring that *every* trial participant receive the "best proven therapy" was deeply problematic. If interpreted literally it actually precluded *any* randomized trial—even an active-controlled trial—once an effective therapy was available. After all, testing the 076 regimen against any newer treatment would have meant depriving the participants receiving the new treatment of "the best proven" treatment, for only the 076 regimen was the *best proven* treatment—the new one was not proven.

However, even if interpreted simply as a requirement *on what control group members must receive*, as many people appear to have interpreted it, the requirement was thought to rule out far too many perfectly acceptable trials.[24] In 2000, after extended international discussion, the declaration was modified but in a way that ultimately reasserted the original strong position.[25] Since then, however, various other significant health policy groups, including UNAIDS, Council for International Organizations of Medical Sciences (CIOMS), the Nuffield Council, and the National Bioethics Advisory Commission (NBAC), have rejected the Helsinki "best proven" requirement, and some have argued that the strong Helsinki view has now emerged as the minority view.[26] However, the debate over what guidelines should replace the "best proven" guideline continues.

The debate just described—which has come to be known as "the standard of care debate"—is one about the *ethics of study design*. It is important to remember this because developing world research raises more questions about ethical study design than just the questions about placebo use described earlier. The particular needs of the developing world challenge the received wisdom about ethical study design on a number of fronts, and it is important that we not let the placebo issue blind us to these other real problems. For example, there are many diagnostic and therapeutic interventions that could be used in research studies, and which for various reasons researchers might wish to use, that are *less effective* than standard interventions employed in developed countries. For instance, in the developed world, response to antiretroviral drugs is measured in terms of CD4 counts or viral loads. But would it be unethical—would it reveal the presence of an objectionable double standard—to use weight gain or other simpler tests in developing countries where the lack of equipment, reliable electricity, and money makes using these laboratory tests difficult or impossible?

In a slightly different vein, although most of the debate has focused on the way in which placebo use in trials like the AZT trials challenges traditional interpretations of the standard of care rule, there are critics who have insisted that such designs pose just as much of a challenge to other traditional rules of ethical study design such as the principle of clinical equipoise.[27] All these varied problems about study design deserve attention in the context of considering which practices are exploitative and which ones are not.

Informed Consent

The second frequent concern voiced about developing world research is that informed consent suffers in these contexts, sometimes to the point of nonexistence. Informed consent is almost universally recognized as a necessary requirement of ethical research. Certainly detailed informed consent is required for all research receiving U.S. government funding, and it is also required for all test results submitted to the Food and Drug Administration (FDA) for approval of a new drug. But critics worry that it will be unusually difficult to obtain meaningful consent from poor, uneducated subjects unfamiliar with the concept of research.

One concern played up by the media is that researchers are not adequately motivated to tackle what is assumed to be an impressively difficult task. In the extreme case, they may even be tempted, once they find themselves far from any oversight bodies, to forgo informed consent altogether.[28] Most parties agree that *if* this occurred it would indeed be problematic. However, there is very little evidence that such extreme behavior is widespread.

More subtle questions arise when we ask whether the consents that are obtained in such settings are really valid. One concern is about *understanding:* perhaps no matter what researchers do, uneducated subjects simply will not be able to grasp what is being presented to them. A different concern is about *voluntariness.* Some critics have claimed that it is impossible for subjects to give truly free consent in such settings. So, for example, one finds claims such as the following:

> I'd argue you can't do studies ethically in a country where there is no basic health care. You can tell a person there that this is research, but they hear they have a chance to get care or else refuse their only good chance at care. How can you put them in that position and then say they are giving informed consent?[29]

> It is difficult to avoid coercing subjects in most settings where clinical investigation in the developing world is conducted. African subjects with relatively little understanding of medical aspects

of research participation, indisposed toward resisting the suggestions of Western doctors, perhaps operating under the mistaken notion that they are being treated, and possibly receiving some ancillary benefits from participation in research, are very susceptible to coercion.[30]

Ultimately, critics have asked "whether a Third World villager who knows little about modern medicine can give informed consent in a way comparable to a Western patient?"[31]

Defenders of these studies counter, in response to the first worry, that being poor and having few health care options does not make a person stupid or unable to understand explanations of clinical research. Indeed, they note that to survive in Africa often requires a great deal of savvy and a keen sense of one's interests and how to realize them. They also note that there are woefully limited empirical data suggesting that research participants in African countries have systematically lower understanding as compared with research participants from developed countries. In *both* developing and developed countries, what little data there are suggest that research participants often fail to understand what *randomization* really amounts to. This suggests that full understanding is hard to achieve *in every setting*. Nonetheless, the data also suggest that subjects often have a relatively good appreciation of the risks and benefits of a study.[32]

Finally, it is pointed out (in response to the second worry) that merely possessing few good options does not undermine the voluntariness of choice. People often confront few options, but nevertheless act voluntarily and autonomously. For instance, individuals who need heart or liver transplants confront a bleak set of options. Yet no one thinks—or should think—that opting for a solid organ transplant is an involuntary or coerced choice.

Reasonable Availability and Fair Compensation

The third common concern about developing world research is that it is unfair to the study participants in particular and to the host communities in general, since in many cases drugs or interventions developed as a result of the research will not be available to either group posttrial because of prohibitive costs.[33] The claim here is that the poor are being used to develop drugs for the rich and that this is itself inherently unethical. Generally, critics have referred to this set of problems as "the problem of reasonable availability," though in fairness there are really *several* issues here as opposed to one. One question is about what is owed to *populations or communities*. The other is about what is owed to *trial participants* once the trial is over. Moreover, labeling the problem as a problem of "reasonable availability" prejudges the question of *what* is owed to communities and participants by implying that what is owed must necessarily be reasonable access to drugs developed through the trial. However, it is possible, as we shall see, to recognize that something is owed, and yet argue that what is owed need not be access to drugs.

The issue of *community* benefit emerged early on as a result of the *International Ethical Guidelines for Biomedical Research Involving Human Subjects (1993)*, published by CIOMS.[34] This document argued:

> As a general rule, the sponsoring agency should agree in advance of the research that any product developed through such research will be made reasonably available to the inhabitants of the host community at the completion of successful testing. Exceptions to this general requirement should be justified and agreed to by all concerned parties before the research begins.[35]

This ethical requirement was reiterated in CIOMS's 2002 revision.[36]

In light of this requirement in the CIOMS guidelines, many criticized the AZT trials because the sponsors did not *guarantee* inhabitants of the countries the AZT posttrial, even if it was proven effective. For instance, Annas and Grodin argued that while the research questions may have been framed with the health needs of developing countries in mind, not nearly enough had been done to guarantee that these populations would receive the drugs actually being tested if they proved effective.[37] Although the trials examined cheaper regimens, there was no pretrial plan agreed to by all involved that laid out how a successful treatment, should one be developed, would be implemented in the host countries. There was no binding commitment from the manufacturer of AZT to make it available at affordable prices, and in most cases the fifty-dollar cost of the short-course AZT regimen would still be unaffordable.

Furthermore, given the poor health care infrastructure of these countries, there was no plan for how to actually distribute the medications. They argued that without binding agreements in place ahead of time, there was no real assurance of reasonable availability, making the AZT trials unethical. In a related article Glantz, Annas, and colleagues summed up their view as follows: "In order for research to be ethically conducted [in developing countries] it must offer the potential of actual benefit to the inhabitants of that developing country. . . . For underdeveloped communities to derive potential benefit from research, they must have access to the fruits of such research."[38] In 2002, the chair and executive director of the United States' NBAC adopted a similar line: "If the intervention being tested is not likely to be affordable in the host country or if the health care infrastructure cannot support its proper distribution and use, it is unethical to ask persons in that country to participate in the research, since they will not enjoy any of its potential benefits."[39]

Critics of the reasonable availability requirement have noted that, as it stands, it is incredibly vague. How is "community" to be defined? Must drugs be provided to every sick member of the host country, or does community not extend as far as national boundaries? And for how long must drugs be provided, particularly if it is clear that the host country will not be able to assume that cost anytime in the near future?

Other critics have gone further and argued that reasonable availability should not be seen as an ethical requirement of research in developing countries.[40] What *is* a requirement is that the host community actually benefit fairly from the conduct and/or results of research. But providing medication posttrial is *not* the only way the community might reap benefits. The important point is to assess the overall net benefits for the community of participating in the research as opposed to focusing exclusively on one particular type of benefit—access to the tested drug.

Moreover, defenders of the view that reasonable availability is not an ethical requirement have pointed out that such a policy makes more sense for various additional reasons. No single trial ever proves or disproves the effectiveness of an intervention. Usually multiple trials are required to persuade the medical community about the effectiveness of drugs and other treatments. Thus, guaranteeing access after only one trial is unrealistic. Furthermore, implementing any particular intervention, even in developed countries, is a haphazard process at best. Adoption of a new drug or technology is not like switching on a light that can occur by an agreement or government fiat. Diffusion of drugs and interventions is a complex social phenomenon that is not under the control of a single sponsor.

Finally, even though all parties appear to agree that benefits (of some sort) must be offered, it is not at all clear why all the responsibility for supplying benefits should rest with *the sponsor* of the research. In many cases, the sponsor, such as the NIH or CDC in the United States, or the Medical Research Council of the United Kingdom (MRC), is legally required to focus on research and not health care implementation. Hence such agencies are legally barred from assuming responsibility for posttrial drug distribution. Many other parties might have ethical obligations for implementing an intervention proven effective by these sponsors, including the host country's government, international aid organizations, or governments in developed countries other than the sponsoring government. So it remains unclear why CIOMS singled out research *sponsors* as being the key ones responsible for assuring reasonable availability.

In addition to concerns about communities, there are also concerns about participants. In particular, what is owed posttrial to participants who are placed on a drug during a study and who benefit from it? For example, in the AZT trials, should someone have undertaken to make AZT available posttrial to the women who participated, and to those children who contracted the virus? This is a particularly charged question in the case of HIV/AIDS trials because antiretroviral treatments are both incredibly beneficial and incredibly expensive. Furthermore, they need to be taken continuously—for the rest of the patient's life—if they are to be effective. There is now an emerging consensus in the international community that such care must be offered, but as with the issue of community benefit, deep questions remain about who exactly is to provide it.[41] Once again, the fact that agencies like NIH are not able, under their mandate, to provide long-term care, makes the question particularly difficult.[42]

Exploitation: The Common Thread

What do worries about standard of care and other aspects of study design, informed consent, and reasonable availability and/or fair benefits all have in common? Exploitation. Underlying each is the worry that poor research participants in developing countries are exploited by research trials sponsored and conducted by developing countries. The real ethical violation of using placebos, or not getting valid consent, or not providing drugs proven effective in the trial or sufficient alternative benefits is that it exploits the people in these developing countries.

The language of exploitation runs throughout the medical literature on these issues.[43] To give just a few examples: After decrying the use of placebos in the maternal-fetal AZT transmission trials, Lurie and Wolfe argued that "residents of impoverished, postcolonial countries, the majority of whom are people of color must be protected from potential *exploitation* in research [our italics]."[44] In her remarks on the same trials, Marcia Angell urged, "Acceptance of this ethical relativism [by which she refers to her opponents' claim that it is permissible for trials to differ based on local differences] could result in widespread *exploitation* of vulnerable Third World populations [our italics]."[45]

Similarly, Annas and Grodin declared that

> unless the interventions being tested will actually be made available to the impoverished populations that are being used as research subjects, developed countries are simply *exploiting* them in order to quickly use the knowledge gained from the clinical trials for the developed countries' own benefit. . . . The central issue in doing research with impoverished populations is *exploitation* [our italics].[46]

However, concerns about exploitation are not limited to clinical research in developing countries. Exploitation is a potential concern in all clinical research. All research "uses" the participants to gain information that, hopefully, will improve the health of others whether directly, or indirectly through additional research. Thus, all research participants are in danger of being exploited. As one South African researcher observed: "The starting point of all clinical trials is the assurance that trial participants will be protected from *exploitation* [our italics]."[47] In a similiar vein it has been claimed that

> [t]he overarching objective of clinical research is to develop generalizable knowledge to improve health and/or increase understanding of human biology; subjects who participate are the means

to securing such knowledge. By placing some people at risk of harm for the good of others, clinical research has the potential for exploitation of human subjects. Ethical requirements for clinical research aim to minimize the possibility of *exploitation* by ensuring that research subjects are not merely used, but are treated with respect while they contribute to the social good [our italics].[48]

However, characterizing the ethical issue at the heart of clinical research as one of exploitation can be both helpful and problematic. It is helpful because it unifies what have often been diffuse, disjointed, and even incoherent concerns about research in developing countries into what seems to be a single, clear ethical issue. It is problematic because the appearance of simplicity is deceiving. Exploitation is itself a diffuse and unclear ethical concept. Hence we run the danger of substituting a vague pile of concerns for an equally vague label—giving it the patina of coherence but without real clarity.

Why is exploitation itself vague and unclear? The problem stems both from the fact that exploitation can be used in morally loaded and morally neutral ways, and from the fact that we often fail to realize that not all "use" of people, despite sounding bad, is morally problematic.

In the most minimal sense, "to exploit" simply means to *use* something to advantage. A weight lifter exploits his muscles to lift weights, a carpenter exploits his tools to build beautiful chairs, a scientist exploits a quirk of nature to make a new cosmological discovery or synthesize a new molecule. In these common cases, the exploitation is not morally worrisome. Moreover, in this simple nonmoral sense, the word quite *naturally* applies to clinical research because research uses human beings to gain generalizable knowledge.

Despite sounding bad, however, use of people, by itself, need not be morally bad, since competent adults need not be *abused* and may consent to being used. Indeed, consent to fair use is what happens in ethical research. A more morally loaded sense of the term, according to which exploitation involves using those who are *vulnerable*, also turns out, when we press on it, to be a description that applies to much ethically justified clinical research on sick people. The problem here is that the notion of "vulnerability," like the notion of "use," is merely a marker for moral concern and not a sure sign of moral infringement. Although it sounds bad to say that we "use those who are vulnerable," it is possible to use those who are vulnerable without taking unfair or inappropriate advantage of their vulnerability. For example, an employer who hires extremely poor workers desperate for a job, and who pays them a decent, livable wage is using those who are vulnerable but without taking unfair or inappropriate advantage of their vulnerability.

Clearly, confusion and misunderstanding can easily arise here. The morally worrisome connotation of exploitation is related to use. But how? That is the tricky question at the heart of most discussions of exploitation. We must address these questions head-on if we are to gain an understanding of current problems in the ethics of clinical research. Specifying what constitutes exploitation is critical not only for correctly labeling a situation or relationship but also for devising the appropriate remedy. Unless we know what the problem is, it is very hard to know what the right solution is. Often the wrong solution will just exacerbate the problem.

The Origin of This Volume and a View of What's Ahead

The essays in this collection emerged from the recognition by members of the Department of Clinical Bioethics of the National Institutes of Health of the centrality of, but also the challenges surrounding, the concept of exploitation. In the spring of 2002 members of the department first convened a seminar series on exploitation and its relationship to research practices in developing countries. This volume of essays is the product of that seminar series, either directly (certain of the essays were written for that series by guest speakers) or indirectly (because the series stimulated additional reflection on the part of individual attendees of the seminar).

Because so much ink has already been devoted to the maternal-fetal HIV transmission studies, and because consequently positions have become entrenched without much openness to deeper reflection, we decided to organize the essays around two different cases that raise many of the important and charged contextual issues in fresh clothes.

The Surfaxin case involves a proposed research study on a new surfactant, a drug sprayed into the lungs of premature infants to increase the pliability of the air sacs and ease breathing. While many natural and synthetic surfactants were already on the market, the pharmaceutical company developing the drug wished to sponsor a randomized controlled study using a placebo, to be conducted in four Latin American countries. The Havrix case, on the other hand, involved the randomized controlled trial of a hepatitis A vaccine in northern Thailand sponsored by the U.S. Army in conjunction with a pharmaceutical company. In this case, the control intervention was not a placebo but a hepatitis B vaccine. Detailed case descriptions are included in this volume, and the authors comment to some degree on one or both of these cases.

Importantly, neither of the two trials we have selected involved HIV/AIDS, and neither trial was conducted in Africa. However, one involved the use of placebos in critically ill infants despite the fact that a known effective intervention already existed. Both trials involved poor participants in developing countries, with researchers coming from the United States. In neither case was it expected that the trial drugs, if proven effective, would be made available any time soon to participants or their communities, though in both cases other types of benefits were offered by the sponsors. One was a government-sponsored study, the other sponsored by a pharmaceutical company.

In addition to the two case studies and the essays that follow, this volume also contains a chapter entitled "Research Ethics, Developing Countries, and Exploitation: A Primer." It has been our aim from the start to make this volume as accessible as possible to people from different disciplines: physicians, clinical researchers, health policy analysts, philosophers, bioethicists, public health students and professors, and health lawyers. Hence, the first half of that chapter provides an introduction to the fundamental concepts of research ethics and the special issues that arise when they are applied to a developing world setting. These include informed consent, randomized controlled trials (RCTs), standard of care, clinical equipoise, and so on. This section is intended for readers who are familiar with ethical theory but less familiar with the peculiar concerns of clinical research. The second half of the chapter provides an overview of the concept of exploitation to help orient those less familiar with philosophy to the various ways in which philosophers have approached the topic. This section will briefly introduce readers to the history of the concept (in particular, its Marxist meaning), as well as provide an introduction to the contemporary non-Marxist conceptions that figure in these essays. The section lays out the central questions about exploitation that remain open for debate.

We hope this volume raises the quality of thought and public deliberation on exploitation by elucidating what really constitutes exploitation and what can be done to mitigate it, all in the context of real situations that confront policy makers, ethicists, government and corporate officials, the media, and the public.

Notes

1. Edward M. Connor et al. "Reduction of Maternal-Infant Transmission of Human Immunodeficiency Virus Type 1 with Zidovudine Treatment," *New England Journal of Medicine* 331 (1994): 1173–80.

2. *Id.*

3. Christine Grady, "Science in the Service of Healing," *Hastings Center Report* 28, no. 6 (1998): 34–38, at 35.

4. Connor et al., *supra* note 1, at 1173.

5. Peter Lurie and Sidney M. Wolfe, "Unethical Trials of Interventions to Reduce Perinatal Transmission of the Human Immunodeficiency Virus in Developing Countries," *New England Journal of Medicine* 337 (1997): 1853–55, at 853.

6. Indeed, 90 percent of all HIV-infected individuals reside in developing countries. These statistics are based on November 2004 figures from the UN-AIDS Web site, http://www.unaids.org/en/resources/questions_answers.asp#II (accessed July 24, 2005).

7. Grady, *supra* note 3, at 35.

8. Robert A. Crouch and John D. Arras, "AZT Trials and Tribulations," *Hastings Center Report* 28, no. 6 (1998): 26–34, at 33.

9. *Id.* at 26; Grady, *supra* note 3, at 35.

10. Crouch and Arras, *supra* note 8, at 26.

11. Grady, *supra* note 3, at 35.

12. World Health Organization, *Recommendations from the Meeting on Mother-to-Infant Transmission of HIV by Use of Antiretrovirals* (Geneva: WHO, 1994).

13. Lurie and Wolfe, *supra* note 5, at 853.

14. *Id.*

15. Marcia Angell, "The Ethics of Clinical Research in the Third World," *New England Journal of Medicine* 337 (1997): 847– 49.

16. Richard Saltus, "Journal Departures Reflect AIDS Dispute," *Boston Globe*, October 16, 1997, A11.

17. Harold Varmus and David Satcher, "Ethical Complexities of Conducting Research in Developing Countries," *New England Journal of Medicine* 337 (1997): 1003– 5.

18. See, e.g., volume 12, issue 4 (1998) of *Bioethics:* David B. Resnik, "The Ethics of HIV Research in Developing Nations," 286-306; Reidar K. Lie, "Ethics of Placebo-Controlled Trials in Developing Countries," 307–11; Udo Schuklenk, "Unethical Perinatal HIV Transmission Trials Establish Bad Precedent," 312–19; Joe Thomas, "Ethical Challenges of HIV Clinical Trials in Developing Countries," 320–27; Carlos del Rio, "Is Ethical Research Feasible in Developed and Developing Countries?" 328–30; see also volume 28, issue 6 (1998) of *Hastings Center Report:* Ezekiel J. Emanuel, "A World of Research Subjects: Introduction," 25; Crouch and Arras, *supra* note 8; Grady, *supra* note 3; Leonard H. Glantz, George J. Annas, Michael A. Grodin, and Wendy K. Mariner, "Research in Developing Countries: Taking 'Benefit' Seriously," 38–42; Carol Levine, "Placebos and HIV: Lessons Learned," 43-48.

19. Lurie and Wolfe, *supra* note 15; Angell, *supra* note 15. The language of "double standards" originates with Lurie and Wolfe.

20. This rule is generally traced to the World Medical Association's (WMA) Declaration of Helsinki, which in turn is a development of the Nuremberg Code, the first formal code of clinical research ethics drawn up in the wake of the Nuremberg trials of the Nazi doctors who conducted horrific human experiments during World War II. However, it is worth noting that although this is a widely recognized norm of medical research, it is not a *binding* rule for much research. It is not, for example, included in the U.S. Federal Code of Regulations (DHHS Title 45, CFR 46) that govern all human subjects research that receives U.S. government funding. Nor is it contained in that part of the U.S. Federal Code (DHHS 21 CFR 50 and 56) that specifies the ethical requirements research must pass if it is to be used to win FDA approval. The current version of Helsinki at the time of this dispute was the one from 1996. However, the relevant passage (paragraph II.3) predates 1996. The 1989 version of the Declaration of Helsinki is reprinted in George J. Annas and Michael A. Grodin, *The Nazi Doctors and the Nuremberg Code: Human Rights in Human Experimentation* (New York: Oxford University Press, 1992), 339– 42.

21. The Declaration of Helsinki, September 1989, par. II.3.

22. Grady, *supra* note 3, at 35.

23. This is significant, because some of the rhetoric surrounding these trials, particularly Marcia Angell's comparison of the AZT trials to the infamous Tuskeegee trials of untreated syphilis, implies that defenders have only the most crude types of utilitarian arguments on their side. The suggestion is that these are people for whom no treatment of subjects is ruled out if it will lead to useful medical knowledge. However, that is not the position of most defenders. See Angell, *supra* note 15, at 847.

24. Robert J. Levine, "The 'Best Proven Therapeutic Method' Standard in Clinical Trials in Technologically Developing Countries," *IRB: A Review of Human Subjects Research* 20 (1999): 5–9; Reidar K. Lie, Ezekiel J. Emanuel, Christine Grady, and David Wendler, "The Standard of Care Debate: The Declaration of Helsinki versus the International Consensus Opinion," *Journal of Medical Ethics* 30 (2004): 190–93.

25. For discussion of the proposed revisions, offered before the final changes occurred, see Brennan, "Proposed Revisions to the Declaration of Helsinki—Will They Weaken the Ethical Principles Underlying Human Research?" *New England Journal of Medicine* 341 (1999): 527–30; Robert J. Levine, "The Need to Revise the Declaration of Helsinki," *New England Journal of Medicine* 341 (1999): 531–34; Kenneth J. Rothman, Karin B. Michels, and Michael Baum, "For and Against: Declaration of Helsinki Should Be Strengthened," *British Medical Journal* 321 (2000): 442–45.

26. See, e.g., Joint United Nations Programme on HIV/AIDS (UNAIDS), *Ethical Considerations in HIV Preventative Vaccine Research* (Geneva: UNAIDS, 2000); Council for International Organizations of Medical Sciences, *International Ethical Guidelines for Biomedical Research Involving Human Subjects* (Geneva: CIOMS, 2002); Nuffield Council on Bioethics, *The Ethics of Research Related to Healthcare in Developing Countries* (London: Nuffield Council on Bioethics, 2002); National Bioethics Advisory Commission, *Ethical and Policy Issues in International Research: Clinical Trials in Developing Countries* (Bethesda, MD: NBAC, 2001). For the claim that a new consensus has emerged that contradicts Helsinki, see Lie, Emanuel, Grady, and Wendler, *supra* note 24.

27. For discussion of this, see chapter 1 in this volume.

28. See, e.g., Howard W. French, "AIDS Research in Africa: Juggling Risks and Hopes," *New York Times*, October 9, 1997; Sharon LaFraniere, Mary Pat Flaherty, and Joe Stephens, "The Dilemma: Submit or Suffer: The Body Hunters, Article III," *Washington Post*, December 19, 2000.

29. George Annas quoted in LaFraniere, Flaherty, and Stephens, *supra* note 28.

30. Nicholas A. Christakis, "The Ethical Design of an AIDS Vaccine Trial in Africa," *Hastings Center Report* 18, no. 3 (1988): 31–37, at 31.

31. LaFraniere, Flaherty, and Stephens, *supra* note 28.

32. Christine Pace, Christine Grady, and Ezekiel J. Emanuel, "What We Don't Know about Informed Consent," *SciDevNet*, August 28, 2003, www.scidev .net/en/opinions/what-we-dont-know-about-informed-consent.html.

33. See, e.g., Glantz, Annas, Grodin, and Mariner, *supra* note 18; Crouch and Arras, *supra* note 8.

34. The Council for International Organizations of Medical Sciences (CIOMS) is an international nongovernmental organization closely tied to the World Health Organization (WHO) and founded by WHO and the United Nations Educational Scientific and Cultural Organization (UNESCO).

35. The Council for International Organizations of Medical Sciences, *International Ethical Guidelines for Biomedical Research Involving Human Subjects* (Geneva: CIOMS, 1993), Commentary on Guideline 15, at 45.

36. The Council for International Organizations of Medical Sciences, *International Ethical Guidelines for Biomedical Research Involving Human Subjects* (Geneva: CIOMS, 2002), Guideline 10, at 32.

37. George J. Annas and Michael A. Grodin, "Human Rights and Maternal-Fetal HIV Transmission Prevention Trials in Africa," *American Journal of Public Health* 88 (1998): 560–63, at 561.

38. Glantz, Annas, Grodin, and Mariner, *supra* note 18, at 39.

39. Harold T. Shapiro and Eric M. Meslin, "Ethical Issues in the Design and Conduct of Clinical Trials in Developing Countries," *New England Journal of Medicine* 345 (2001): 139–42, at 139. Also see National Bioethics Advisory Commission, *Ethical and Policy Issues in International Research*, chap. 4.

40. Participants in the 2001 Conference on Ethical Aspects of Research in Developing Countries, "Fair Benefits for Research in Developing Countries," *Science* 298 (2002): 2133–34; and "Moral Standards for Research in Developing Countries: From 'Reasonable Availability' to 'Fair Benefits,'" *Hastings Center Report* 34, no. 3 (2004): 17–27, reprinted as chapter 9 of this volume.

41. Christine Grady, "The Challenge of Assuring Continued Post-trial Access to Beneficial Treatment," *Yale Journal of Health Policy, Law, and Ethics* 5, no. 1 (2005): 425–35.

42. See, e.g., *NIH Guidance for Addressing the Provision of Antiretroviral Treatment for Trial Participants Following Their Completion of NIH-Funded Antiretroviral Treatment Trials in Developing Countries* (Bethesda, MD: National Institutes of Health, Office of Extramural Research, 2005), available at http://grants.nih.gov/grants/policy/antiretroviral/QandA.htm#Purpose.

43. Indeed, the examples in the text barely scratch the surface. Other instances in which the issues have been framed in terms of exploitation include Emanuel, *supra* note 18; Glantz, Annas, Grodin, and Mariner, *supra* note 18;

Grady, *supra* note 3; Ronald Bayer, "The Debate over Maternal-Fetal HIV Transmission Prevention Trials in Africa, Asia and the Caribbean: Racist Exploitation or Exploitation of Racism?" *American Journal of Public Health* 88 (1998): 567–70; Salim S. Abdool Karim, "Placebo Controls in HIV Perinatal Transmission Trials: A South African's Viewpoint," *American Journal of Public Health* 88 (1998) 564–66; Isabelle de Zoysa, Christopher J. Elias, and Margaret E. Bentley, "Ethical Challenges in Efficacy Trials of Vaginal Microbicides for HIV Prevention," *American Journal of Public Health* 88 (1998): 571–75; Resnik, *supra* note 18; Lie, *supra* note 18; del Rio, *supra* note 18; Barry R. Bloom, "The Highest Attainable Standard: Ethical Issues in AIDS Vaccines," *Science* 279 (1998): 186–88; Brennan, *supra* note 25; Udo Schuklenk and Richard Ashcroft, "International Research Ethics," *Bioethics* 14, no. 2 (2000): 158–72; Solomon R. Benatar, "Avoiding Exploitation in Clinical Research," *Cambridge Quarterly of Healthcare Ethics* 9 (2000): 562–65; Solomon R. Benatar and Peter M. Singer, "A New Look at International Research Ethics," *British Medical Journal* 321 (2000): 824–26; Mary Pat Flaherty and Doug Struck, "Life by Luck of the Draw: The Body Hunters, Article VI," *Washington Post*, December 22, 2000; Shapiro and Meslin, *supra* note 39; Paquita de Zulueta, "Ethical Imperialism or Unethical Exploitation?" *Bioethics* 15 (2001): 547; Ruth Macklin, "After Helsinki: Unresolved Issues in International Research," *Kennedy Institute of Ethics Journal* 11 (2001): 17–36; Michael Specter, "The Vaccine: Has the Race to Save Africa from AIDS Put Western Science at Odds with Western Ethics?" *New Yorker*, February 3, 2003, 54–65.

44. Lurie and Wolfe, *supra* note 5, at 855.

45. Angell, *supra* note 15, at 848.

46. Annas and Grodin, *supra* note 37.

47. Karim, *supra* note 43, at 565.

48. Ezekiel J. Emanuel, David Wendler, and Christine Grady, "What Makes Clinical Research Ethical?" *Journal of the American Medical Association* 283 (2000): 2701-11.

Research Ethics, Developing Countries, and Exploitation: A Primer

JENNIFER S. HAWKINS

As the AZT trials demonstrated, questions about the ethical conduct of clinical research in developing countries are anything but simple. Informed judgments about the cases in this book, and about future directions for policy, require familiarity with both the details of clinical research and significant moral distinctions. This chapter aims to provide some background material relevant to understanding the complexities of the current debates.

The first section provides a basic overview of the fundamental concepts of research ethics as they relate to developing country research—informed consent, randomized controlled trials (RCTs), standard of care, and clinical equipoise. It is intended for readers who are familiar with ethical theory but less familiar with the peculiar concerns of clinical research. It aims to familiarize them with the concepts and clearly articulate the disputed questions currently relevant for the discussions of international research that follow.

The second section provides an overview of the concept of exploitation to help orient those less familiar with philosophy to the ways in which philosophers have approached the topic. Exploitation is commonly associated with Marxism, but there is, in addition to the Marxist tradition, a robust tradition of non-Marxist accounts of exploitation of which the essays in this book are representative. This section will briefly introduce readers to both the Marxist and the non-Marxist understandings of the concept, and set out the central questions about exploitation that remain open for debate.

Brief Background to Clinical Research Ethics

Medical research aims to generate knowledge that will hopefully, in turn, lead to improvements in medical practice. It is a long process. Often there is an initial phase of basic scientific research conducted in laboratories. Animal studies are then usually conducted before new agents are tried out in a human body. "Clinical research" refers to the later phases of medical research, when human bodies enter the equation. Even here there are multiple stages. "Phase I" is the name traditionally given to the first studies of an agent in humans. Such studies are usually very small, and hence cannot reveal anything general about how effective an agent is at curbing disease. Instead, the aim is to first learn about "toxicity, metabolism, and other drug dynamics."[1] Many such studies are carried out on healthy volunteers, though research on new cancer drugs is an exception.

Phase II and Phase III studies are generally randomized controlled trials where the new agent is compared with something else. Unlike Phase I trials, they are usually conducted on subjects with the illness for which an improvement in treatment is being sought. Phase II studies are generally much smaller than Phase III, and still largely concerned with gaining understanding about safety and side effects. It is the large Phase III clinical trials that enroll hundreds and sometimes thousands of human subjects that aim to determine whether a new agent will indeed prove to be a useful general treatment for the illness in question. The controversies described here are all related to the conduct of Phase III trials.

Informed Consent

Informed consent is almost universally recognized as a requirement for the ethical conduct of clinical research. Indeed, the more common danger in discussions of research ethics is for people to reduce all moral concerns about research to concerns about consent. While consent is important, it is only one of the key components of ethical research.[2]

Valid informed consent has four requirements. First, only those potential subjects who pass the requirements for decision-making competence should be asked to give consent. When it is necessary to enroll incompetent subjects, consent must be obtained from an appropriate surrogate. Three additional requirements must be satisfied with respect to either the competent subject or the incompetent subject's surrogate. There must be full disclosure of all the relevant information, the subject or surrogate must understand the information, and he or she must then consent freely or voluntarily. Force, coercion, and undue inducement are all recognized as undermining the voluntariness, and hence the validity, of informed consent.

In the context of research in developing countries, a number of distinct and sometimes contradictory concerns have been raised about informed consent. Most recent discussion has emphasized the difficulties of obtaining genuine informed consent in developing countries. Another, older concern is that informed consent may not be culturally appropriate in all parts of the world. Whereas the first group is concerned that consent is not being obtained often enough, the second thinks that consent may not even be necessary. Let us consider first the concerns of those who think genuine consent is not obtained often enough.

Some of the concerns that arise here are concerns about *understanding*. In 1997, for example, a *New York Times* article that focused specifically on one of the controversial AZT trials in Côte d'Ivoire sponsored by the National Institutes of Health (NIH) and the Centers for Disease Control (CDC) raised worries about the true level of subject understanding.[3] One subject singled out by the reporter clearly did not understand the concept of a placebo despite repeated explanations and questionings. She is quoted as saying:

> They gave me a bunch of pills to take, and told me how to take them. Some were for malaria, some were for fevers, and some were supposed to be for the virus. I knew that there were different kinds, but I figured that if one of them didn't work against AIDS, then one of the other ones would.[4]

Although there is no evidence to suggest that this woman's poor level of understanding is a widespread phenomenon, such anecdotal evidence is understandably troubling to those who see full understanding among subjects as a central requirement for ethical research. No doubt the challenges of obtaining informed consent among poor, uneducated populations can be daunting. There are often significant language barriers. Not only must the information be translated, but many languages lack words for important medical-scientific concepts.[5] It can be extremely difficult to find a way to explain randomization or the concept of a placebo. In authoritarian cultures, it may also be difficult to get subjects to appreciate that they really are free not to participate, and that their health care will not be jeopardized if they refuse.[6] Then there is the problem—familiar from developed world settings as well—of the therapeutic misconception. This is the tendency of some patients to believe, despite being told otherwise, that the research has a therapeutic purpose.[7]

Perhaps the most pressing theoretical question with relation to informed consent and understanding is that of *how much* understanding must be achieved if research is to go forward while remaining ethical. For this reason, the requirement of understanding is one of the more worrisome, and hence contentious, aspects of the traditional analysis. At one extreme is the view that understanding is not actually necessary for consent to be valid.[8] At the other end is the equally extreme view that complete understanding of all details is required. Taken literally, this view would lead to the conclusion that much clinical research—not just clinical research conducted in developing countries—is unethical, because what evidence we have suggests that full understanding is rarely achieved in *any* setting. Most theorists appear to accept a view somewhere in the middle. But where to draw an appropriate line remains troubling.

Another set of extremely common concerns are those about *voluntariness*. For example, in a newspaper article detailing some of the worries about consent to research in developing countries, the law professor and bioethicist George Annas is quoted as saying:

> I'd argue you can't do studies ethically in a country where there is no basic health care. You can tell a person there that this is research, but they hear they have a chance to get care or else refuse their only good chance at care. How can you put them in that position and then say they are giving informed consent?[9]

Although Annas does not say precisely what it is that undermines informed consent in these cases, his reference to the *choice* subjects face suggests that he is worried about voluntariness. He also suggests not just that obtaining informed consent is difficult but that, because of the circumstances in developing countries, it is actually *impossible*. This suggests, in turn, that he must either believe that all offers made in such circumstances are necessarily coercive, *or* that all such offers necessarily count as undue inducement. However, neither claim has any merit.

Unfortunately, it is not uncommon for theorists to assume that whenever a person facing a grim set of alternatives makes a choice—even if she chooses what under the circumstances is clearly in her best interests—it must be coerced.[10] Such misconceptions are further ingrained because we often speak loosely of the "force" of circumstances. However, the identification of coercion proper requires that we consider two features: the choice set of the agent (B), and the actions (if any) of other parties (A) that have unfairly created that choice set. The first requirement for coercion is that B's set of options be altered unfavorably in the sense of being narrowed. This much is common to many cases of being "forced by circumstances." The second, equally important requirement for coercion, however, is that some agent A (the coercer) must have deliberately brought about the narrowing of the set *so as* to get B to do what he wants. This may come about as a result of A forcibly eliminating options from B's set. Alternatively (and much more commonly), it involves A threatening to make B worse off if B does not do as A wishes. (Here the *threat* serves to narrow the set of "good" options B has by altering the payoffs associated with them.) It is this second crucial condition that distinguishes coercion from mere harsh choice situations.

Once we abandon the simplistic equation of coercion with harsh choice situations, there is no reason to suppose that the offers researchers extend to potential subjects in developing countries are *necessarily* coercive as Annas suggests. There is simply no evidence to suggest that researchers routinely force or threaten subjects. They simply make them offers that are, in the sad context where subjects have few options for good health care, extremely attractive.

Those who think genuine informed consent is impossible in impoverished settings might, alternatively, be worried that all such transactions—made against a backdrop of poverty and desperation—constitute *undue inducement*. For example, in a recent policy brief, Lindegger and Bull note that "economic factors" may undermine voluntary consent. In particular, if subjects have few other options for health care, these authors worry that research may be *too attractive*.[11] They give as an example the following statement from a Thai subject who claimed:

> The study staff gives good advice and when this project is over I hope I can enroll in another study. For that matter, I hope there will be new studies for me to participate in all the time. If there would be no more studies, I don't know if I would have the strength to go on, as I would not know where to get drugs outside of clinical trials.[12]

The idea behind undue inducement is that some offers are excessive and hence irresistible in a way that is morally problematic. But how are we to understand this more precisely? While it is sometimes claimed that an offer is excessive whenever it leads a person to choose something she would not otherwise choose, this is a highly implausible account of the badness of undue inducement. That would suggest that every case of accepting a job for a good salary would count as undue inducement.[13] A better account of what is morally problematic with undue inducement is that certain highly attractive offers may lead individuals to make choices that are not in their long-term interests, by, for example, leading them to accept risks that are not really worth it. However, if that is correct, it is hard to see how the offers made in developing world research necessarily induce in a bad way. For in the cases that concern us, the sad fact is that, by participating in research, subjects really are choosing something that does—given their current options—serve their long-term interests.[14] As Annas admits in the quotation from earlier, it may be their only chance for effective care.

In short, since there is no reason to believe that either coercion or undue inducement is a *necessary* feature of offers made to subjects in developing countries, there is no reason to think that voluntary informed consent is impossible to obtain.

Let us now consider briefly the claims of those who think that informed consent in developing countries may not be ethically required and may even be culturally inappropriate. In the years prior to the dispute about the AZT transmission trials, a number of commentators argued that, for cultural reasons, individual informed consent might not be a necessary ethical requirement of research in developing countries.[15] The claim was that informed consent is a uniquely Western ideal, one grounded in the peculiarly Western fascination with personal autonomy understood generally as individual decision making.[16] Where this value is not shared, it was argued, it may be inappropriate to impose such practices. This does not seem to be a widely held view, and it has been explicitly challenged.[17] But it does reflect genuine concerns people have had about how to approach informed consent in cultures where the practice does not neatly fit with local norms. Without being able to settle the issues here, it is worth making a few points about the general weakness of such arguments. The problem derives from placing too much emphasis on the autonomy-based justification for informed consent, as if that were the *only* reason to obtain informed consent. However, there are other justifications for the practice besides that one.

First, *even if* informed consent is a Western practice reflecting Western values, it is worth remembering that RCTs are also a Western practice that reflect Western values. Assuming that people are interested in importing the practice of RCTs, it may not be inappropriate to insist that informed consent be imported along with RCTs. At any rate, we should not take the mere fact that individuals in other places find the practice odd or cumbersome to be reason for giving it up. Their puzzlement may simply reflect their unfamiliarity with the realities of research as opposed to treatment. Informed consent is part of the apparatus developed in the West for safeguarding participants in a particular type of Western practice that strongly resembles but nonetheless differs from the practice of medicine. If it makes sense to think that ethical practices develop in accordance with the prevailing nonethical context, it would not be surprising to discover that a community with no tradition of research will have had no prior need to develop a practice of individual consent. But it would be too hasty to assume that it would not benefit from having a practice such as informed consent in place when it begins to participate in research.

Second, such arguments assume that the only ethical considerations that speak in favor of informed consent are considerations pertaining to decision making. In essence, the claim is that if individuals in a particular community do not value the opportunity to make decisions for themselves, then there is no need to obtain individual informed consent. This argument assumes that informed consent is merely a vehicle for allowing people to exercise decision-making power.

However, informed consent is much more than that, as experience even in the West has shown. Numerous empirical studies have shown that people in the developed world are frequently not as interested in making decisions for themselves as theorists assume.[18] Yet they are still frequently interested in being informed about what is going on, even when they are letting someone else decide for them.[19] It is important that people understand what is going on, even if they defer decision-making authority. There is more that matters to people than simply being able to exercise choice. It is at least possible, therefore, that informed consent serves an ethical function, even in cases where people are quite happy to defer the final decision about whether to participate to someone else (perhaps a senior family member or a community leader). Having the practice of individualized consent in place simultaneously serves to offer those few who might want to make a decision for themselves the opportunity to do so, while ensuring that those who do not care as much about exercising choice are still well-informed about what is happening.

Finally, the practice of obtaining informed consent serves another important function that is all too often ignored. These are the benefits that derive from transparency. The practice of informed consent can benefit subjects indirectly because of the ways it influences the behavior of researchers. It is plausible to suppose that the general transparency that results when each subject has to be carefully informed of all aspects of the research heightens the awareness and sensitivity of the researchers. Knowing that others know what you are doing, and why, can be a useful way of instigating a sense of accountability that may itself serve to reinforce ethical conduct among researchers.

Randomized Controlled Trials

Theorists frequently like to point out that the history of human subjects research is longer than often supposed—that human beings have been trying things out on one another for a long time. While this is certainly the case, it is also true that the modern era of clinical research using randomized controlled trials is breathtakingly new. This is particularly amazing when we consider the sheer volume of such trials occurring in the world today. Yet, according to one expert, this era of RCTs only really began "in the early 1950s with the evaluation of streptomycin in patients with tuberculosis."[20]

A randomized controlled trial involves dividing subjects into groups, or "arms," each of which will be treated in a different way for the sake of controlled comparison. The subjects are assigned to particular arms randomly—by lottery, as it were—in order to ensure that unacknowledged bias does not lead researchers to cluster similar people together in groups. If all or most of the people with a particular medically significant characteristic are clustered in one arm of a trial, then differences in the responses of subjects in that arm cannot be reliably attributed simply to the general difference in study drug or intervention. The differences might also have arisen because all of these people differ from the general population in some important way. Because bias can creep in in very subtle ways, randomization is considered extremely important for arriving at generalizable comparisons of one group to another.

In most cases, RCTs are also "double blinded," which means that neither individual subjects *nor researchers* know, during the course of the trial, who is in which group. Only certain members of the research team, who have no interactions with subjects, have the information that links particular subjects with particular interventions. To accomplish a truly blind trial, the different interventions being studied must be made to appear identical. To give a rather trivial example, if a study drug is given as a set of five pink pills, then any other medications used in other arms of the trial (or a placebo, if there is one) would also be presented to subjects as five pink pills.

The point of such elaborate hiding of information is to control for placebo effects. It is well documented that many people will experience some level of improvement whenever they believe they are receiving an effective treatment (whether or not they are). In other words, the epistemic state of the subject has a measurable effect that is not part of the effect a drug produces on its own. Hence, it is important to ensure that all participants are in the same epistemic state, so that any measured differences in subject response can be reliably attributed to differences in the medical efficacy of the different intervention agents. To accomplish this, researchers ensure that all participants are in an epistemic state of ignorance.

Placebo-Controlled Trials and Active-Controlled Trials

One of the key disputes in discussions of research ethics concerns study design. While clinical trials can, for various reasons, assume a bewildering variety of forms, only two basic designs need concern us here: placebo-controlled trials (PCTs) and active-controlled trials (ACTs), sometimes referred to as equivalency trials. For the sake of simplicity, I shall assume that we are always dealing with trials with only two arms. In reality, many trials have multiple arms, and in some cases incorporate both placebo and active controls. Also for the sake of simplicity, I will write as if all RCTs are trials of single drugs, though of course RCTs are used to test novel drug combinations, novel drug regimens (as in the AZT trials, where AZT itself was not new), vaccines (as in the Havrix case presented in this volume), and all sorts of medical procedures, even including complex forms of surgery. The term "drug" is more convenient than the correct but cumbersome phrase "investigational agent or intervention."

An active-controlled (or equivalency) trial compares a test drug to an already established drug that has been used successfully for the same condition. In an ACT, the question being asked is: Is the new drug better than, or at least equivalent to, the existing drug? An ACT compares two types of treatment to one another, usually on the assumption that, if the new drug is not at least as good as the old, the new one will not be worth developing.[21] Of course the "goodness" of a drug (or any intervention) is not as simple as I am making it seem here, for it is an "all-things-considered" assessment on the basis of efficacy, safety, and side effects. However, keeping this important qualification in mind, it is still true that *if* the new drug is not (all things considered) as good as the old, it would not be used in a context where the old drug is readily available.

An ACT is not designed to answer the question, for less effective drugs, whether those drugs are still *better than nothing*. All it tells us is whether or not the new drug is at least as good as the old. In cases where the new drug is not as good as the old, there is no direct way, with an ACT, to gauge how *much better* than nothing the new drug is. Of course it is sometimes possible to answer such a question *indirectly* with data from an ACT if one *also* possesses data from a PCT of the old therapy.

But it must be possible to generalize from one trial to the other (if too many variables are different, this may cause problems), and of course this also assumes that a PCT was once done. This is not always true; many standard therapies have never been tested against placebo.

Placebo-controlled trials are RCTs in which one arm of participants receives a placebo (i.e., some type of *medically* inert substance). A well-conducted placebo-controlled trial enables researchers to answer the question: Is the test drug more effective than nothing, and if so, how much better is it? The idea that one is comparing a drug to *nothing* is not literally correct. But, as we shall see, it is a simplifying fiction that need not undermine the basic rationale for such trials.

The reason it is not *nothing* is that placebos have a measurable effect. Indeed, controlling for this effect is what makes having some form of control important. Placebo effects appear to have attitudinal (mental) origins, and as such they will enter into the active arm of the trial anyway. Hence, the use of a placebo arm is preferable to just giving the test drug to a bunch of people and observing how well they respond compared with the general population. Researchers want to control for those observable health improvements that are simply the result of changes in participant attitudes (i.e., placebo effects). In many cases, it is important to answer the question: To what degree are observed beneficial effects attributable to the test drug *alone*—as opposed to other factors, *whatever these may be*? This matters, as it is only the benefits of the drug itself that should be considered when deciding whether the drug is worth developing and distributing.

As a general rule, placebo controls are not used in the developed world, once some form of effective therapy exists for a condition. However, many people think that there are ethically justified exceptions to this rule. A large part of its rationale is to ensure against inadequate attention to individual subject welfare. In many cases, attention to welfare is extremely important either because the welfare of the particular subjects in question is independently quite fragile (as in the case of very sick people used as research subjects), or because the research drug itself places individual welfare at high risk, or for both reasons together. But not all research is like this, and many RCTs are not very dangerous. For example, Emanuel and Miller point out that in trials involving conditions such as baldness, or some types of headaches, it may be perfectly okay to use placebo controls.[22] The real issue arises when the health risks involved are significant. It is easy to forget such points precisely because the cases that attract the attention of research ethicists are usually the dramatic cases in which life itself is at risk.

Furthermore, it is often the case that PCTs, because of their design, involve fewer subjects overall than ACTs. In some cases, this fact itself can, arguably, make it ethical to use placebos. For example, where the health dangers of being assigned to placebo are not too great, and the health profile of a new drug is highly uncertain (there is some chance that it will have quite negative side effects), it may well be *better* to test the new drug against placebo, since by doing so you will expose many fewer people to the unknown risks of the test drug. Emanuel and Miller explain the point well:

> Equivalence trials which evaluate the hypothesis that one drug is equivalent to another, typically require larger samples to achieve sufficient power because the delta or the difference between the rates of response to the two drugs is likely to be smaller than that between the rates of response to an investigational treatment and placebo. Consider an equivalence trial in which an investigational drug is compared with a standard drug that is known to have a 60 percent response rate. With a delta of 10 percent (if they were equivalent the difference between the standard and investigational drugs would be less than 10%) and a one-sided statistical test to show equivalence, each group must contain 297 participants. Conversely, if a placebo is hypothesized to have a 30% response rate and the investigational drug a 60% response rate, then only 48 participants are needed in each group. With the sample required for the equivalence trial—larger by a factor of six than the sample required for the equivalence trial—many more subjects will be exposed to an investigational drug that may be ineffective or even more toxic than the standard drug.[23]

These examples serve to remind us that the issue of placebo use is quite complex. Not all trials pose significant risks to subjects. Moreover, it is not always safe to assume that the risks posed to subject well-being by nontreatment are greater than the risks posed by new treatments.

Standard of Care

Two important principles—the principle of standard care and the principle of clinical equipoise—have traditionally guided thinking about the ethics of RCTs. Both were originally formulated in the context of developed world medicine, and both are intended to apply to all research conducted on subjects who suffer from the condition for which improved treatment is sought. Moreover, these two principles have come under renewed scrutiny as a result of the controversies over developing world research. Developing world research has challenged the general understanding of these norms, and some fear that it may challenge the continuing validity of the principles themselves.

In this section I focus on the first principle: *the principle of standard care*. It requires that members of a control group be given whatever is the current standard of care for the condition being studied. Hence, the principle is *comparative:* it requires that researchers consider how subjects in a trial fare in relation to people outside the trial. The touchy question arises when we try to specify further the appropriate outside reference point for the comparison. Is it local or global? Is it a comparison with how things actually are (locally or globally) or a comparison with how they medically ought to be?[24]

One major issue in the discussion of the AZT trials was how to interpret the principle of standard care. Paragraph II.3 of the pre-2000 Declaration of Helsinki is the traditional source for this principle.[25] It states, "In any medical study, every patient, including those of a control group, if any, should be assured of the best proven diagnostic and therapeutic method." The problem, however, is that it is not beyond dispute what exactly the original drafters of the declaration intended when they wrote paragraph II.3. Does it merely require that one give the control group whatever is best from what is generally available locally? That is one way to understand the phrase "standard of care."[26] On this model, the AZT trials satisfied the principle. Alternatively, the phrase might be understood to refer to a medical standard of judgment. This would not be an interpretation of "standard" in terms of what is actually done (either locally or globally) but an interpretation of "standard" in terms of medical consensus about what is medically best (globally).[27] On this model, the AZT trials do not satisfy the principle. The real question, however, is not what Helsinki says but which interpretation makes the most moral sense.

To an ethicist it seems most natural to try to resolve this issue by taking a step backward and considering the moral rationale that led to the adoption of the principle in the first place. Do we have a good understanding of that rationale? Is it possible to depart from the principle while remaining true to the underlying moral rationale? If not, how committed are we to the particular moral values enshrined in the principle of standard care? Might we, on occasion, think that other moral purposes trump those served by the principle? These questions can be answered only if we first say what the underlying moral purpose is.

However, when it comes to the principle of standard care, there is disagreement even about this. A good first attempt to explain the principle might go as follows: as a society we value research, but we value the rights of individuals *more*. We do not want to pursue research at just any cost. Clearly there are some kinds of knowledge that could be gained by sacrificing the interests of a few individuals, but we do not wish to be that kind of society, and hence we will not conduct such research, even if some (albeit rare) individuals were to volunteer to make such sacrifices. We will not ignore the welfare of a few for the sake of the many.

The preceding explanation is very similar to the ones most often given. It is, at its core, a rejection of crude forms of utilitarian thinking in research ethics—forms that recognize no constraints on the pursuit of a worthy end.[28] For example, in her criticism of the AZT trials, Marcia Angell, in addition to citing Helsinki on what control group subjects should get, also cites the following line: "In research on man, the interest of science and society should never take precedence over considerations related to the well-being of the subject."[29]

However, the passage cited is no more transparent than anything we have seen so far. It tells us we must show concern for the well-being of subjects and not ever let the temptations of research lead us to lower our level of concern from its normal, appropriate level. But what is the normal, appropriate level? What does "concern for well-being" even mean?

On one view, showing concern for the well-being of others simply means taking care to ensure that one's own actions do not *negatively* affect the well-being of others, for example, by injuring them or allowing them to be injured. Employers show concern for the well-being of employees by making sure that the workplace is safe, thereby preventing harm. But there is another, more active sense of showing concern for well-being. In this sense, I show concern for your well-being only if I do something to enhance or improve it. It is somewhat natural to fall into this second mode of thinking when considering sick people and the treatments they need, particularly if one views researchers as having all the same therapeutic obligations as physicians. Still, it is important to recognize that, relative to their baseline condition of sickness, treatment is a positive improvement.

Hence, even the idea that researchers must never allow the goal of achieving a greater common good to erode concern for subject well-being has (at least) a couple of interpretations. On the one hand, it could be interpreted to mean that researchers must never do anything that (prospectively) they expect would make a subject worse off than she otherwise would have been had she not participated. On the other hand, if we think of the obligations of researchers in a more medicalized sense, then we might interpret the principle as requiring that researchers never (knowingly) deny a sick person treatment. On the first reading AZT passes; on the second it fails.

Hence, deciding which interpretation of the principle of standard care makes sense requires confronting a difficult question at the core of research ethics: To what extent are the obligations of researchers similar to the obligations of physicians? Do researchers have an obligation to treat? As we shall soon see, similar issues arise in connection with the second important principle of clinical research ethics, the principle of clinical equipoise.

Questions about standard of care are deep questions about the foundations of research ethics. Yet it is easy to see why these issues might not have been resolved (or in some cases even appropriately recognized) prior to the crises in developing world research. For in the context of the developed world, people who interpret the principle of standard care in these two distinct ways will still, for the most part, differentiate between ethical and unethical trials *in the exact same way*. This is because in the developed world there is widespread access to the best medical treatment. In such an environment, those who adopt the more minimalist reading of "standard of care"—according to which it simply requires not making any subject worse off than she otherwise would have been—will insist that control group subjects get the best care because that is what the subjects would otherwise get outside of a trial. To offer them less in such a context is to ask them to sacrifice their well-being (in the sense of lowering it) for the sake of research. Those who adopt the more robust reading of "standard of care"—according to which it requires not denying the most effective treatment to any research subject—will also insist that the control group get the best care, but for different reasons. In short, in these environments different underlying understandings of the moral rationale for the principle of standard care will be hidden by superficial agreement on cases. The developing world cases, on the other hand, bring out the conflict vividly.

Clinical Equipoise

The second important principle that has traditionally defined the ethics of RCTs is the *principle of clinical equipoise*. It states that it is ethical to enroll subjects in an RCT only if there is genuine uncertainty within the medical-scientific community about which arm of a trial will be more beneficial for subjects.[30] It applies to either a PCT or an ACT. This principle is also comparative, but here it is intratrial comparison of one arm to another that matters.

The underlying moral rationale for the principle is the idea that researchers are also physicians. They are thus thought to have *therapeutic obligations* to their subjects.[31] Historically, the principle was introduced to help resolve a problem of role conflict in research, a problem that appeared to be particularly acute in the case of RCTs. A doctor has an obligation to do the best she can medically for her patients with the resources she has. Fulfilling this obligation, however, can potentially conflict with the goal of gaining generalizable knowledge, since, at times, knowledge can best be furthered by doing *less* than what is therapeutically best for a patient.

RCTs appear particularly problematic from this standpoint. How can a physician-researcher, obligated qua physician to provide the best care, justify to her patient-subject leaving the ultimate choice of therapy completely up to chance? Is there any way to view "flipping a coin" as compatible with doing one's best? The answer, supposedly enshrined in the principle of equipoise, is that an individual physician-researcher *may* be justified in doing this if, prospectively, the medical-scientific community is unable to agree whether one arm of the trial will be better for the subjects. The idea is that, if there is no consensus on this matter within the medical-scientific community, then the individual physician-researcher is not violating any therapeutic obligation by employing randomization. The important point to stress, however, is that equipoise, in this tradition, is always conceived of as a principle based on a physician's obligation to do her best for her patients.

It is easy to misunderstand the principle of equipoise. Consider, for example, what it means to think that one arm of a trial will be *better* for subjects. For a novice it would be natural to construe "better" merely in terms of efficacy. The usual patient wants to know: Just how likely is this to cure or ameliorate my condition? However, the notion of the "best" arm is an all-things-considered judgment. It represents, in Benjamin Freedman's phrase, an estimation of the "net therapeutic advantage" of an intervention after distinct variables such as safety and effectiveness have been balanced against one another.[32] Equipoise properly understood requires that the medical-scientific community be epistemically indifferent with respect to the question which arm of the trial will be "best" in terms of *net therapeutic advantage*. That is compatible with thinking that one arm is likely to be more effective than another at, for example, preventing the transmission of a virus.

So did the AZT trials satisfy the principle of equipoise? That turns out to be hard to decide. Some defenders of the trials pointed out that AZT was known to exacerbate anemia. Since the populations in which the trials were to be conducted have high levels of malnutrition and anemia, it could not be determined ahead of time how safe AZT would be. Hence it has been argued that, as between low-dose AZT and placebo, equipoise held because even though low-dose AZT was expected to be more effective, it was genuinely not possible to know ahead of time whether this effectiveness would outweigh other real dangers associated with the drug.[33] However, critics of these trials such as Marcia Angell denied that the evidence was sufficient to license any concerns about safety. Hence, she claimed the trials failed equipoise.[34] This dispute is about the interpretation of specific data, and to this day there is no agreement on the answer.

However, whatever the truth may be in the AZT case about the expected net therapeutic advantages of low-dose AZT as compared with placebo, there is a deeper controversy over the understanding of equipoise that we can lose sight of if we focus too much on the details of the anemia/safety debate. To get clear about this controversy, it is helpful to step back for a moment and consider *in isolation* two questions that most theorists of equipoise consider together.

First, given that clinical equipoise has, as its underlying rationale, the goal of allowing doctors to fulfill their obligations to patients, let us consider for a moment—in isolation from concerns about research—the nature of a physician's obligations in the face of uncertainty. Since we are ultimately interested in the idea of being evenly divided about the net therapeutic advantages of two (or more) treatments and so, as it were, "on the fence" about a decision, we might frame the clinical question that interests us as follows: Under what circumstances is a physician really justified in allowing a treatment decision between two options to be made by flipping a coin? When does uncertainty put her in the position where flipping the coin really is *as good as any other way* of deciding the matter, and so in a position where deciding by the flip of a coin will not violate her therapeutic obligations?

Presumably there are some norms that guide physicians in making such choices. Here we are interested not so much in the actual norms that guide actual doctors (which may vary a lot and sometimes in ways that are problematic), but in the ideal set of such norms—the ones that *ought* to guide physicians' thinking about such cases. These are the norms than an ideally informed and reflective community of physicians would be guided by in making choices for patients. In what follows, I shall simply refer to this ideal set as the set of *therapeutic choice norms*. There are two significant things to notice about these norms. First, if we take seriously the underlying moral rationale for equipoise—the aim of ensuring that a researcher fulfills her physician obligations—then these ideal therapeutic choice norms (whatever they turn out to be) should define clinical equipoise in research. Second, it is important to notice that there is room for reasonable disagreement about the precise formulation of these norms. In other words, while not just any answer would be acceptable, there is some wiggle room here. As we shall see shortly, the fact that there is room for reasonable disagreement is itself significant.

The second important question to consider is a complex one about when running a clinical trial is morally worthwhile. Let us momentarily consider this question in isolation from therapeutic concerns. Clinical trials are designed to eliminate or reduce uncertainty about some matter. But such trials, precisely because they involve human subjects, always have human costs. Hence, not every improvement in clinical knowledge—not every reduction or elimination of uncertainty—is worth pursuing. That will depend on the value of the knowledge gained and how this relates to the human costs. On the *knowledge* side, value depends both on the *degree* of certainty to be gained by the proposed trial and on the *type* of knowledge it is. Overall, the trial must reflect an appropriate balancing of gains against costs: the value of what is to be gained must be able to justify the real costs to the subjects, whatever these may be.[35]

I want to focus for the moment on questions about the *appropriate degree* of certainty. That this is an important determinant of value in a trial is reflected in the common requirement that, at the outset, there must actually be a significant degree of *uncertainty* about the relative net therapeutic merits of the interventions to be compared (including placebo as a possible "intervention"), and that the trial as designed must actually be able to reduce or eliminate that uncertainty. However, certainty is a matter of degree. Knowledge is best thought of as an asymptote—a limit that over time we approach nearer and nearer to, but never actually reach. This is just to say that it is always *possible* to gain greater degrees of certainty about a general conclusion. At a certain point, however, we are satisfied with the degree of certainty attained and view the search for greater certainty as not worth it. In the case of clinical research, a large part of what determines when it is no longer worth pursuing additional certainty is the human costs. Whether we are aware of it or not, or whether we explicitly frame such decisions to ourselves in this way, some such judgments (about how to appropriately balance human costs against greater certainty) implicitly lie behind the judgments we make about which clinical trials are morally worth running.

Presumably there is some ideal set of norms that would tell us how to balance these various concerns in order to arrive at judgments about which trials are worth running. Without trying to define these norms here, we can refer to the ideal set (whatever it turns out to be) as the set of *overall balancing norms*. As with therapeutic choice norms, we should note that there is room for reasonable disagreement over what the ideal set of overall balancing norms would be.

These two questions—(1) which therapeutic choices can legitimately be made by the flip of a coin and (2) which trials are morally worth running, all things considered—are distinct. The majority of theorists, however, make the answer to the second question depend on the answer to the first. One way of deciding when there is a sufficient degree of scientific uncertainty about the relative merits of two or more interventions to justify running a clinical trial is to say that we have the appropriate degree of uncertainty if and only if a physician, contemplating treatment choices for a patient and guided by the ideal set of therapeutic choice norms, would be indifferent as between these interventions. I shall call this *the alignment approach*. The deeper controversy about equipoise (alluded to earlier) arises because there is more than one way to arrive at alignment.

To see this, imagine a hypothetical case involving a drug D that has been shown by previous research to be extremely helpful in high doses for a serious condition Z. High-dose treatment with D is unavailable in the developing world and will be for a long time to come, despite the wide prevalence of Z in some countries. These countries therefore have an interest in knowing whether low doses of D are effective and if so just *how* effective they are. There is no evidence to suggest (as some people thought there was in the AZT case) that D might pose a danger to the particular population. There are, of course, health differences between the two groups, as there are between any two populations. But given what is already known about D from earlier trials of the high-dose regimen— in particular what is known about how the body handles D— there is no reason to expect that these health differences predict any difference in the toxicity of D for the two populations. Hence, investigators are contemplating running a trial of low-dose D against placebo.

Would this proposed trial satisfy the principle of clinical equipoise? It is actually hard to say. Some would argue that the trial violates the therapeutic intent of equipoise *and*, therefore, is not worth running. It arguably violates the therapeutic intent because it seems that an ideal physician adhering to ideal therapeutic choice norms would have good reason to prefer low-dose D over placebo. After all, given how effective high-dose D is known to be, it seems reasonable to suppose that low-dose D will still be *more effective* than placebo. Moreover, given what is known about how people process high-dose D, is seems reasonable to suppose that low-dose D will be at least as safe as high-dose D. Finally, it is significant that Z is a serious illness, where the consequences of doing nothing are bleak. Ideal therapeutic choice norms are presumably sensitive to such facts. Most physicians faced with a serious illness in their patient would be *more* willing to proceed despite great uncertainty about the benefits and safety of a proposed treatment than they would in a similar case where the patient's illness was not as severe. Indeed, on one reasonable view, the ideal therapeutic choice norms say that a physician contemplating treatment for a particular patient with Z and faced with only the choice between low-dose D or nothing would be *obligated* to offer low-dose D.

Of course, the evidence for safety and effectiveness of low-dose D is extremely thin (that is why others want to run a trial). But it is at least within the realm of reasonable views to think that a physician guided by the ideally specified therapeutic choice norms would not be *indifferent* as between low-dose D and placebo. If one adopts a vision of therapeutic choice norms that gives this result, *and* one believes in alignment, then one will also view a trial comparing low-dose D to placebo as ethically unjustifiable. A theorist who approaches the topic this way allows her semi-independent sense of the appropriate therapeutic choice norms to shape her views about the types and degrees of scientific uncertainty worth eliminating.

There is, however, a different kind of alignment theorist. These are people who hold *both* that such trials satisfy the therapeutic intent of equipoise *and* that such trials are morally, all things considered, worth running. Such a theorist might argue that there is really no good *therapeutic* reason for preferring low-dose D over placebo at this point. After all, no one has ever tested low-dose D for the treatment of Z. With respect to efficacy, all we have to go on is a very loose inference from the fact that high-dose D is effective to the conclusion that low-dose will *probably* be at least *somewhat effective* as well. And with respect to safety, all we have to go on is a very loose inference from the fact that high-dose D was not toxic in one population to the conclusion that low-dose will *probably* be safe in a very different population. But such inferences have been known to fail in the past. Precisely because they have sometimes failed in the past, because Z is such a serious illness, and because we are contemplating giving thousands of people low-dose D for Z, we want to make sure low-dose D really works and really is safe. On such a view, there cannot be a therapeutic obligation to provide a treatment in the absence of a certain degree of certainty about its safety and effectiveness, a degree of certainty that is lacking here. So a trial comparing low-dose D and placebo cannot be said to violate a therapeutic obligation.[36] Moreover, given how important it is to know that low-dose D is better than placebo, such a trial is well worth running.

The theorist who adopts this view agrees that therapeutic obligations place a limit on the kinds of research that are permissible. However, her sense of what the ideal therapeutic choice norms are is not, in this case, fully independent of her views about the type and degree of scientific uncertainty it is important to eliminate. Nor is such a viewpoint obviously flawed. It can seem natural to reason from the fact that we lack a significant degree of scientific certainty about the relative merits of two treatments, to the conclusion that a physician would therefore have no good therapeutic reason to prefer one to the other, and hence no obligation to decide the matter in any other way than by flipping a coin. This is to let one's sense of significant scientific uncertainty shape one's appreciation of the appropriate therapeutic choice norms.

In short, because there is room for reasonable disagreement about what the ideal therapeutic choice norms are and also various ways of aligning the answers to questions (1) and (2), there are different possible views about when equipoise is satisfied. Given that, for the majority of theorists, satisfying equipoise is a necessary requirement for an ethically justifiable trial, it turns out that there are correspondingly different ways of distinguishing between acceptable and unacceptable trials.

There is a third possible position to adopt in relation to equipoise, albeit a minority view. This view rejects alignment altogether, that is, rejects the attempt to use the notion of therapeutic indifference to settle the question of which trials are morally worth undertaking. Since equipoise in research is designed to ensure that researchers satisfy their obligations as physicians, equipoise depends on the notion of therapeutic indifference. So to give up on the idea that therapeutic indifference will settle the matter of which trials are morally acceptable is to give up on the principle of clinical equipoise. This view has been defended in other contexts, though not specifically in relation to developing world trials.[37] But one might think that the specific problems raised by developing world second-best alternative trials make this option appear even more attractive than it otherwise might.

What might motivate such a move? One motivation is that each of the two quite different ways of reaching alignment has drawbacks. Consider first the position of those who argue that such trials fail equipoise and are therefore impermissible. Such a view of therapeutic choice norms coupled with a commitment to alignment has profound consequences for one's view of many developing world trials, in particular those that seek information about second-best treatment alternatives. Such a view will rule out not only a trial comparing low-dose D to placebo *but also* a trial comparing low-dose D to high-dose D. In the AZT case, Angell famously suggested substituting the proposed placebo-controlled trials of low-dose AZT with trials comparing low-dose AZT to the 076 regimen.[38] But, as several critics pointed out, such a trial would *also* fail equipoise as Angell appears to understand it.[39] In her proposed alternative, there will be a reasonable therapeutic preference for the 076 regimen over low-dose D. In many instances, this kind of view will rule out any trial (placebo or active) of an intervention expected from the outset to be less effective than some other known intervention.

The alternative way of reaching alignment sketched earlier avoids this unfortunate outcome. But it may seem to some theorists that it does so by stretching beyond plausibility the notion of ideal therapeutic choice. In other words, it is at least reasonable to think that ideal *therapeutic choice norms* really are closer to the kinds of norms Angell appeals to. But perhaps this need not mean that a trial is therefore unethical. Perhaps this just shows that ideal therapeutic choice norms cannot always be used as a reliable measure of when a trial is ethically justifiable. If one pursues this line of thought, one must also question whether it makes sense to see researchers as having all the same therapeutic obligations as physicians. However, abandoning the view that researchers have the obligations of physicians is not necessarily abandoning the view that they have significant obligations to their subjects. What these obligations are remains to be spelled out, but it does not imply an "anything goes" approach to research ethics.

Equipoise has always been a contentious topic. Problems with the understanding of equipoise—problems that stem from the fact that there is room for reasonable disagreement about both the ideal therapeutic choice norms and the ideal justifiability norms—arise even in developed countries. However, the kinds of cases that have come up in developing countries have made these existent tensions all the more visible and urgent. Trials like AZT, which seek to discover the effectiveness of what are expected to be second-best treatment alternatives, pose interesting challenges to the common commitment to seeing the justifiability of research as dependent on fulfillment of therapeutic obligations.

History and Meaning of "Exploitation"

The most general meaning of the term "exploitation" is "advantageous use" of something or someone. This broad definition includes nonmoralized meanings of the term as, for example, in the claim "A exploited the hill to get a good view of the ocean." However, the sense that interests moral philosophers is the sense in which a *person* (or group of persons) is used. Furthermore, the use must be *unfair* or *morally problematic* in some sense. Different theories of exploitation are different accounts of what is morally problematic with certain ways of using people.

It is primarily through the influence of Marx and his followers that exploitation became a familiar moral term, and for that reason people often assume that the term has application only within a Marxist framework. There is, however, a robust and growing contemporary literature that seeks to develop non-Marxist accounts of exploitation. This volume is best viewed as a contribution to this (relatively) new stream of thought. Nonetheless, in thinking about exploitation, it is helpful to know a bit about the history of the term, including Marx's use, because many of the central questions of the current debate have been shaped by the Marxist tradition.

Marxist Exploitation

In Marx, "exploitation" is used both descriptively and normatively in ways that are sometimes in tension with one another. This has led to lively debate among Marxist scholars about the best, most authentic account of Marxist exploitation. For the sake of simplicity, I shall focus on one view here: that of Jon Elster.[40]

Marxist exploitation requires first that an individual labor more than is strictly necessary to meet his or her own needs and hence more than would strictly be required to sustain his or her labor over time. When the product of this surplus labor is appropriated by another person (who is thereby enabled to work less than he or she strictly would have to in order to meet his or her needs), we have exploitation.[41] This technical, descriptive account, however, does not tell us what (if anything) is morally problematic about exploitation. Moreover, it is possible to imagine cases that would fit the technical, descriptive definition but would not strike us as morally problematic at all.[42]

Despite the apparent tensions between Marx's descriptive account and the term's normative meaning, Elster argues (convincingly, I think) that Marx intended to use the word in a normatively loaded sense. In short, Marx took exploitation to be fundamentally *unjust*.[43] It is true that Marx failed to notice that some unobjectionable cases might fit his descriptive definition, but it is easy enough to see why he might have overlooked this fact. The cases he primarily focused upon and which inspired his work—nineteenth-century cases of extremely poor people working under horrific conditions for subsistence wages, even as their employers became incredibly wealthy—did have all the outward marks of deep injustice.[44]

Those unfamiliar with Marx may be surprised to learn that Elster must *argue* for the claim that Marx thought exploitation was unjust. However, this *is* required because of the way in which Marx himself framed the issues. He was deeply distrustful of moral language because he believed that the meaning of moral terms is shaped by the concerns of the most powerful social class. In order not to have the success of his arguments depend upon agreement about moral terminology, Marx simply refused to use the terminology of morality and justice. Elster plausibly insists, however, that we understand Marx better, overall, if we view him as a *moral* philosopher who unwisely ceded the meanings of important words to his rivals, but who was nonetheless motivated by a passionate sense of the injustice of the institutions of his day.[45]

While it is easy to see the link between Marx's sense of the term "exploitation" and the general idea of unfair use, it is also true that Marx's account is of little practical help when it comes to the concerns of this book. Indeed, that is true in connection with many contemporary debates where we might want to analyze charges of exploitation. Marx's account is both too narrow (it is concerned only with the uncompensated use of a person's excess labor) and too broad (since it applies to the vast majority of wage labor transactions in a capitalist society). If we are to use the term without at the same time engaging in a wholesale critique of capitalism, we need an analysis that allows us to single out particularly egregious uses of persons, while maintaining the background assumption that not *all* exchanges under capitalism are egregious. Furthermore, we want to examine the idea that transactions other than labor agreements may be exploitative. We need an account that applies to both personal and commercial transactions, as well as one that can help us think about not only the morality of exchanging familiar market commodities but also the morality of exchanging items not usually viewed as *commodities* in quite the same sense: items such as women's procreative labor, kidneys (or other organs), or the use of one's body for medical research.[46]

Contemporary Non-Marxist Approaches to Exploitation

The contemporary non-Marxist approach to "exploitation" begins with the idea that one person (A) exploits another person (B) when A takes advantage of B in a morally inappropriate way, where the emphasis on *appropriateness* is intended to underscore the fact (too often overlooked) that not all instances of taking advantage are problematic.[47] All the authors in this collection share at least this minimal account of exploitation. In addition, they agree about the answers to the following three significant questions: (1) Must exploitation be involuntary? (2) Must exploitation be harmful for the exploitee? (3) Does it follow from the fact that a practice is exploitative that it ought to be prohibited?

Consider first the question: *Must exploitation be involuntary?* The authors collected here agree that the answer is no.[48] This marks a significant point of departure from the Marxist tradition.

Marxists frequently maintain the opposite: namely, that exploitation is never voluntary because whenever workers agree to sell their labor to capitalists, their decision is *coerced*. This thesis is underwritten, in turn, by the Marxist account of the historical origin of the circumstances that make it appealing for workers to accept subsistence-level wages. As emphasized earlier, coercion is importantly different from cases in which individuals are "forced" to choose something by harsh circumstances. Coercion is present only when A forcibly narrows B's option set *or* threatens to make B worse off if B does not do as A wishes. Bad circumstances are not *in themselves* coercive, as long as A did not create the circumstances in the first place.

If this is correct, then it might seem that Marxists are simply guilty of confusing harsh choice situations and coercion. Workers usually agree to accept subsistence wages from capitalists because they are poor, and because subsistence wages are better than nothing. But (in the usual case at least) no one threatens to make them worse off if they refuse to work for these wages. Hence, it would seem they are not *coerced*. However, Marx believed that the background circumstances against which subsistence wage offers tend to look good to workers *have themselves been unjustly constructed by capitalists*.[49] Hence, the decisions of the workers are coerced in the first sense of the term: namely, one party has forcibly narrowed the option set of the other. Only against this broad historical assumption does it make sense to see *all* choices to accept low wages as involuntary.

There is consensus among the authors in this collection that while exploitation *may* be involuntary, lack of voluntariness is neither necessary nor sufficient to create exploitation. On the one hand, a transaction may be fully voluntary and yet morally problematic in some *other* way that supports the charge of exploitation. Of course, different theorists offer different accounts of what the moral problem with a voluntary transaction might be. Perhaps, as Alan Wertheimer suggests (in chapter 3), a fully voluntary transaction between A and B is exploitative if the division of the benefits and burdens created through the transaction is distributively unfair.[50] Or perhaps, as Alisa Carse and Margaret Little argue (in chapter 7), a voluntary transaction counts as exploitative if A takes advantage of a deep vulnerability of B's and this vulnerability is one that, given A's normative role, A has *special* moral reason *not* to press.[51] On the other hand, a transaction may be *involuntary* but still not exploitative, as, for example, when A paternalistically forces B to do something for her own good, but A gains nothing thereby.

Consider next the question: *Must exploitation be harmful for the exploitee?* Once again, the consensus answer is no.[52] Exploitation *may*, but need not, be harmful.

Over time, many people, Marxists and non-Marxists alike, have been tempted to assume that exploitation involves harm.[53] This is partly driven by the thought that the harmfulness of exploitation must be what explains its badness. Indeed, some people seem to fear that without harm there will be nothing for an exploitee to complain *of.* This mode of thinking is also partly reinforced by the fact that there is a loose sense of "harm" in which "harm" is just a synonym for wrong. Clearly, if exploitation wrongs a person, and wrongs are harms, then exploitation harms. However, it is worth keeping the loose sense of "harm" distinct from the more substantive notion according to which a person suffers harm when her welfare-related interests are lowered relative to some appropriately specified baseline. In this sense, it is quite possible for one to be wronged without being harmed. The earlier examples can be used to illustrate this point as well: distributive unfairness in the outcome of a transaction may be present even when both parties benefit to some extent. And again, a person may be used in ways that seem particularly worrisome even though she is not made worse off welfare-wise by the transaction. Indeed, some of the authors in this collection would maintain that some of the most troubling kinds of wrongs are those that occur in the absence of direct harm.

Consider, finally, the third question: *Does it automatically follow from the fact that a practice is exploitative that it ought to be prohibited?*[54] The consensus answer is that this does *not* follow. There is wide disagreement among this group about which actual practices under which circumstances *count* as exploitative, and disagreement about which (if any) of these practices should be prohibited. Still, everyone agrees that not all morally troubling actions are appropriately regulated by the state or (in international contexts) by international governing agencies. Some aspects of morality are rightly made into law, but others are appropriately left to individual conscience and the milder regulation of public opinion. Hence, even if certain clinical research practices turn out to be exploitative, additional argument is needed to establish that they should be prohibited.

Notes

1. Robert J. Levine, *Ethics and Regulation of Clinical Research*, 2nd ed. (New Haven, CT: Yale University Press, 1986), 6.

2. Ezekiel J. Emanuel, David Wendler, and Christine Grady, "What Makes Clinical Research Ethical?" *Journal of the American Medical Association* 283 (2000): 2701–11.

3. Howard W. French, "AIDS Research in Africa: Juggling Risks and Hopes," *New York Times*, October 9, 1997.

4. *Id.*

5. E.g., Grace Malenga, a medical researcher in Malawi, discusses the difficulties of explaining the concept of a placebo (for which there is no direct translation) in Sharon LaFraniere, Mary Pat Flaherty, and Joe Stephens, "The Dilemma: Submit or Suffer," article 3 of "The Body Hunters," *Washington Post*, December 19, 2000, A01.

6. Quarraisha Abdool Karim et al., "Informed Consent for HIV Testing in a South African Hospital: Is It Truly Informed and Truly Voluntary?" *American Journal of Public Health* 88, no. 4 (1998): 637–40.

7. Paul S. Appelbaum et al., "False Hopes and Best Data: Consent to Research and the Therapeutic Misconception," *Hastings Center Report* 17, no. 2 (1987): 20–24; Paul S. Appelbaum, Loren H. Roth, and Charles W. Lidz, "The Therapeutic Misconception: Informed Consent in Psychiatric Research," *International Journal of Law and Psychiatry* 5 (1982): 319–29.

8. Gopal Sreenivasan, "Does Informed Consent to Research Require Comprehension?" *Lancet* 362 (2003): 2016–18.

9. This quotation from Annas appears in LaFraniere, Flaherty, and Stephens, *supra* note 5. Also see George J. Annas and Michael A. Grodin, "Human Rights and Maternal-Fetal HIV Transmission Prevention Trials in Africa," *American Journal of Public Health* 88, no. 4 (1998): 560–63.

10. For example, consider the following quotation: "It is difficult to avoid coercing subjects in most settings where clinical investigation in the developing world is conducted. African subjects with relatively little understanding of medical aspects of research participation, indisposed toward resisting the suggestions of Western doctors, perhaps operating under the mistaken notion that they are being treated, and possibly receiving some ancillary benefits from participation in research, are very susceptible to coercion." Nicholas A. Christakis, "The Ethical Design of an AIDS Vaccine Trial in Africa," *Hastings Center Report* 18, no. 3 (1988): 31–37, at 31. For more extensive discussion of common

confusions about coercion in clinical research, see Jennifer S. Hawkins and Ezekiel J. Emanuel, "Clarifying Confusions about Coercion," *Hastings Center Report* 35, no. 5 (2005): 16–19.

11. Graham Lindegger and Susan Bull, "Ensuring Valid Consent in a Developing Country Context," *SciDevNet*, November 1, 2002, www.scidev.net /en/policy-briefs/ensuring-valid-consent-in-a-developing-country-con.html.

12. The HIV Netherlands Australia Thailand Research Collaboration, *A Model for HIV-AIDS Clinical Research in a Developing Country* (Geneva: UNAIDS, 2000), cited in Lindegger and Bull, *supra* note 11.

13. Ezekiel J. Emanuel, "Ending Concerns about Undue Inducement," *Journal of Law, Medicine and Ethics* 32 (2004): 100–105, at 100.

14. Emanuel further points out that when all the other standard requirements for ethical research are met (favorable risk-benefit ratio, IRB review, etc.), then by definition undue inducement has been ruled out, since trials that present excessive risks will have been eliminated. This does not serve to show that undue inducement never occurs, but it does serve to show that it is *possible* to eliminate it, by ensuring that the other requirements of ethical research are met. See Emanuel, *supra* note 13, at 102.

15. Christakis, *supra* note 10; Robert J. Levine, "Informed Consent: Some Challenges to the Universal Validity of the Western Model," *Law, Medicine and Health Care* 19 (1991): 207–13; Carl E. Taylor, "Clinical Trials and International Health Research," *American Journal of Public Health* 69, no. 10 (1979): 981–83.

16. Lawrence O. Gostin, "Informed Consent, Cultural Sensitivity and Respect for Persons," *Journal of the American Medical Association* 274 (1995): 844–45.

17. Carel B. Ijsselmuiden and Ruth R. Faden, "Research and Informed Consent in Africa—Another Look," *New England Journal of Medicine* 326 (1992): 830–34; Marcia Angell, "Ethical Imperialism? Ethics in International Collaborative Clinical Research," *New England Journal of Medicine* 319 (1988): 1081–83.

18. Leslie F. Degner and Jeffrey A. Sloan, "Decision-Making during Serious Illness: What Role Do Patients Really Want to Play?" *Journal of Clinical Epidemiology* 45 (1992): 941–50; Jack Ende et al., "Measuring Patients' Desire for Autonomy: Decision-Making and Information Seeking Preferences among Medical Patients," *Journal of General Internal Medicine* 4 (1989): 23–30; Robert F. Nease Jr. and W. Blair Brooks, "Patient Desire for Information and Decision-Making in Health Care Decisions: The Autonomy Preference Index and the Health Opinion Survey," *Journal of General Internal Medicine* 10 (1995): 593–600; H. J. Southerland et al., "Cancer Patients: Their Desire for Informa-

tion and Participation in Treatment Decisions," *Journal of the Royal Society of Medicine* 82 (1989): 260–63; William M. Strull, Bernard Lo, and Gerald Charles, "Do Patients Want to Participate in Medical Decision-Making?" *Journal of the American Medical Association* 252 (1984): 2990–94.

19. Indeed, this is a *kind* of choice, and for some people it *may* represent a strategy for maintaining ultimate veto power. In other words, many people may be quite happy to let others make certain kinds of choices, as long as they know what is going on. For by remaining informed, the individual leaves open the possibility of asserting herself later, if for some reason she comes to believe that the wrong decision has been made.

20. Eugene Passamani, "Clinical Trials—Are They Ethical?" *New England Journal of Medicine* 324 (1991): 1589–92, at 1589.

21. Although there is a clear sense in which there is no good *medical* reason to develop a new drug that is not as effective (all things considered) as one already available, there may be *financial* reasons for doing so, particularly if one can hide from others the fact that the new drug is not as effective. For this reason, in the developed world pharmaceutical companies often prefer to test a new drug against a placebo *if they can*, because such a trial will reveal whether the new drug is effective without thereby revealing how it compares to existing drugs. Companies are allowed to do this only when the health effects for subjects of receiving placebo are not too dire. There are, of course, other reasons for wanting to use placebos—for example, in cases such as depression research, where the illness under study is known to have a high rate of spontaneous remission—but in cases where these sorts of methodological reasons are absent, one might wonder why placebos are allowed. Under current U.S. law the FDA only requires companies to demonstrate *efficacy*, not *superior or equivalent efficacy*. On this topic, see Marcia Angell, *The Truth about the Drug Companies* (New York: Random House, 2005), 75.

22. Ezekiel J. Emanuel and Franklin G. Miller, "The Ethics of Placebo-Controlled Trials—A Middle Ground," *New England Journal of Medicine* 345 (2001): 915–19, at 916.

23. *Id.*

24. A good account of the contrast between descriptive and normative notions of medical standards and their implications for this debate is provided by Alex John London, "The Ambiguity and the Exigency: Clarifying 'Standard of Care' Arguments in International Research," *Journal of Medicine and Philosophy* 25 (2000): 379–97.

25. Declaration of Helsinki, September 1989, para. II.3.

26. Robert J. Levine, "The 'Best Proven Therapeutic Method' Standard in

Clinical Trials in Technologically Developing Countries," *IRB: A Review of Human Subjects Research* 20, no. 1 (1998): 5–9.

27. Peter Lurie and Sidney M. Wolfe, "Unethical Trials of Interventions to Reduce Perinatal Transmission of the Human Immunodeficiency Virus in Developing Countries," *New England Journal of Medicine* 337 (1997): 853–55.

28. It is important to emphasize that what is being rejected is a crude form of utilitarian thinking. Many more sophisticated forms of utilitarian thinking, or of consequentialist thinking more generally, embrace theories of rights and try to maximize beneficial consequences within the constraints imposed by those (consequentially justified) rights.

29. Marcia Angell, "The Ethics of Clinical Research in the Third World," *New England Journal of Medicine* 337 (1997): 847–49, at 847; reference to para. III.4 of the 1989 version of the Declaration, *supra* note 25.

30. Benjamin Freedman, "Equipoise and the Ethics of Clinical Research," *New England Journal of Medicine* 317 (1987): 141–45.

31. For example, in "Equipoise and the Ethics of Clinical Research," Freedman makes frequent references to the duties of a clinician. For a detailed overview of the links between equipoise and the view of a researcher as simultaneously a clinician with all the duties of a clinician, see Franklin G. Miller and Howard Brody, "A Critique of Clinical Equipoise: Therapeutic Misconception in the Ethics of Clinical Trials," *Hastings Center Report* 33, no. 3 (2003): 19–28.

32. Benjamin Freedman, "Placebo-Controlled Trials and the Logic of Clinical Purpose," *IRB: A Review of Human Subjects Research* 12, no. 6 (1990): 1–6. The phrase "net therapeutic advantage" is introduced on p. 2.

33. Harold Varmus and David Satcher, "Ethical Complexities of Conducting Research in Developing Countries," *New England Journal of Medicine* 337 (1997): 1003–5, at 1004; Christine Grady, "Science in the Service of Healing," *Hastings Center Report* 28, no. 6 (1998): 34-38 at 36; M. H. Merson, "Ethics of Placebo-Controlled Trials of Zidovudine to Prevent the Perinatal Transmission of HIV in the Third World" (editorial), *New England Journal of Medicine* 338 (1998): 836; R. J. Simonds, M. F. Rogers, and T. J. Dondero, "Ethics of Placebo-Controlled Trials of Zidovudine to Prevent the Perinatal Transmission of HIV in the Third World" (editorial), *New England Journal of Medicine* 338 (1998): 836–37.

34. Angell, *supra* note 29, at 848.

35. The metaphor of balancing can falsely suggest that *any* cost to subjects no matter how high can be justified by enough gain on the "other side." However, almost everyone writing about research ethics would disagree with that and insist that there are absolute limits to the total costs we are willing to impose on human subjects. There is a limit beyond which further gains in knowl-

edge cannot justify proceeding. In the text, for ease of exposition, I take this to be understood. Even so, the balancing metaphor remains a useful way of picturing the kinds of decisions that have to be made: those decisions where the contemplated human costs are still within the permissible range. For even within this range, if particular costs are to be justified, it must be true that the costs are appropriately balanced against the type and degree of certainty to be gained.

36. For example, I believe this is the view of equipoise held by Christine Grady, supra note 33.

37. See, e.g., Miller and Brody, *supra* note 31.

38. Angell, *supra* note 29, at 847.

39. See, e.g., Reidar K. Lie, "Ethics of Placebo-Controlled Trials in Developing Countries," *Bioethics* 12 (1998): 307–11; Alex John London, "Equipoise and International Human-Subjects Research," *Bioethics* 15 (2001): 312–32.

40. Jon Elster, *An Introduction to Karl Marx* (New York: Cambridge University Press, 1986), chap. 5; also Jon Elster, "Exploitation, Freedom and Justice," in *Marxism* (*Nomos* 26), ed. J. Roland Pennock and John W. Chapman (New York: New York University Press, 1983), 277–304, reprinted in *Exploitation: Key Concepts in Critical Theory*, ed. Kai Nielsen and Robert Ware (New York: Humanities Press, 1997), 27–48.

41. Elster, *An Introduction to Karl Marx, supra* note 40, at 80.

42. This is true no matter which account of the wrongness of Marxist exploitation one favors. For the rival conceptions of what is morally wrong with Marxist exploitation, see note 43 below.

43. This is really two claims: first, that exploitation is a *moral wrong*, and second that the moral wrong is a form of *injustice*. Some Marxists insist the Marx's critique of capitalism was not a value-based critique at all; that Marx was not in the business of moral assessment. Others allow that Marx saw moral flaws with capitalism, but that injustice was not one of them. Allen Wood, in "The Marxian Critique of Justice," *Philosophy and Public Affairs* 1 (1972): 244–82, defends the former, more radical view. Among those who see Marx as engaged in moral criticism of capitalism, there are two views about the wrongness of exploitation. Some locate the wrongness in the lack of freedom of those who are exploited: in the fact that they are forced to labor for the capitalist class. See, e.g., Nancy Holmstrom, "Exploitation," *Canadian Journal of Philosophy* 7 (1977): 353–69; Jeffrey Reiman, "Exploitation, Force, and the Moral Assessment of Capitalism," *Philosophy and Public Affairs* 16 (1987): 3–41; Justin Schwartz, "What's Wrong with Exploitation?" *Nous* 29 (1995): 158–88. Others have argued that the wrongness of Marxist exploitation (even if exploitation is typically brought about by force) must be understood primarily in terms of distributive

justice. For variants of this view, see Richard Arneson, "What's Wrong with Exploitation?" *Ethics* 91 (1981): 202–27; John E. Roemer, "Should Marxists Be Interested in Exploitation? *Philosophy and Public Affairs* 14 (1985): 30–65; G. A. Cohen, "The Labor Theory of Value and the Concept of Exploitation," in *History, Labour, and Freedom* (Oxford: Clarendon Press, 1988), 209–38.

44. Elster, *An Introduction to Karl Marx, supra* note 40, at 92.

45. *Id.* at 92–93.

46. The literature on these other topics is vast. However, an interesting recent attempt to relate exploitation to commercial surrogacy, kidney sales, and other body commodification debates is Stephen Wilkinson, *Bodies for Sale: Ethics and Exploitation in the Human Body Trade* (New York: Routledge, 2003).

47. This is common ground among the contemporary non-Marxist theorists, including Joel Feinberg, *Harmless Wrongdoing* (New York: Oxford University Press, 1990), chaps. 31 and 32; Robert Goodin, "Exploiting a Situation and Exploiting a Person," in *Modern Theories of Exploitation*, ed. Andrew Reeve (London: Sage, 1987), 166–200; Hillel Steiner, "A Liberal Theory of Exploitation," *Ethics* 94 (1984): 225–41; Alan Wertheimer, *Exploitation* (Princeton, NJ: Princeton University Press, 1996); Ruth J. Sample, *Exploitation: What It Is and Why It's Wrong* (New York: Rowman and Littlefield, 2003).

48. All the authors mentioned in note 47 above also agree that exploitation need not be involuntary.

49. For example, "Marx argued that the English enclosures from the sixteenth to the eighteenth century were partly carried out with a view to drive the small peasants from the land, thus coercing them into selling their labor power." Elster, *An Introduction to Karl Marx, supra* note 40, at 82–83.

50. See also Wertheimer, *supra* note 47.

51. This is only one kind of case that counts as exploitative on their view.

52. Once again, this view is also shared by all the authors mentioned in note 47 above.

53. For example, Allen Buchanan, *Marx and Justice* (Totowa, N.J.: Rowman and Littlefield, 1982), 44.

54. This question is central to Wertheimer's project in *Exploitation*.

Case Studies: The Havrix Trial and the Surfaxin Trial

The Havrix Trial

Thailand
Population: 65.4 million (2005)
Government type: constitutional monarchy
Previous colonial rule: none
GDP: $181 billion (2005) $545.8 billion (purchasing power parity 2005)
Health expenditure as % of GDP: 6%
GDP per capita: $8,300 (purchasing power parity 2005)
Health expenditure per capita (PPP): $349
Life expectancy at birth: 70 (M), 74 (F)
Infant mortality rate: 20.5 per 1,000 live births
Physicians per 100,000 population: 30
Corruption Perception Index (2004): 3.6, country number 64

Data from CIA World Book, WHO Countries Report, and Transparency International's Annual Report

Havrix is an inactivated hepatitis A vaccine that was tested in 1990 among schoolchildren from Kamphaeng Phet province in northern Thailand.[1] The study was a collaboration of Walter Reed Army Institute of Research (U.S. government), SmithKline Beecham Biologicals, and Thailand's Ministry of Public Health. Initially, there was a randomized, double-blind Phase II study involving 300 children, primarily family members of physicians and nurses at the Kamphaeng Phet provincial hospital. After demonstration of safety and a hepatitis A–neutralizing antibody response, a randomized, double-blind Phase III trial with a hepatitis B vaccine control involving 40,000 children aged one to sixteen was initiated.

The study was conducted in Thailand for several reasons. First, there was increasing hepatitis A infection during adolescence and adulthood, when morbidity was greater, including more hepatitis A outbreaks at schools, such as at the National Police Academy in 1988. Second, while hepatitis A transmission was focal, there was a sufficiently high transmission rate—119 per 100,000 population—in rural areas to assess vaccine efficacy. Third, the area had been the site of a prior Japanese encephalitis (JE) vaccine study.[2] Ultimately, the JE vaccine was registered in Thailand in 1988 and included in the Thai mandatory immunization policy in 1992.

Importantly, there was no formal, prior agreement to make Havrix widely available in Thailand. Due to competing vaccination priorities, especially for implementation of hepatitis B vaccine, the cost of a newly developed hepatitis A vaccine, and the available health care budget in Thailand, it was unlikely that in the foreseeable future Havrix would be included in Thailand's national immunization program in which vaccines are provided to the population at no cost. In addition, SmithKline Beecham Biologicals made no commitment to provide free Havrix to Thailand. However, the company did verbally commit to pursue Havrix registration in Thailand, anticipating a permissive use recommendation by the Ministry of Public Health with sales limited to the private market. While there was no promise of pricing for the private market, SmithKline Beecham Biologicals had previously utilized tiered pricing. Registration and sales on the private market would enable the Ministry of Public Health to use Havrix to control hepatitis A outbreaks at schools and other institutes. Nevertheless, at the start of the trial, all collaborators recognized that the largest market for Havrix would be travelers from developed countries to developing countries.

There were benefits for Thailand from the Havrix trial. First, by design, all 40,000 children in the trial would receive the hepatitis B vaccine and, if it proved effective, the hepatitis A vaccine. Second, medical services were augmented. The research team contracted with community public health workers to examine all enrolled children absent from school at their homes, to provide necessary care, and, if appropriate, to arrange transfer to the district or provincial hospital.

There were also benefits for the population. Public health stations throughout Kamphaeng Phet province that lacked adequate refrigeration to store vaccines, medicines, and blood specimens received new refrigerators. Similarly, those lacking reliable access to the existing FM wireless network linking the health stations with the provincial hospital's consultants were joined to the network. In the six schools that had hepatitis A outbreaks during the study, the research team arranged for inspection of the schools and identification of deficiencies in toilet facilities, hand-washing facilities, and water storage. At each school, the researchers contracted to have recommended improvements implemented. In addition, the public health workers were provided with unlimited stocks of disposable syringes and needles, as well as training on measures to reduce the incidence of blood-borne diseases. Hepatitis B vaccinations were provided to all interested government personnel working on the trial, including approximately 2,500 teachers, public health workers, nurses, technicians, and physicians. Since all the deaths of enrolled research participants were tracked and investigated, the research team identified motor vehicle accidents, especially pedestrians struck by cars, as a major cause of mortality in the province and recommended corrective measures.[3] Finally, although there was no long-term commitment made by SmithKline Beecham at the time to the population, the training of Thai researchers and experience in conducting the Havrix trial may have facilitated subsequent trials, including the current HIV vaccine trials in Thailand.

In initiating and conducting the trial there were extensive consultations in Kamphaeng Phet province. The provincial governor, medical officer, education secretary, and hospital director provided comment before granting their approval. In each of the 146 communities that participated in the study, researchers made public presentations about the study and held briefings for interested parents and teachers. Each school appointed a teacher to maintain liaison with the research team. Parental and community support appeared to be related to the provision of hepatitis B vaccine to all participants, since it was perceived to be a major health problem and the children lacked access to the vaccine. Furthermore, the protocol was reviewed by the Thai Ministry of Public Health's National Ethical Review Committee as well as two institutional review boards in the United States. The Ministry of Public Health appointed an independent committee composed of thirteen senior physicians and ministry officials to monitor the safety and efficacy of the trial.

Several Thai scientists objected to participation in the Havrix trial, raising four arguments. First, some argued that Thailand had no interest in the hepatitis A vaccine or expectation of deploying it. Consequently, the trial did not address a pressing health need of the country in a manner appropriate to the country but did address a health interest of the U.S. Army. Thus, the Thai children who participated were used as "testing material" for the benefit of the U.S. Army and others from developed countries. Second, there was insufficient technology transfer. In particular, there was no training of Thai researchers to conduct testing for antibody to hepatitis A and other laboratory skills. Third, it was claimed, there was inadequate respect or capacity development accorded to the Thai researchers collaborating on the vaccine study. Not only were Thai researchers not the principal investigators on the study, but a contested claim suggested that none of the Thai investigators were individually named in the original protocol but were simply referred to as "Thai researchers." Only after protests were they individually identified. Finally, if the vaccine was proven safe and effective, there was no provision to ensure it would be made available to Thailand at a reduced cost. The sentiment against Thai participation in the trial was summarized by a prominent vaccine researcher: "Journalists in the country have accused the government and medical community of a national betrayal in allowing Thai children to be exploited. . . . The role of Thailand in rounding up its children for immunization was hardly seen as a meaningful partnership in this research aim. In private, government ministers agreed with this, but the sway of international politics and money was too persuasive."[4] Indeed, there was an attempt to persuade the Ministry of Public Health, and especially the National Ethical Review Committee, not to approve the study.

The Surfaxin Trial

Bolivia
Population: 8.86 million (2005)
Government type: constitutional republic
Previous colonial rule: Spain

GDP: $10.1 billion (2005) and $23.6 billion (purchasing power
   parity 2005)
GDP per capita: $2,700 (purchasing power parity)
Health expenditure as % of GDP: 7.0%
Health expenditure per capita: $179
Life expectancy at birth: 63 (M), 68 (F)
Infant mortality rate: 53 per 1,000 live births
Physicians per 100,000 population: 73
Corruption Perception Index (2004): 2.2, country number 122

Data from CIA World Book, WHO Countries Report, and Transparency International's
   Annual Report

Respiratory distress syndrome (RDS) is a common and potentially fatal
disease in premature infants that is caused by insufficient surfactant in
the lungs. Surfactant is a protein fluid that reduces alveolar surface tension, enabling proper lung inflation and aeration. In most full-term infants, surfactant ensures soft and pliable lungs that stretch and contract
with each breath. Premature infants have underdeveloped lungs that are
stiff and do not inflate as easily, and as a result they are more likely to
have RDS.

The use of surfactant replacement therapy as the standard treatment
for RDS in the Western world has produced a 34 percent reduction in
neonatal mortality in randomized trials.[5] Nevertheless, RDS remains
the fourth leading cause of infant mortality in the United States and is
responsible for up to half of all infant mortality in developing countries,
where babies do not typically have access to surfactant therapy or ventilator support.

Surfactant therapy has been approved for use in Latin America, but
its high cost (about U.S. $1,100–2,400 per child) precludes it as a viable
option for most infants in Latin America, where per capita annual health
spending ranges from U.S. $60 to $140. In Bolivia, Ecuador, and Peru,
where only a privileged minority has access to surfactant therapies and
adequate prenatal monitoring, RDS continues to be responsible for at
least 30 percent of neonatal deaths.[6]

Four surfactants have been approved by the U.S. Food and Drug Administration (FDA) since 1990. The first, Exosurf, was a synthetic product approved in 1990 for the prevention of RDS in infants with birth
weights less than 1,350 grams, and for treatment of heavier infants who

have evidence of incomplete lung development and/or have developed RDS. Approval for these uses was made on the basis of placebo-controlled trials. In these trials, all children received mechanical ventilation. Exosurf was delivered into the ventilator in a spray form, whereas the "placebo" control was a spray of air.

In 1991, a new surfactant drug derived from cow lung surfactant, called Survanta, was approved for the prevention and treatment of RDS in premature babies weighing between 600 and 1,700 grams. Approval of Survanta was also based on placebo-controlled prevention and treatment trials. Another surfactant, Infasurf, was approved in 1998 on the basis of its superiority to Exosurf on various clinical measures in two trials, one of treatment and one of prophylaxis. There was also a treatment trial for RDS comparing Infasurf to Survanta showing no apparent difference, and a comparative randomized trial for the prevention of RDS in premature infants less than twenty-nine weeks of age, in which Infasurf was inferior to Survanta. Infasurf was approved for the prevention of RDS in premature infants less than twenty nine weeks of age, despite its inferiority to Survanta.[7] None of the Infasurf trials involved a placebo arm. One subsequent surfactant, Curosurf, was approved in 1999 on the basis of two trials, one comparing single versus multiple doses of Curosurf, and the second comparing single-dose Curosurf to disconnection from mechanical ventilation and administration of manual ventilation for two minutes. Superiority of multiple-dose Curosurf was shown.

In 2000 a private U.S. drug company, Discovery Labs, planned a study to demonstrate the efficacy of a new synthetic surfactant called Surfaxin for the treatment of RDS in a Phase III study. The drug company deliberated with the FDA about an acceptable study design. Although a trial designed to demonstrate the superiority of Surfaxin to Exosurf would have been accepted by the FDA as evidence of Surfaxin's effectiveness, the sponsor did not think it could succeed with such a trial. Based on its experience with previous surfactant studies, the FDA concluded that a noninferiority trial of Surfaxin against Survanta could not yield data that would support the approval of Surfaxin. Survival, prevention of RDS, and various clinical measures used in effectiveness studies had proven, individually, to be insufficiently consistent to identify a credible "noninferiority margin"[8] for surfactant drugs in a noninferiority trial, despite the clear overall evidence of effectiveness of surfactants.

After some deliberations, a multicenter, double-blinded, randomized, two-arm, placebo-controlled trial was proposed, involving 650 premature infants with RDS to be conducted in Bolivia. The hospitals chosen for participation in the study generally did not have surfactant available for the treatment of RDS. The sponsor agreed to provide endotracheal tubes, ventilators, and antibiotics for all study participants. It was also proposed that a team of American neonatologists would be sent to supervise the study and help train local health care personnel.

In participating research centers, parents of infants showing symptoms of RDS would be asked to give consent for their babies to participate in the study. The infants would then be intubated with an endotracheal tube and either given air suffused with Surfaxin or air without any drug. The proposed study end points were all-cause mortality and mortality due to RDS.

The sponsor agreed to set up a data safety and monitoring board, as well as a steering committee composed of host-country members to ensure that appropriate safety standards would be met. The principal target market for the drug was the United States and Europe, and the sponsor had no specific plans for marketing Surfaxin in Latin America. However, the sponsor engaged in some preliminary discussions with the participating hospitals about making Surfaxin available to them at reduced cost if it proved to be efficacious in the trial. No firm agreement was reached in these negotiations.

The Bolivian hospitals were selected because they could not routinely provide surfactant treatment for RDS yet were of sufficient quality to support and run the more elaborate intensive care unit facilities that the sponsor had promised in return for its participation. In the study, although half the infants with RDS would not have access to surfactant, they would not be denied a treatment to which they now have access. The ventilator support that both the surfaxin and "placebo" patients would receive in the proposed study was known to improve survival and was better than the treatments generally available to both groups prior to the study.

Notes

1. B. L. Innis et al., "Protection against Hepatitis A by an Inactivated Vaccine," *Journal of the American Medical Association* 271 (1994): 1328–34.

2. C. H. Hoke et al., "Protection against Japanese Encephalitis by Inactivated Vaccines," *New England Journal of Medicine* 319 (1988): 608–14.

3. C. A. Kozik et al., "Causes of Death and Unintentional Injury among School Children in Thailand," *Southeast Asian Journal of Tropical Medicine and Public Health* 30 (1999): 129–35.

4. "Interview with Professor Natth," *Good Clinical Practice Journal* 6, no. 6 (1999): 11.

5. R. F. Soll, "Synthetic Surfactant for Respiratory Distress Syndrome in Preterm Infants," in *The Cochrane Library*, issue 4, (Oxford: Update Software, 2000).

6. RDS is thought to be responsible for about 30 percent of infant deaths in Bolivia, Ecuador, and Peru.

7. www.fda.gov/cder/foi/label/1998/20521lbl.pdf.

8. International Conference on Harmonization, "Choice of Control Group in Clinical Trials," *Federal Register* 66 (2001): 24390–91.

3

Exploitation in Clinical Research

ALAN WERTHEIMER

Introduction

Many bioethicists have claimed that clinical research in underdeveloped societies is vulnerable to the charge of exploitation. Here are some typical statements:

1. "Unless the interventions being tested will actually be made available to the impoverished populations that are being used as research subjects, developed countries are simply exploiting them in order to quickly use the knowledge gained from the clinical trials for the developed countries' own benefit."[1]

2. ". . . the placebo-controlled trials are exploitative of poor people, who are being manipulated into serving the interests of those who live in wealthy nations. . ."[2]

3. ". . . there is always the nagging possibility that the assurances of such benefits may offer inordinate inducements to poor and impoverished populations and thus represent another form of exploitation."[3]

4. "If the knowledge gained from the research in such a country is used primarily for the benefit of populations that can afford the tested product, the research may rightly be characterized as exploitative and, therefore, unethical."[4]

5. "If the results of a clinical trial are not made reasonably available in a timely manner to study participants and other inhabitants of a host country, the researchers might be justly accused of exploiting poor, undereducated subjects for the benefit of more affluent populations of the sponsoring countries.[5]

6. "Residents of impoverished, postcolonial countries, the majority of whom are people of color, must be protected from potential exploitation in research. Otherwise, the abominable state of health care in these countries can be used to justify studies that could never pass ethical muster in the sponsoring country."[6]

7. "... it is a fundamental ethical principle that those involved in research in developing countries ... should not take advantage of [exploit?] the vulnerabilities created by poverty or a lack of infrastructure and resources."[7]

As these statements suggest, many commentators seem to accept what I call the *exploitation argument*. Reduced to its essentials, that argument maintains something like this:

(1) If a practice is exploitative, it should not be permitted.
(2) Placebo-controlled trials (PCTs) such as the Surfaxin trial are exploitative.
(3) Therefore, PCTs should not be permitted.

As it stands, the exploitation argument moves much too quickly. First, it is not clear when a practice is actually exploitative as in (2). Although commentators advance accusations of exploitation with relative ease, they rarely provide an account of exploitation on which their accusation rests. Second, and more important, it is not clear whether we should accept (1). I shall argue that it is plausible to argue that some sorts of exploitation should not be prohibited. Indeed, I shall argue that efforts to interfere with (allegedly) exploitative research may be deeply misguided.

The purpose of this chapter is threefold. First, I develop some analytical distinctions about the concept of exploitation and the essential elements of exploitation. Second, I explore the *moral force* of exploitation and, in particular, the arguments for prohibiting exploitative transactions or relations. Third, I try to bring those analyses to bear on the ethical issues that arise in conjunction with PCTs such as the Surfaxin trial and the Havrix trial. Two caveats. First, for present purposes, I shall confine my remarks to the Surfaxin trial because I do not think there are important moral distinctions between the cases and because it has generated more extensive critical commentary. Second, I propose to set aside all questions as to whether PCTs such as the Surfaxin trial are compatible with any set of standard principles of biomedical research, as exemplified by the Declaration of Helsinki, or the *International Ethical Guidelines for Biomedical Research Involving Human Subjects*, (by the Council for International Organizations of Medical Sciences [CIOMS]), and so forth. The question here is whether and why a practice is justifiable, not whether it is (in)compatible with any existing document.

The Concept of Exploitation

The word "exploitation" can be used in a nonmoral or nonderisive sense, where it means simply to "use" or "take advantage of." So we might say, "The basketball player exploited his great jumping ability." We are interested in wrongful exploitation. At the most general level, A exploits B when A takes unfair advantage of B.[8] One problem with such a broad account is that there will "be as many competing conceptions of exploitation as theories of what persons owe to each other by way of fair treatment."[9] To make more progress, consider a few examples that might be thought to involve exploitation.

> *Student Athletes*. A, a major university, provides B with a scholarship to play on its football team. A gains considerable revenue, but like most athletes, B gets little education, does not graduate, and does not go on to play professional football.[10]
> *Kidneys*. A, who is affluent, offers to pay B $25,000 for one of his kidneys for purposes of transplantation. B, who is poor, agrees in order to better provide for her family.[11]
> *Surrogacy*. A pays B $10,000 to become impregnated with A's sperm (through artificial insemination) and to waive her rights to the child after birth.[12]
> *Psychotherapy*. A, a psychotherapist, proposes to B, his patient, that they have sexual relations. B, who is infatuated with her therapist, agrees.[13]
> *Lumber*. There has been a hurricane in Florida. A, a lumber retailer, triples his price for lumber. B, who needs lumber to rebuild, pays A's price.

Lecherous Millionaire. B's child will die unless she receives expensive surgery for which the state will not pay. A, a millionaire, proposes to pay for the surgery if B will agree to become
his mistress. B agrees.

With such examples in mind, let us stipulatively refer to a statement
that A's interaction with B is wrongfully exploitative as an *exploitation
claim*. The first task of a theory of exploitation is to provide the truth
conditions for an exploitation claim. For example, does A exploit B in,
say, Lumber? Why or why not? Interestingly, the truth of an exploitation
claim settles less than is often thought. For even if A wrongly exploits B
in Lumber, it does not follow as a matter of moral logic that we should
prohibit or regulate the transaction between A and B. And so the second task of a theory of exploitation is to provide an account of its *moral
force*. In particular, we must determine on what grounds we are justified
in prohibiting or regulating exploitative transactions.

What are the truth conditions of an exploitation claim? When is a
transaction exploitative? Consider the following proposed definitions of
exploitation:

1. "[T]o exploit a person involves the *harmful, merely instrumental
utilization* of him or his capacities, for one's own advantage or for the
sake of one's own ends [emphasis added]."[14]

2. "It is the fact that the [capitalist's] income is derived through
forced, unpaid, surplus [wage] labor, *the product of which the workers do not
control*, which makes [wage labor] exploitive [emphasis added]."[15]

3. "Exploitation necessarily involves benefits or gains of some kind
to someone. . . . Exploitation resembles a zero-sum game, viz. what the
exploiter gains, the exploitee loses; or, minimally, for the exploiter to gain,
the exploitee must lose."[16]

4. "Exploitation [in exchange] demands . . . that there is no reasonably eligible alternative [for the exploitee] and that the consideration or
advantage received is incommensurate with the price paid. One is not
exploited if one is offered what one desperately needs at a fair and reasonable price."[17]

5. "Common to all exploitation of one person (B) by another (A) . . .
is that A makes a profit or gain by turning some characteristic of B to

his own advantage. . . . [E]xploitation . . . can occur in morally unsavory forms without harming the exploitee's interests and . . . despite the exploitee's fully voluntary consent to the exploitative behavior."[18]

6. "Persons are exploited if (1) others secure a benefit by (2) using them as a tool or resource so as (3) to cause them serious harm."[19]

7. "An exploitative exchange is . . . an exchange in which the exploited party gets less than the exploiting party, who does better at the exploited party's expense. . . . [T]he exchange must result from social relations of unequal power . . . exploitation can be entered into voluntarily; and can even, in some sense, be advantageous to the exploited party."[20]

8. "[E]xploitation is a psychological, rather than a social or an economic, concept. For an offer to be exploitative, it must serve to create or to take advantage of some recognized psychological vulnerability which, in turn, disturbs the offeree's ability to reason effectively."[21]

All these accounts are compatible with the general claim that "A wrongfully exploits B when A takes unfair advantage of B," but there are some important differences among them. Some accounts are technical definitions of exploitation that are specific to a Marxist approach. Some accounts invoke the Kantian notion that one wrongfully exploits when one treats another instrumentally or merely as a means (1, 6). On some accounts, the exploited party must be harmed (1, 2, 3, 6), whereas others allow that the exploited party may gain from the relationship (4, 5, 7). On some accounts, the exploited party must be coerced (2, 4) or exhibit a defect in the quality of the consent (8), whereas other accounts maintain that exploitation can be fully voluntary or consensual (5, 7).

I think it best not to put rigid constraints on what counts as exploitation. While some exploitative transactions are harmful to the exploitee, as is likely in Psychotherapy, we often refer to cases in which the alleged exploitee seems to gain from the transaction as exploitative, as exemplified by almost all the other examples, such as Student Athletes, Surrogacy, Kidneys, Lumber, and Lecherous Millionaire. For these reasons, it will be useful to make two sets of distinctions. First, we can distinguish between *harmful exploitation* and *mutually advantageous exploitation*. By mutually advantageous exploitation, I refer to those cases in which both parties (the alleged exploiter and the alleged exploitee) reasonably expect to gain from the transaction as contrasted with the pretransaction status quo. We can similarly distinguish between *nonconsensual exploitation* and *consensual exploitation*. By nonconsensual exploitation, I refer to cases in which the exploitee does not token consent at all or does not give sufficiently voluntary, informed, or competent consent. Consensual exploitation refers to cases where the exploited party has given voluntary and appropriately informed consent to the transaction. Although the two sets of distinctions are not equivalent, they do overlap, and so to simplify matters, I shall generally presume that mutually advantageous transactions are also consensual.[22]

It might be argued that it begs the question to assume that exploitation can be mutually advantageous or consensual. On this view, if the alleged exploitee benefits and consents in Lumber or Lecherous Millionaire, then she has no complaint and has not been exploited. As a substantive claim, the objection fails. Even if we were to grant that the *word* "exploitation" is best limited to cases in which the exploitee is harmed (and I would not so grant), we would *still* have to ask whether there are important moral distinctions between those cases that are (*ex hypothesi*) wrongly referred to as mutually advantageous *exploitation* and those mutually advantageous transactions that are regarded as fair and nonexploitative. It would remain an open question as to whether some mutually advantageous and consensual arrangements, such as Lumber and Lecherous Millionaire, are wrongful and why they are wrongful. And it would remain an open question as to whether such transactions should be prohibited.

The Elements of Exploitation

Let us start with the claim that A exploits B when A takes unfair advantage of B. Taking unfair advantage could be understood in two ways. First, it may refer to some dimension of the *outcome* of the exploitative act or transaction, that is, the transaction is substantively unfair. And this, it seems has two elements: (1) the benefit to A and (2) the effect on B. We may say that the benefit to A is unfair because it is wrong for A to benefit at all from his act (e.g., by harming B) or because A's benefit

is excessive relative to the benefit to B. Second, to say that A takes unfair advantage of B may imply that there is some sort of defect in the
process by which the unfair outcome comes about, for example, that A
coerces B into giving (apparent) consent or that A deceives B or fails to
provide B with relevant information. In the final analysis, I believe that
a moral defect in the outcome is both necessary and sufficient to support
an exploitation claim. Nonetheless, because there are important moral
distinctions between consensual and nonconsensual exploitation, it is
crucial to consider defects in consent as well.

The Outcome of a Transaction

In assessing the exploitativeness of a transaction, we must consider two
dimensions: its effect on A and its effect on B.

BENEFIT TO A

A cannot take *unfair* advantage of B unless A gets some *advantage* from
the transaction with B. It follows that A does not exploit B when A does
not, in fact, benefit from the transaction. Recall Student Athletes. If a
university loses money on its athletic programs, we cannot say that it exploits its athletes, although it may mistreat them nonetheless.

We can see the relevance of the "benefit to A" by contrasting exploitation with other forms of wrongdoing, such as discrimination or oppression. If A refuses to hire B solely because of B's race, then it would be
odd to say that A exploits B, for A does not gain from the wrong to B.
Let us say that A oppresses B when A deprives B of freedoms or opportunities to which B is entitled. If A gains from the oppressive relationship, as when A enslaves B, then A may both oppress and exploit B. But
if A does not gain from the oppression, the oppression is wrong but not
exploitative. A father may oppress his children without exploiting them.

Although A exploits B only when A gains from the transaction with
B, we can be relatively open-ended as to what counts as a benefit to A.
A may gain money or sexual pleasure or a child or scientific knowledge.
Given our present concern, it is important to stress that A can exploit B
while trying to serve perfectly benevolent ends. A university may exploit

its athletes in order to build a better library. Medical researchers may exploit experimental subjects for the benefit of others.

A transaction or interaction with A may affect B in three ways. It may have no effect on B. It may be harmful to B. It may be advantageous to B. Let us consider each.

No Effect. There are cases in which B is not directly affected by A's utilization of B, what Feinberg refers to as "harmless parasitism," as when A follows B's taillights in a dense fog. A uses B to his own advantage, but does not render B worse off (assume that B is not bothered by A's headlights in B's mirror).[23] These cases raise some interesting questions, but I shall not pursue them here.

B Is Harmed. It is relatively uncontroversial that exploitation can be harmful to B, as in slavery, extortion, and fraud, where A gains by imposing a harm on B. While harmful exploitation is typically morally worse than mutually advantageous exploitation, it does not raise as many interesting theoretical issues, and so I propose to set it aside.

B Gains. In cases of mutually advantageous exploitation, the transaction appears to benefit both A and B, as may be true of Student Athletes, Lumber, Surrogacy, Kidneys, and Lecherous Millionaire. I say "appears to benefit" because it is not always clear whether the transaction is beneficial to B. In assessing the effect of a transaction on B, it is important to keep the following considerations in mind.

First, in asking how A's action affects B's interests, we must be careful to adopt an *all-things-considered* point of view. There are, after all, negative *elements* in virtually all uncontroversially beneficial transactions. Paying money for a good that is clearly worth the price is still a negative element in the transaction. If A and B enter into a cooperative agreement where A gives B $100 for a book that is worth a lot to A (because it completes a collection) but is worth little to B, we do not say that B has been harmed by the transaction just because B no longer possesses her book any more than we say that A has been harmed because the transaction required A to pay $100. Similarly, even if the sale of a kidney has significant negative elements, it is *possible* that the value of the gains to the seller exceed the value of the costs.

Second, in assessing the effects of a transaction on B, we should generally adopt an *ex ante* rather than an *ex post* point of view. Suppose that A enters into a type of business transaction with B, where B expects (*ex ante*) to gain 80 percent of the time and lose 20 percent of the time, as when A sells B land on which B hopes to find oil. I suppose that we can say that these are harmful transaction in those cases where B fails to find oil, but we do not regard it as harmful in any morally significant way if B's *ex post* utility is negative but B's *ex ante* utility is clearly positive.

Third, we should *not* assume that a mutually advantageous transaction is unfair or exploitative simply because A takes advantage of B's vulnerabilities or desperate situation to strike a deal. Consider the following examples:

> *Generic.* A proposes to sell B the generic version of a lifesaving drug for a fair price. B accepts.
> *Surgery.* A proposes to amputate B's leg for a fair fee. Because B will die unless she agrees to the amputation, B authorizes A to perform the surgery.

Although B has no reasonable alternative to accepting A's proposal in both Generic and Surgery, A does not exploit B in either case because a transaction is exploitative only if the distribution of the benefits is *unfair*. Indeed, even if B's present situation is unjust and not merely unfortunate, it does not follow that the transaction between A and B is exploitative. Even if B's condition in Surgery results from C's culpable negligence, A's transaction with B may be beyond reproach. To put the point in slightly different terms, it is important to distinguish between the claim that A is *taking unfair advantage* of B and the claim that A is *taking advantage* of B's unfortunate or unfair circumstances. A may take advantage of unfairness to B without taking unfair advantage of B.

Fourth, we should resist the temptation to say that a transaction is harmful to B because it involves a more abstract or moral form of harm. Contemporary discussions of exploitation are often intertwined with allusions to the Kantian mantra that one should never treat another merely as a means to one's own ends, but always as ends in themselves. Along these lines, Allen Buchanan argues that exploitation occurs "whenever persons are harmfully utilized as mere instruments for private gain," and adds that this could apply to business transactions between two affluent bankers—"Each harmfully utilizes the other as a mere means to his own advantage."[24]

It is not clear what to make of this view. First, on one plausible reading of the Kantian maxim, one treats another as a mere means only when one treats "him in a way to which he could not possibly consent," as in cases of coercion and fraud, where A seeks to undermine B's capacity as an autonomous decision maker.[25] On this view, the bankers may be treating each other as a means to their own ends, but they are not treating each other *merely* as a means to their own ends because each banker's treatment of the other banker requires the other banker's consent. Second, even if we thought that treating another as a means was a way of harming her, we would still want to distinguish between those cases in which B is harmed *apart* from being treated as a means from those in which B is not harmed apart from the harm that derives from being treated as a means. So the Kantian view does nothing to deny the distinction between harmful exploitation and mutually advantageous exploitation.

When Are Mutually Advantageous Transactions Unfair? It seems better simply to grant that some allegedly exploitative transactions are mutually advantageous and go on to ask what makes a mutually advantageous transaction *unfair*. Unfortunately, there is no nonproblematic account of fair transactions.[26] Here are several possibilities.

We might say that a transaction is unfair when the goods exchanged are "incommensurable," as might be thought of the exchange of a bodily organ for money—"You can't put a price on a kidney." There are two problems here. First, it is not clear whether and when goods are ultimately incommensurable. As Ruth Chang has argued, incommensurability claims are more difficult to support than is often supposed.[27]

Second, if goods are incommensurable, it is not why an exchange of those goods is unfair. We typically say that an exchange is unfair when the exploitee receives too little. If we cannot compare what the parties receive, how can we claim that the alleged exploitee receives too little and thus that the exchange is therefore unfair?

Second, assuming that we can compare the gains of the parties, it is frequently suggested that a transaction is exploitative when A gains much more than B. But how should we measure their relative gains? If we measure the parties' gains by reference to the utility they receive as compared with the baseline in which there is no transaction at all, then the alleged exploitee may well gain *more* than the exploiter. If a doctor overcharges for lifesaving surgery that only he can perform, the patient still gains much more than the doctor. The doctor gets some money; the patient gets her life. Indeed, and on closer inspection, the exploiter's power over the exploitee typically stems precisely from the fact that the exploiter does not stand to gain too much. The exploiter can easily walk away from the transaction, whereas the exploitee cannot. So unequal benefit is a problematic criterion of exploitative transactions.

This suggests that we cannot evaluate the fairness of a transaction solely by comparing how much utility the parties receive from the transaction. Rather, we must measure the fairness of their gains against a *normative standard* as to how much the parties *ought* to gain. That standard is not easy to specify, and thus there may be reasonable disagreement as to whether a transaction is, in fact, unfair. I have elsewhere suggested that we might use a "hypothetical market" criterion of a fair transaction, where the terms are fair if they were the terms that would be agreed to by rational informed bargainers in a competitive market environment.[28] Although I think that approach is helpful, it is also vulnerable to criticisms that I shall not pursue here.

We appear to be stuck. Although I cannot produce a nonproblematic theory of fair transactions, I remain convinced that some mutually advantageous transactions are quite unfair and exploitative. I am reluctant to mimic Justice Potter Stewart's view of pornography with respect to exploitation ("I shall not attempt to further define pornography, but I know it when I see it"). First, I believe that our intuitions are often erroneous, that we view some transactions as unfair when they are eminently fair (say, given the costs or risks involved). For example, we may think it unfair for a lender to charge a high rate of interest to a penurious borrower, but it is possible that such rates are necessary to compensate the lender for the high risk that the loan will not be repaid. Second, I remain hopeful that an adequate theory of fair transactions can be developed, even if I cannot now provide such a theory. For present purposes, however, I will simply assume that some mutually advantageous transactions are unfair by reference to an appropriate normative standard and that A exploits B when A gains more than A should (or B gains less than B should) from the transaction.

DEFECTS IN CONSENT

Although I have suggested that exploitation can be perfectly consensual, the claim that A exploits B is often associated with the claim that B does not token or signal consent to the transaction at all or that B's token of consent is not sufficiently voluntary, informed, or competent—in a word *valid*. At first glance, it seems plausible to argue that A does not exploit if B voluntarily agrees to what might otherwise be a maldistribution of advantages, as when B voluntarily decides to make a gift of goods or labor to A. It would, for example, be odd (although perhaps not impossible) to claim that a hospital exploits its volunteer workers. But intentional altruism aside, an unfair transaction is arguably exploitative even if B's decision is well informed and rational, given the objective situation in which B finds herself.

Yet consent matters. Even though exploitation can be consensual, there are important moral distinctions between consensual and nonconsensual exploitation. I will assume that valid consent by a participant or her surrogate is generally necessary for the ethical conduct of research. There are, of course, many cases where consent fails yet there is no question of exploitation. Suppose, for example, that A is conducting an active-controlled trial (ACT) in which patients receive the standard care or an experimental treatment and that the researchers simply neglected to provide adequate information. The researchers are not *exploiting* the participants, but the trial may be unethical nonetheless.

Consent matters in the present context for the following reason. Even though the truth of an exploitation claim does not presuppose any defect in consent, the *moral force* of an exploitation claim may turn on whether the exploitation is consensual or nonconsensual, if only because the absence of valid consent is often a good indication that the transaction is a case of harmful exploitation rather than mutually advantageous exploitation. In addition, there may be reason to prohibit nonconsensual exploitation, but to *permit* consensual exploitation. And so it is crucial to determine whether an arguably exploitative transaction is or is not sufficiently consensual.

There are some instances of alleged exploitation in which the exploitee does not give the slightest token of consent, where the exploitee may be entirely passive. A may sell photographs of B without B's knowledge, or rob a purse from a sleeping B, or inject B with a drug. In some cases of alleged exploitation, B tokens consent, but B's consent is arguably not valid because there are defects in voluntariness, information, or competence. Let us briefly consider these potential defects in B's consent.

Voluntariness. We generally say that consent is voluntary when it is not coerced. But what does that mean? In general, A coerces B to do X only if A proposes (threatens) to make B worse off with reference to some baseline condition if B chooses not to do X.[29] If A gets B to pay A $100 per week by threatening to bomb B's store if he does not pay up, then A coerces B into paying $100 a week. By contrast, if A gets B to pay A $100 per week by proposing to clean B's store each night, then A has made a noncoercive (or inducive) offer to B.

The previous cases are easy because the baselines by which we evaluate the distinction between proposing to make someone worse off and better off are quite clear. Other cases are more difficult, because specifying the appropriate baseline against which to evaluate a proposal can be a complicated matter. We can ask, for example, whether A proposes to worsen B's situation relative to B's pre-proposal status quo or where B has a *right* to be, what I have referred to as B's moralized baseline.[30] Consider the following:

> *Lifeguard.* A is a professional lifeguard at B's country club. B is drowning in the swimming pool. A proposes to help B if and only if B agrees to pay A $1,000. B agrees.
>
> *Immunity.* A, a prosecutor, tells B that he will prosecute B for a felony unless B turns state's evidence and testifies against C. If B does so, A will give B immunity. B agrees.

Is B's agreement voluntary in these cases? Now B's status quo or pre-proposal situation in Lifeguard is that B is drowning. Relative to that baseline, A does not propose to make B worse off if B refuses A's proposal. Nonetheless, if B has a right to be rescued by A (or if A has a duty to try to rescue B), then A's "declared unilateral plan"—what A proposes to do if B does not accept A's proposal—is to violate B's rights. Hence we may say that B's consent is coerced and that his agreement with A is not binding. By contrast, we are not inclined to regard B's agreement in Immunity as coerced. Although A is proposing to render B worse off than B's pre-proposal or status quo baseline (where B is not charged), and even though A has placed B in a situation in which she faces prosecution, A's declared unilateral plan would *not* violate B's rights, and thus we would not regard A's testimony as coerced. Rather, we might say that A is making a noncoercive offer to B. In my view, the moral status of A's declared unilateral plan is the key to determining whether A's proposal is coercive and whether B's agreement is appropriately consensual.

If we apply this view to some of my hypothetical cases, it is arguable that A does *not* coerce B in cases such as Lumber, Lecherous Millionaire, Surgery, Kidneys, or Surrogacy. For A does not propose to violate B's rights if B rejects A's proposal in any of these cases. Consider a more difficult case:

> *Rescue.* A, a tug, encounters a ship (B) in distress and proposes to take it in tow for a fee that greatly exceeds the normal market price for such services. B agrees. B then sues to recover the fee on the grounds that he agreed under duress.

Rescue is more difficult, because it is not clear whether B has a right to be rescued by A or whether A has an obligation to rescue B. In any case, these cases show that the mere fact that B may have no acceptable alternative to accepting A's proposal does *not* entail that B's decision is coerced or that B's consent is not valid. We would not, for example, say that A commits a battery in Surgery just because B has no choice but to agree to surgery. Moreover, even if B's background situation is unjust, it does not follow that A's proposal is coercive. Recall Lecherous Millionaire. Even if a just society would enable B to pay for her daughter's surgery, B certainly has no right that A pay for her surgery.[31] A's declared unilateral plan would not violate B's rights.

To put the previous discussion slightly differently, it is crucial to distinguish between moral defects in B's *background situation* and moral defects in the transactions that occur within that situation. In my view, we often focus on the wrong target. Although we often have moral reason to object to both the background situation and the transaction, the relative invisibility of background situations (as contrasted with transactions) and our relative helplessness with respect to people's unfortunate or unjust background situations may lead us to wrongly object to transactions that are themselves relatively unobjectionable given those background situations.

Information. The validity of B's consent can also be undermined by defects in B's information such that B's decision is not likely to advance B's interests considered from an *ex ante* and *all-things-considered* point of view. In some cases, B's informational deficiencies may be due to fraud, as when A deliberately sets back the odometer in a car that he is selling. In other cases, A may withhold or fail to disclose information that A has an obligation to provide. And so B's consent to purchase a home from A may be invalid if A fails to tell B that the roof leaks. And in the paradigmatic medical context, B's consent to surgery is not valid if A fails to inform B of the risks that are involved. It is not clear what level of information is required by valid consent in one context or another (for example, commercial, sexual, or medical) or what to do about cases in which A provides information, but B does not understand it. Nonetheless, valid consent always requires some level of information or the absence of some forms of deception.

Competence. Even if A provides B with all the relevant information, B may not have the competence to process that information. We often assume that minors and those with mental impairments or deficiencies do not have the cognitive or emotional capacities to give valid consent to some interactions or transactions. Similarly, those who lack adequate education may be unable to make reasonable evaluations of the alternatives. Moreover, B's competence can be temporarily disturbed, as in Psychotherapy, where an (otherwise) competent B may be in the grips of transference. Furthermore, B's judgment can also be distorted when A makes what I call a *seductive offer*, where the lure of short-term benefits causes B to excessively discount the long-term costs and to make a decision that does not serve her long-term interests, as *may* be true of cases such as Kidneys and Surrogacy. In my view, seductive offers are not coercive, because A does not propose to violate B's rights if B rejects A's proposal, but they can seriously compromise the quality and validity of B's consent nonetheless.[32]

Consensual Exploitation. All that said, there are numerous cases of alleged exploitation where B would not have agreed under better or perhaps more just background conditions, where A has played no direct

causal role in creating those circumstances, where A has no special obligation to repair those conditions, and where B is fully informed as to
the consequences of various choices and fully capable of making such
choices. Without wanting to prejudge the various cases, I suggest that
such conditions *may* obtain in Kidneys, Surrogacy, Lecherous Millionaire, and Lumber. Precisely because B's objective situation is what it is,
it may be reasonable for B to agree to proposals to which those who are
better situated would not agree. Although it would not be rational for
an affluent American to sell a kidney for $25,000, it does not follow that
it is irrational for an impoverished Egyptian to do so. We must be careful. I do not deny that A's transaction with B may be wrong even if B
gives valid consent. Moreover, I do not preclude the possibility that a
transaction should be prohibited even if it is consensual. Perhaps people
should not be able to sell their kidneys even if they can and do give valid
consent to do so, say, because bodily parts simply should not be for sale.
The present point is that we should not presume that B's consent is invalid on grounds of coercion, information, competence, or rationality,
just because we think the transaction is morally objectionable.

What Is the Moral Force of Exploitation?

Let us assume that an interaction is properly described as exploitative.
What justifies interfering with an exploitative transaction? The moral
force of harmful and nonconsensual exploitation is relatively unprob-
lematic. There may be a question as to whether a transaction is actually
harmful or nonconsensual, but there is certainly at least a prima facie
case for prohibiting A from acting in ways that harm B or to which B
does not consent.

Mutually advantageous and consensual transactions present a more
difficult set of problems. Even if a transaction between A and B is unfair, it might be thought that there can be nothing *seriously* wrong about
an agreement from which both parties benefit and where A has no obligation to enter into any transaction with B. I do not see why this is so.
Recall Rescue and Lumber. Even if A is under absolutely no obligation
to transact with B, we might still think A has moral reason to be fair to

B given that A benefits from the interaction with B. Suppose that the following represents the gains of A and B in Rescue:

	A's payoff	B's Payoff
(1) No transaction	0	0
(2) Unfair transaction	10	1
(3) Fair transaction	5	5

One might think that the wrongness of A's behavior must track the outcome for B, such that A's behavior in (1) must be worse than A's behavior in (2) because B is worse off in (1) than in (2). Nonetheless, I believe it is possible that A's behavior is morally worse in (2) than in (1) even though B is better off in (2) than in (1). I say it is *possible* because the morality of transactions is a complicated and underanalyzed moral issue.

Wrongness is one thing, and interference is another. Those who argue that a practice is exploitative are not solely concerned to offer a moral critique of the practice. Rather, they typically assume that exploitation provides a reason for intervention. Thus, when critics argue that commercial surrogacy exploits the birth mothers, they also typically argue that surrogacy contracts should be unenforceable or entirely prohibited. Similar things are said about the sale of bodily organs. Those who make such arguments do frequently claim that the transactions are nonconsensual or harmful, but some seem prepared to argue for intervention even if the transactions are consensual and mutually advantageous. That line of argument is more difficult to sustain. After all, even if A's behavior is seriously wrong in such transactions, it might be argued that it would be wrong to interfere with or prohibit transactions that are beneficial to both parties and to which both parties consent. Consider, once again, the payoff structure of Rescue as described earlier. Suppose A proposes (2) (where A gets 10 and B gets 1). B counters that they should agree on (3) (where A gets 5 and B gets 5). A rejects (3) and tells B that it is either (1) (no transaction) or (2) (unfair transaction). Given these options, B is prepared to accept (2). At first glance it seems that society is not justified in preventing B from accepting (2), its unfairness notwithstanding. If B prefers to allow A to act wrongly, it is arguable that *we* have no justification for interfering.

On what grounds might we justify interfering with consensual and mutually advantageous exploitative transactions? In the following sections, I shall briefly discuss six lines of argument for intervention. I do not think that all these arguments are successful, but it will prove useful to distinguish among them.

Paternalism

We sometimes interfere with transactions on paternalistic grounds, in order to protect B from making a decision that does not advance her own interests. But a paternalistic argument for interference simply does not apply in the present context. Even if we think it legitimate to interfere with someone for her own good (as when we require people to wear seat belts), we cannot justify intervention on paternalistic grounds if the exploitative transaction is advantageous to the exploitee and if interference is not likely to result in a transaction that is more beneficial to B. So we can set paternalism aside.

Harm to Others (Negative Externalities)

We might interfere with mutually advantageous and consensual transactions because they give rise to harm to others or have negative externalities. For example, even if commercial surrogacy is beneficial to the participants directly involved, such activities might have negative effects on the way in which society perceives and treats women or children.[33] And even if Lecherous Millionaire were beneficial to B, a system that allows some to take advantage of society's reluctance to provide health care may postpone the day in which society chooses to do so. So preventing B from improving *her* position in this case may, in the future, benefit other persons in similar situations. Three points about this line of argument. First, if intervention has positive effects (or reduces negative effects) on others, the case for intervention is relatively easy to make. Second, it is an empirical question—and often an extraordinarily complex empirical question—as to whether interfering with a practice would actually have positive effects on others. Asserting that a practice such as surrogacy has harmful effects on children and women does not show that it does. Third, this line of argument for intervention has *nothing* to do with exploitation per se. The point is not to protect the exploitee but to protect others.

Strategic Intervention

Recall the payoff structure of Rescue, where A can make a credible threat to opt for (1) (no transaction) rather than (3) (fair transaction) and so get B to agree to (2) (unfair transaction). Interestingly, however, if we *prohibit* A from entering into transaction (2) with B, it is possible that A will propose (3) rather than (1). After all, A benefits from (3), and so has no reason to opt for (1) if we take (2) off the table. This may occur when A and B are in a bilateral monopoly as in Rescue, where A is the only seller and B is the only buyer. If we prohibit A from charging an exorbitant price for his services, then A might offer his services for a reasonable price rather than walk away. The strategic argument would not justify interfering in cases such as Lumber. For if B did not want to contract with A at A's proposed price, A will find other buyers. Still, there may be numerous situations in which such strategic arguments can work.[34] In effect, such situations present a prisoners' dilemma or collective action problem among the potential targets of proposals. In the absence of a prohibition on such proposals, it may well be better and perfectly rational for each to accept an exploitative proposal. Yet it would be better for all if they were prevented from agreeing to exploitative proposals, for then they would receive less exploitative proposals. It is precisely this sort of rationale for intervention to which labor unions often appeal. It may be perfectly rational for each individual employee to accept a low wage rather than no wage at all, but it is better for all (or most) if none are allowed to accept a low wage, for they may then be offered a higher wage.

Prophylactic Arguments

There may be a type of situation in which it is difficult to determine whether the transaction is, in fact, mutually advantageous or whether B is giving rational informed consent. Given these epistemological difficulties, it may make sense to prohibit all such transactions because the expected harms associated with the "bad" transactions outweigh the expected benefits associated with the "good" transactions. Something like this may occur in situations like Psychotherapy. It is, after all, distinctly possible that *some* psychotherapist-patient interactions are perfectly benign. Indeed, some have resulted in happy marriages. Still, given that many such interactions are harmful and nonconsensual, it may be better to prohibit all such transactions.

A BRIEF INTERLUDE: THE PRINCIPLE OF PERMISSIBLE EXPLOITATION

Before considering two additional arguments for interfering with mutually advantageous and consensual transactions, it is worth noting that the previous four arguments share a common feature. At the most basic level, they are all *person-affecting arguments*. All attempt to justify interfering with transactions on the grounds that interference is better for *someone*. That raises an interesting question: Could we justify interfering with mutually advantageous and consensual transactions when interference is *better for no one*? That is more difficult. To get a clear grip on the problem, let us make the following assumptions:

1. A is under no obligation to transact with B on any terms.
2. A proposes to transact with B on terms X.
3. A's transaction with B on terms X is to A's benefit (or to the benefit of someone other than B) and also serves B's *ex ante* and all-things-considered interests (setting aside paternalistic arguments).
4. B makes a voluntary, informed, and rational decision to transact with A on terms X, and we can reliably determine that B's decision is voluntary, informed, and rational (setting aside prophylactic arguments).
5. If A is not allowed to transact with B on terms X, A will choose not to interact with B on terms that are more favorable to B. Rather, A will choose not to transact with B at all (setting aside strategic arguments).
6. Preventing A from transacting with B on terms X will not have any significant positive consequences for anyone else (setting aside harm to others).

I do not know how often these conditions exist. But if such conditions do obtain, then we must ask whether we could have moral reason to prevent a transaction that is good for the parties involved, is worse for no one else, and to which the parties consent. Note that the question is *not* whether B could reasonably refuse to participate in the transaction even though it would serve B's interests to do so, in which case condition 4 would not hold. People often refuse to participate in transactions from which they might benefit because they regard the terms as unfair, and I am reluctant to say that they are being unreasonable. The question for us is whether the state or anyone else could justifiably prevent B from entering into an unfair transaction with A that achieves the best possible result for them (that is, condition 5 is true), worse for no one else, and to which they both consent. Let us refer to the claim that it would be wrong to interfere with such transactions as the *principle of permissible exploitation* (PPE).

Justice

With this interlude behind us, there are at least two possible arguments for rejecting PPE. A deontological argument would maintain that we are justified in prohibiting a transaction simply because it is unfair or unjust. Although I do not think it *incoherent* to claim that there might be deontological reasons to reject PPE, such a view is difficult to justify. One cannot reject PPE by appealing to some of the traditional arguments against consequentialism. PPE does not claim that we should allow any action that has better aggregate consequences, where the advantages to some outweigh the losses to others. In Rawlsian terms, PPE does not fail to take seriously the distinctions between persons. PPE says that we should allow a transaction whenever it would be better for all parties to the transaction and worse for no one else. Moreover, because PPE precludes intervention only when the parties consent to the transaction, one cannot easily reject PPE on the grounds that it allows A to use B as a mere means to his own ends. For, as I have argued, it is at least plausible to maintain that A does not treat B as a *mere* means if B's valid consent is a necessary condition of any transaction between A and B.

A Symbolic Argument

Finally, a symbolic argument maintains that we are justified in prohibiting unfair but mutually advantageous transactions as a way to symbolize or express the view that the exploiters are behaving wrongly. Now to the extent that such expressions motivate people to transact more fairly, then the symbolic argument is actually a species of the strategic argument or the harm-to-others argument. It would not violate PPE. A pure symbolic argument requires that the symbolization have no effect on anyone's behavior. As with the deontological argument, I do not think the symbolic argument is incoherent. But I think it very difficult to make a case for symbolic expressions when the symbolism does not make anyone better off and makes some worse off.

Although I lack a knockdown argument for PPE, I suspect that PPE is a plausible principle of *nonideal* moral theory. Whereas ideal moral theory aims to provide the principles for a just society and a just world, nonideal moral theory aims to provide the principles by which individuals should act under unjust or nonideal moral conditions and, among other things, the principles that should underlie societal sanctions on individual behavior under nonideal moral conditions.[35] Although Rawls restricts himself to developing an ideal theory of a just society, he notes that the problems of nonideal theory "are the pressing and urgent matters. These are the things that we are faced with in everyday life."[36] Just as we must ask how things should be, we must also ask what we should do given that things are not as they should be.

The ethics of clinical research in underdeveloped countries is a problem of nonideal moral theory. In a more just world, these nations would not be so underdeveloped. But just because a transaction would not occur under ideal or just conditions, it does not follow that it is wrong for it to occur under nonideal conditions. Given the nonideal background conditions under which people find themselves, there should be a very strong presumption in favor of principles that would allow people to improve their situations if they give appropriately robust consent, if doing so has no negative effects on others, and this even if the transaction is unfair, unjust, or exploitative.

An Interim Summary

Before considering exploitation in clinical research, let us take stock. In the preceding sections, I have argued for the following:

1. Exploitation can be harmful and nonconsensual or mutually advantageous and consensual.

2. We must distinguish the question as to whether a transaction is exploitative from the moral force of that exploitation. We should not assume that we are justified in prohibiting or regulating transactions just because they are exploitative.

3. A does not exploit B simply because A takes advantage of B's vulnerabilities to transact with B. A transaction is exploitative only if the terms of the agreement are unfair.

4. To say that a transaction is unfair requires an account of unfairness. If a transaction were unfair only when the exploiter gains more than the exploitee, many allegedly exploitative transactions would not be unfair.

5. The voluntariness and rationality of consent are not vitiated by objective background situations that make it rational for people to make choices that they would not make under better conditions.

6. There are several arguments for interfering with mutually advantageous and consensual transactions on grounds of exploitation. The most plausible arguments are the strategic argument and the prophylactic argument.

7. As a principle of nonideal moral theory, there should be a strong presumption against interfering with transactions that are better for the parties concerned and worse for no one else, that is, what I have called the principle of permissible exploitation.

Exploitation in Clinical Research

Let us now return to the issue of clinical research in developing countries by focusing on the possible use of PCTs such as the Surfaxin trial. As I noted at the outset, it is often claimed that clinical research must not be exploitative if it is to pass ethical muster. To recall our starting point, many commentators advance a version of what I called the exploitation argument. That argument maintains something like this:

(1) If a practice is exploitative, it should not be permitted.
(2) Placebo-controlled trials such as the Surfaxin trial are exploitative.
(3) Therefore, PCTs should not be permitted, or should be permitted only if the exploitation can be nullified or sharply reduced.

On closer inspection, and as evidenced by the quotations with which we began, those who advance something like the exploitation argument actually have in mind several distinct but related arguments and several different prescriptions for nullifying or reducing the alleged exploitation. Because there is little unity among the arguments and prescriptions, it will prove useful to consider them separately through the lens of the analysis I have advanced. Two preliminary observations: First, I hope that the previous analysis shows that (2) is more difficult to support than is often supposed, because we lack a nonproblematic theory of the distinction between exploitative and nonexploitative transactions. Nonetheless, for the sake of argument, I am prepared to accept that (2) may well be true in the present context. Second, I hope to have shown that (1) is false. If a practice involves consensual and mutually advantageous exploitation, there is good reason to allow it to go forward unless one of the arguments for intervention can be sustained.

The discussion of these arguments for intervention will prove most interesting if we make three assumptions. First, I assume that all participants receive care that is at least as good as and probably better than if the trial had not been conducted at all. After all, even those who receive the placebo may be receiving better (and certainly no worse) than normal care in, say, Bolivia.[37] Second, I shall assume that there are plausible—not necessarily compelling—scientific or economic reasons to prefer a PCT to an ACT. It might be thought that it is legitimate to prefer a PCT on grounds of scientific validity but not on grounds of cost. I disagree, but I will not pursue that issue here. Rather, in order to bring the ethical issues into sharper relief, it is better to make the problem harder for ourselves. If we assume that there are at least plausible reasons to want to conduct a PCT, the question then becomes whether those reasons are outweighed by ethical reasons to reject such a study. Third, and with reference to my discussion of PPE, I shall assume that if the sponsor is not permitted to conduct a PCT in Bolivia, it is possible that the sponsor will either abandon the study or go elsewhere. I do *not* mean that the sponsor would merely *threaten* to abandon the investigation as a bargaining tactic to secure what it regards as a better arrangement. Rather, I mean that the sponsor might in fact abandon the investigation or go elsewhere if it is not allowed to conduct a PCT in Bolivia.[38] With these assumptions in mind, let us now consider the various claims and prescriptions that are frequently linked with the exploitation argument.

Standard of Care

It may be thought that one way to avoid exploitation in clinical research is to insist that all participants be offered at least the normal standard of care. The Declaration of Helsinki states that "in any medical study, every patient—including those of a control group, if any—should be assured of the best proven diagnostic and therapeutic method."[39] The Surfaxin trial seems to be incompatible with this principle, unless one fudges with the notion of the "best proven . . . method" by arguing that we should adopt a "local" standard, under which the best proven method is no treatment at all. The real question is whether we should accept the principle. Discovery Labs would have been forced to comply with this provision if the study had been undertaken in the United States, if only because participants would not consent to receive a placebo rather than the normal standard of care. But if Discovery Labs is not required to provide any care at all to Bolivians, why should we insist that it provide at least the normal standard of care to participants in the study?

We can consider the standard care principle in terms of the *strategic argument* for intervention. In the *developed* world, if we insist that ACTs be used whenever a standard therapy exists and whenever there are no very strong scientific reasons for preferring a PCT, there is little risk that the research will simply go away. Although the drug companies might prefer PCTs because they are cheaper, the potential subjects in the developed world are collectively helped by rules that force researchers to treat patients better than they otherwise might. By contrast, that argument does not work so easily in the developing world, because the companies will just go elsewhere if too many constraints are placed on research. If that is right, interference cannot be justified as the best strategy for improving the lot of potential research subjects in Bolivia, since it may not in fact improve their lot. The justification that exists for the standard care principle in the developed world may simply not hold in the developing world.

It is worth noting here that analogues to the standard care principle in clinical research can also arise in nonmedical contexts.[40] Just as we can ask whether we should permit a PCT in Bolivia, we can ask whether U.S.-based corporations can offer low wages (by American standards) to Bolivian workers. In principle, it is hard to see that there is any fundamental distinction between alleged exploitation in medical research and alleged exploitation in wages, labor, or any other sort of transaction. If Nike has no obligation to provide those that it employs with a "living" wage (however that is defined), it is hard to see why researchers have an obligation to provide the subjects with the normal standard of care. And if researchers do have such an obligation, it is arguable that Nike has a comparable obligation.

Whatever we conclude about Nike, it may be argued that the standard care principle reflects the view that physicians have special moral obligations to their patients that are not replicated in other contexts. Here I raise two points. First, the "standard care" principle is not self-justifying. It needs to be defended, particularly in contexts where its application may not promote the welfare of the subjects. I do not say that we should necessarily reject the standard care principle as a universal maxim for medical research. I say only that we should not accept it uncritically as a moral given. Second, even if we were to accept something like the standard care principle as a requirement for *medical care*, the ethical principles that govern clinical research need not be identical with or entailed by the principles of medical ethics that apply to relations between physicians and patients. Suppose a researcher says this to a prospective subject:

> Although I am trained as a doctor, you are not my patient. I am conducting a trial. If you are selected to receive Surfaxin, then you will receive care that we think will prove beneficial. If you are se-

lected to receive a placebo, then your baby will not receive such care. If you don't want to participate with us on those terms, that's fine. But I don't want you to think that I regard your baby as my patient.

There may or may not be good reasons to reject this view, but here, too, those reasons must be given. And, for what it is worth, this author does not see why the principles that we think should govern physician-patient relations should automatically be applied to relations between researchers and subjects even if the researchers happen to be trained physicians.

Unequal Benefits

Bracketing the previous issue, it may be argued that the Surfaxin trial is exploitative and should not go forward because it is wrong for citizens in a developed society to gain large benefits from trials conducted on citizens of underdeveloped societies who may not benefit at all. In effect, we must ask whether this is a case of mutually advantageous exploitation (if it is exploitation) and whether it is a case of *exploitation*, assuming that the transaction is mutually advantageous. Here I want to raise five issues. First, it is arguable that there is an important sense in which the Surfaxin trial is actually beneficial to *all* trial participants, not just those who receive Surfaxin. In the previous section I argued that we ordinarily view the terms of a transaction from an *ex ante* rather than an *ex post* perspective. From an *ex ante* perspective, it is arguable that all participants benefit, even if half of the participants will not benefit *ex post*. This is not a conceptual trick. Consider how we think about standard medical treatments. If B has an illness for which the standard therapy works 50 percent of the time, we would not object to A's providing the treatment. If we extend that perspective to participation in the trial rather than treatment itself, it is not a large stretch to claim that it is not wrong to offer an opportunity from which participants can expect to benefit 50 percent of the time.

Second, it is not clear how to measure the parties' relative benefits. If we evaluate their benefits in something like "utility gain" relative to their status quo, the expected utility gain of participants in Bolivia, who would normally receive no medical care at all, is quite substantial and may actually be *greater* than the expected utility gain of any citizen in a developed society who, after all, can afford the standard therapy even if Surfaxin should prove superior.[41] I do not say that "comparative utility gain" from the status quo is the best way to assess the fairness of a distribution of benefits. At the same time, the claim that a distribution of benefits is unfair must also be defended.

Third, we do well to remember that the people in developed societies that may benefit from the Surfaxin trial are innocent and medically (if not economically) needy infants. Whatever exploitation there may be, it is not as if affluent American adults are decorating their oversized living rooms with oriental rugs handmade in sweatshops by the children of Afghanistan.[42] Even if Discovery Labs is the primary beneficiary, we should not let the language of exploitation obscure the moral status of the ultimate recipients or the benefits that they may hope to receive, namely, a superior or less costly lifesaving treatment.

Fourth, and related to the previous point, we must ask how much moral weight we should place on the benefits that accrue to the researchers or to the citizens of the developed society as contrasted with the effects of the trials on the participants. Consider the hypothetical *Murfaxin* trial, which is similar to the Surfaxin trial, except that the sponsor is the National Institutes of Health rather than a pharmaceutical company and that the U.S. government was prepared to provide Murfaxin without cost to all needy Americans (but not Bolivians) if the trial should prove successful. It is arguable that the Murfaxin trial is less exploitative than the Surfaxin trial because the sponsors do not benefit financially and the beneficiaries are not affluent. But if we are concerned with the welfare of the *participants* and not the gain to the sponsors, then the ethical statuses of the two trials stand or fall together and the language of exploitation does not perspicuously capture our concern.

Fifth, it may be thought that there is something particularly obnoxious about a practice in which the affluent entice the poor to provide a service that will primarily benefit the rich when it is perfectly feasible for the affluent to provide this service for themselves. There may be something unseemly about such a practice, but I do not see why we should regard medical research as particularly different from a wide variety of practices that fit this description, such as hiring nannies, gardeners, domestics, coal miners, construction workers, or volunteer (professional) soldiers. Perhaps there is something morally special about hiring others to serve as subjects for medical research, but it is hard to see what it might be.

Consent

Assume, arguendo, that the Surfaxin trial is a case of mutually advantageous exploitation. I have argued that whereas we should generally prohibit nonconsensual exploitation, we often have reason to permit consensual exploitation. There are two questions that we can raise here: (1) Do the participants in studies such as the Surfaxin trial actually give valid informed consent? (2) Is it possible that such participants *can* give valid informed consent?

Clearly, the answer to both questions will turn on our criteria for valid consent. Although we cannot resolve that here, I think it entirely possible that the answer to (1) is no. David Rothman notes that even in developed countries such as the United States, informed consent is often problematic with respect to treatment, much less clinical trials.[43] It may or may not be feasible to resolve these sorts of cognitive deficiencies, but, if not, it would not follow that the research would be impermissible. If prospective subjects are not themselves capable of giving informed consent to participate, it is still possible that they *would* (hypothetically) consent if they were capable. And it is also possible that a proxy or surrogate, such as the government or its representatives, can supplement their consent by insisting that participation in the study actually serves their interests just as parents serve as surrogates for their children who are not capable of giving informed consent.

We should distinguish between these sorts of cognitive deficiencies in a subject's consent and worries that are often advanced about the *voluntariness* of the subject's consent. It is often argued that one's consent is not voluntary just in case one has "no acceptable alternative." And, it may be said, impoverished parents who would ordinarily have no medical care available to treat their infants with respiratory distress syndrome have no choice but to participate in a study in which they have a *chance* of obtaining medical care for them.

I argued earlier that we should resist this line of argument. I have argued that A's proposal is coercive only if A proposes to violate B's rights if B rejects the proposal. The central fact is that the sponsors do not propose to violate a potential subject's rights in the Surfaxin trial should a potential subject decide not to participate. In principle, there is little distinction between a choice between (1) amputation surgery and death and (2) participation in a trial and no medical care. Just as a rational person would choose surgery over death, a rational person might choose participation in a trial over no medical care, and if we do not think that the prospect of death undermines valid consent, there is no reason to think that the prospect of receiving no medical care does so.

There may be other worries about consent. As I also argued earlier, a proposal might constitute a seductive offer even if it is not coercive and thus compromise consent in a different way. The CIOMS worries that the offer of medical care may "induce prospective subjects to consent to participate in the research against their better judgment." Here it is important to distinguish between two claims: (1) the inducements constitute a seductive offer that distorts the judgment of the subjects and motivates them to consent to participate when doing so does not advance their interests; (2) given the subject's objective circumstances, the inducements make it rational for the subjects to participate. In the latter case, the inducements are large enough to render participation compatible with the participants' better judgment, although participation would have been against their better judgment in the absence of those inducements. When (1) is true, there is good reason to regard consent as invalid, but there is no reason to regard consent as invalid when (2) is true.

In my view, the real tragedy of poverty is not that poverty renders (1) sometimes true, but that it often renders (2) true. And if (2) is true in a given case, we do not respect subjects' humanity or rationality by denying their capacity to make their lives less miserable than they already are. We should not confuse our moral worries about the objective circumstances in which people find themselves with worries about their capacity or right to make decisions about their lives within those circumstances. David Rothman writes that "abject poverty is harsh enough without people having to bear the additional burdens of serving as research subjects."[44] But the point could easily go the other way. We might say, after all, that abject poverty is harsh enough without denying people the opportunity to make their lives somewhat less miserable by participating in biomedical research and receiving benefits that they would not otherwise receive.

Community Consent

Some commentators have argued that medical research such as the Surfaxin trial not only requires the consent of the participants (or their surrogates), but also requires the consent of the community. In other words, the Surfaxin trial could be a case of individual consensual exploitation but community nonconsensual exploitation. Broadly speaking, there seem to be three arguments for this view. First, some commentators reject what they regard as a "highly individualistic" conception of rights and duties that underlies the significance of informed consent, one that allegedly assumes an "atomistic view of the person" that they find wanting. This is a large topic that I shall not pursue. Suffice it to say that I regard individuals—not communities—as the ultimate locus of moral value, and I believe such a conception is compatible with a robust social or political communitarianism. Suppose, for example, that one wants to *reject* the provision of the Declaration of Helsinki that states that "considerations related to the well-being of the human subject should take precedence over the interests of science and society" on the grounds that this principle does not give sufficient weight to the interests of society. One hardly need reject moral individualism to do so. After all, to what does the "interests of . . . society" refer, if not the interests of other individuals? The declaration's claim that the interests of experimental subjects should take precedence over the interests of those individuals who are not subjects may or may not be correct, but it has nothing to do with a conflict between individualism and communitarianism.

Second, it may be argued that a community's consent can be required because its present and future members have interests that must be protected and that these interests are not identical with the interests of the individual subjects. Such a requirement is perfectly reasonable to the extent that the community has such interests, but it is another question as to what sorts of alleged interests justify overriding the consent of the participants. Charles Weijer observes that "providing information on disease treatment may negatively affect beliefs regarding traditional healing."[45] No doubt this is true. But whether a community's interest in preserving a false and dangerous set of beliefs justifies preventing its citizens from receiving (or potentially receiving) efficacious medical care is rather doubtful.

Third, it may be argued that the community or its government is well positioned to screen the quality of the individual's consent, given the sorts of cognitive deficiencies I noted previously. I see nothing untoward in this form of "soft paternalism," if there is good reason to think that the community can and will make decisions on behalf of persons whose competence is suspect.[46] But this raises a difficulty that has gone somewhat unnoticed. Suppose a community decides to accept the Surfaxin trial because it believes that half a loaf is better than none. If we take seriously the community's authority to reject the Surfaxin trial on behalf of its members, then it is difficult to justify ignoring its acceptance of the Surfaxin trial. As I have argued, there may be strategic reasons to prohibit PCTs if doing so will prevent a "race to the bottom" among the societies that might be used for such studies and if so doing will result in studies that provide better care for the participants. Whether such an argument will work in the present context depends on the facts, on what will happen if the sponsors are not allowed to conduct a PCT. But bracketing such reasons, it will be difficult to argue that a trial should not be permitted if both the experimental subjects and the community's representatives consent to it, unless it can be shown that doing so has negative externalities that outweigh the interests of the subjects and their society.

Suppose that the strategic argument would work in Bolivia. The sponsors would most prefer to conduct a PCT, but given the choice between an ACT and abandoning the research, it will opt for an ACT. Interestingly, even under these conditions, it is still not clear whether we should insist upon an ACT. Here I return to the issue of costs. Suppose that the sponsors make the following proposal: (1) we can do an ACT rather than a PCT, in which case all participants will receive Surfaxin or the present standard of care; (2) we can do a PCT and will provide 75 percent of the money we save from such a study to your public health ministry. Although a decision to require an ACT rather than a PCT will better serve the interests of the participants, it may not better serve the medical interests of Bolivians writ large. Accommodating the experimental subjects might deprive the society of resources that could better be used elsewhere. Here, as everywhere, there is no free lunch. In the final analysis, there may be reason to prefer the interests of trial participants to other people in need of medical care, but it is hard to see why that is so.

Reasonable Availability

As I noted at the outset, worries about exploitation in clinical research often focus not just on the treatment of the experimental subjects themselves but on the benefits to the community when the study is over. Although the commentators have not been precise about this, they may be arguing (1) that the research would not be exploitative if the products that result from such studies were to be made available to present or future citizens of the host country, or (2) that whatever exploitation is inherent in the research, it would be counterbalanced and the research rendered permissible if the results were reasonably available to present or future citizens of the host country. There are at least two sorts of arguments for the *principle of reasonable availability* (RA). First, it may be thought that RA is somehow linked to the validity of the participants' consent: "Thus a good ethical working rule is that researchers should presume that valid consent cannot be obtained from impoverished populations in the absence of a realistic plan to deliver the intervention to the population."[47] Second, it may be thought that this is a matter of distributive justice. If the people in a developing country assume risks by participating in biomedical research, but cannot afford the drugs, vaccines, and other biomedical products when they become available, then they may be exploited for the benefit of people in the developed countries that sponsored the research. To avoid exploitation there must be some reasonable assurance that products derived from the research in which citizens of developing countries participated will be available in that country.

The first argument is deeply problematic whether it refers to participant consent or community consent. I do not see why the validity of a potential *participant's* consent should be at all related to a decision to make a product available to others in the posttrial environment. There may be reasons not to treat her consent as sufficient to justify the study, but those reasons have little to do with the validity of her consent. And if the *community's* consent is at issue, then the argument is still problematic. For the community's representatives might rationally consent to allow their citizens to participate in a trial so that those citizens can reap the benefit of their participation even if no other citizens are likely to benefit posttrial.

The distributive justice argument has a nice ring and is widely endorsed, but it is actually quite problematic for several reasons. First, if the principles of medical ethics are primarily interested in the way in which patients or subjects are treated, I do not see why the availability of drugs to *other* persons has much bearing on the ethical status of a study.

Second, it is not clear why *national boundaries* are of moral significance. Why must the product be made available in "that country"? Even if we thought it important that the benefits of a study that used Bolivians be made available to other impoverished persons, why is it morally significant that these other persons are Bolivians? Perhaps a good argument can be made on behalf of the moral relevance of national boundaries, but once again, it is not clear why such boundaries are important in the present context or what weight they should carry.

Third, it is not clear why the burden of providing products to the citizens of the host country or any other population should fall on those who are conducting the research. Suppose, for example, that the Surfaxin trial were being conducted by a struggling Indian pharmaceutical company and that neither the firm nor the Indian government has the resources to make the drug widely available. Under these conditions, it seems strange to think that the study should not go forward because RA cannot be implemented but that it can go forward when RA is feasible, say, when it is sponsored by a large multinational corporation.

Fourth, it is a mistake to assume that the world is divided into the very poor and the very rich. Suppose, for example, that a PCT seeks to test the efficacy of a drug that could be provided to many patients in a moderately poor nation but would be unaffordable in a very poor nation. Should we regard the study as objectionable because it is conducted in a very poor nation rather than a moderately poor nation?

Fifth, to the extent that RA is motivated by principles of distributive justice, we must be careful not to conflate valid concerns about the distribution of medical resources in the world with concerns about the relationship among the participants or the nations involved in particular studies. It is possible that insisting upon RA, when feasible, will generate a shift of resources from the more affluent persons of the world (through their governments) to the less affluent. But if RA is not feasible, then insisting on RA as a precondition of a trial will result in no study at all, and will result in less redistribution, not more.

In this connection, it is also important to distinguish between the claim that the distribution of resources in the world is unjust and the claim that a sponsoring nation (or the home country of the sponsors) is causally responsible for the injustice, that is, that it results from exploitation. Crouch and Arras argue that the misery of people in underdeveloped societies "must be due in no small measure to the flagrantly unjust behavior of the former colonial powers, which plundered their natural resources and subjugated their peoples."[48] I am sure that they are sometimes right, but I am equally sure that they are often wrong. The poorest societies of the world are those that have had the least economic contact with the highly industrialized nations. They have suffered not because imperialism has made them worse off but because the affluent nations have "found too little there to be exploited."[49] Of course, even if the industrialized nations have not *caused* the poverty of the underdeveloped society, they may still have an obligation to *ameliorate* that poverty. But even assuming that the industrialized nations do have such an obligation, it is not clear that insisting on RA is the best way to fulfill it.

Relativism and Double Standards

Many commentators have argued, in effect, that to allow a PCT in an underdeveloped society that would not be permitted in a developed society is to countenance moral relativism or a double ethical standard— "Acceptance of a standard of care that does not conform to the standard in the sponsoring country results in a double standard in research."[50] If the Surfaxin trial would not be permitted in the United States, then it should not be permitted in Bolivia; we should not use "the abominable state of health care in [impoverished] countries . . . to justify studies that could never pass ethical muster in the sponsoring country."[51] As Marcia Angell puts it, we must avoid an "ethical relativism" that would allow for research programs in Third World populations that "could not be carried out in the sponsoring countries."[52]

Now a justification for a PCT in an impoverished society need not appeal to ethical relativism, and I know of no serious arguments on behalf of PCTs that make such an error. Rather, an argument for something like PPE maintains that it should be universally applied, but its application will have different implications in different contexts, just as the principle "serve food that your guests will like" is a universal principle the application of which will yield different results for different guests.[53] If, for example, it would be irrational for Americans to consent to participate in a PCT but it would not be irrational for Bolivians to do so, then insisting that only "rational" consent can be taken as valid will have different implications in the two societies, but there is no relativism here.

If the specter of moral relativism is a red herring, so, too, are polemical references to "double standards." The question is not whether we use different standards in different contexts but whether the use of different standards is justifiable. We do not use a "double standard" in any objectionable sense when we allow sixteen-year-olds to drive, but not to drink or vote, whereas we would be using an objectionable double standard if we allowed sixteen-year-old males to drive but not sixteen-year-old females. The present question is whether the best moral principles render it justifiable to transact with members of a poor society on terms that would not be justifiable in affluent societies. It may or may not, but reference to "double standards" will not resolve that question.

If, to misquote someone (I know not whom), "there's nothing like the prospect of a hanging to focus a man's mind," then there is also nothing like the prospect of desperately ill infants with few prospects of receiving any medical care to focus our mind on the question as to what are the best ethical principles for medical research in the nonideal conditions under which so many people clearly live. Lurie and Wolfe have written that "the provision of placebo . . . to the 325 infants in the control group will result in the preventable deaths of 16 infants."[54] Maybe so. But it may also be true that not engaging in the study at all will result in the preventable deaths of numerous infants or that using an ACT when the extra resources might be better spent elsewhere will also result in the preventable deaths of numerous infants. There are preventable deaths all around us, and if the goal is solely to reduce their number, it is not clear what strategy will best achieve it. References to "preventable deaths" should not be used as an argumentative club.

Prophylactic Arguments

Let us suppose that the principle of permissible exploitation (PPE) is roughly correct and that a perfectly flawless application of PPE will yield different implications for medical research under different socioeconomic conditions, such that studies that would pass ethical muster in Bolivia would not pass ethical muster in the United States. Although few commentators have put their arguments in these terms, it is possible that lurking behind their defense of one of the principles we have considered is a version of the prophylactic argument. It is possible that whereas a flawless application of PPE would justify what appear to be double standards, there is good reason to think that the application of PPE will be far from flawless and that the moral gains consequent to the correct application of PPE will be outweighed by the costs consequent to their erroneous application and to the general weakening of important ethical considerations. This argument would exemplify a well-known strategy of adopting relatively "absolute" ethical rules such as the "standard care" or "reasonable availability" principles even when first best ethical principles would allow for greater flexibility. Three points: First, it is an empirical issue as to whether such arguments work in the present context. Second, it is entirely possible that they do work and that they provide a sound defense for relying on one or more of the principles I have discussed. Third, this line of defense for those principles is not an argument for the "intrinsic rightness" of those principles.

Conclusion

I began by discussing what I called the exploitation argument. The crucial moral premise of that argument maintains that if a practice is exploitative, then it should not be permitted. I have not resolved the question as to whether research such as the Surfaxin trial is properly described as exploitative. I have argued that this requires an account of unfair transactions and also involves complex empirical investigations. But even if the Surfaxin Trial is properly described as exploitative, I have argued that the crucial moral premise should be rejected. For in the absence of good reasons to the contrary, we should generally permit mutually advantageous and consensual exploitation to go forward, although it may turn out that there are good reasons to intervene in the present case.

If I am right, we will not resolve questions as to the justifiability of studies such as the Surfaxin trial by appeal to the derisive language of exploitation. We will resolve them by the rigorous examination of arguments and by the painstaking study of the relevant data. Interested parties should withdraw some of their heavy rhetorical artillery and begin the hard work of deliberating about the best ethical principles for the decidedly nonideal conditions that we encounter.

Acknowledgments

The author wishes to thank Bob Taylor and Pat Neal for their comments on a very early version of this chapter. I also want to thank the editors for their detailed and helpful comments on later versions. It would take too many footnotes to indicate the places in which I have used their suggestions and even their language.

Notes

1. George Annas and Michael Grodin, "Human Rights and Maternal-Fetal HIV Transmission Prevention Trials in Africa," *American Journal of Public Health* 88 (1998): 560–63, at 561.

2. Ronald Bayer, "The Debate over Maternal-Fetal HIV Transmission Prevention Trials in Africa, Asia, and the Caribbean: Racist Exploitation or Exploitation of Racism?" *American Journal of Public Health* 88 (1998): 567–70, at 569.

3. Z. Ahmed Bhutta, "Ethics in Internatonal Health Research: A Perspective from the Developing World," CMH Working Papers, Commission on Macroeconomics and Health, 13.

4. Council for International Organizations of Medical Sciences, *International Ethical Guidelines for Biomedical Research Involving Human Subjects*, (Geneva: CIOMS, 2002).

5. Robert Crouch and John Arras, "AZT Trials and Tribulations," *Hastings Center Report* 28, no. 6 (1998): 26–34, at 29.

6. Peter Lurie and Sidney Wolfe, "Unethical Trials of Interventions to Reduce Perinatal Transmission of the Human Immunodeficiency Virus in Developing Countries," *New England Journal of Medicine* 33 (1997): 853–56, at 855.

7. Nuffield Council on Bioethics, *The Ethics of Research Related to Healthcare in Developing Countries* (London: Nuffield Council on Bioethics, 2002).

8. Allen Wood has argued that exploitation need not involve unfairness, that A exploits B when A uses something about B for A's own ends. See "Exploitation," *Social Philosophy and Policy* 12 (1995): 136–58. It is not clear whether Wood's account is as fairness-free as he thinks, for he goes on to say that A exploits B when A uses B for A's own ends "by playing on some weakness or vulnerability, in that person." This implies that A does not (wrongfully) exploit B if A uses B for A's own ends when A does not play on a weakness or vulnerability, that is, when the transaction is fair.

9. Richard Arneson, "Exploitation," in *Encyclopedia of Ethics*, ed. Lawrence C. Becker (New York: Garland, 1992), 350.

10. The president of Stanford University claimed that big-time college athletics "reeks of exploitation," because the universities gain a great deal of revenue from the services of the athletes while the athletes (whose graduation rate is much lower than that of nonathletes) gain little from their college experience. Donald Kennedy, "So What If College Players Turn Pro Early?" *New York Times*, January 19, 1990, B7.

11. *USA Today* featured an article advocating the legalization of organ sales, whereby a person could be paid cash for a kidney. One reply maintained that such a policy would "open wide the door to exploitation." September 14, 1991.

12. One commentator observed that "one of the most serious charges against surrogate motherhood contracts is that they exploit women." Martha Field, *Surrogate Motherhood* (Cambridge, MA: Harvard University Press, 1989), 25.

13. The code of the American Psychiatric Association states that "the psychiatrist's ethics and professional responsibilities preclude his/her gratifying his/her own needs by exploiting the patient." From American Psychiatric Association, "Principles of Medical Ethics with Annotations Especially Applicable to Psychiatry," 1985, cited in *Ethical Issues in the Professions*, ed. Peter Y. Windt et al. (Englewood Cliffs, NJ: Prentice-Hall, 1989), 567.

14. Allen Buchanan, *Ethics, Efficiency, and the Market* (Totowa, NJ: Rowman and Allanheld, 1985), 87, emphasis added.

15. Nancy Holmstrom, "Exploitation," *Canadian Journal of Philosophy* 7 (1997): 353–69, at 357, emphasis added.

16. Judith Farr Tormey, "Exploitation, Oppression and Self-Sacrifice," *Philosophical Forum* 5 (1974): 206–21, at 207–8.

17. Stanley Benn, *A Theory of Freedom* (Cambridge: Cambridge University Press, 1988), 138.

18. Joel Feinberg, *Harmless Wrongdoing* (Oxford: Oxford University Press, 1988), 176–79.

19. Stephen Munzer, *A Theory of Property* (Cambridge: Cambridge University Press, 1990), 171.

20. Andrew Levine, *Arguing for Socialism* (London: Verso, 1988), 66–67.

21. John Lawrence Hill, "Exploitation," *Cornell Law Review* 79 (1994): 631–99, at 637.

22. Most consensual transactions are mutually advantageous and vice versa.

23. Feinberg, *supra* note 18, at 14.

24. Allen Buchanan, *Marx and Justice* (Totowa, NJ: Rowman and Allanheld, 1984), 44.

25. Christine Korsgaard, "The Reasons We Can Share," *Social Philosophy and Policy* 10 (1993): 24–51, at 40.

26. See Alan Wertheimer, *Exploitation* (Princeton, NJ: Princeton University Press, 1996), chap. 7.

27. See her introduction to *Incommensurability, Incomparability, and Practical Reason*, ed. Ruth Chang (Cambridge, MA: Harvard University Press, 1997).

28. See Wertheimer, *supra* note 26, 230–36.

29. For an extended analysis, see my *Coercion* (Princeton, NJ: Princeton University Press, 1987).

30. *Id.* chaps. 12 and 13.

31. Indeed, we can imagine that B makes the identical proposal to A in order to fund her daughter's surgery, in which case B's options would remain the same (no surgery + no sex vs. surgery + sex), but it would be preposterous to claim that A had coerced her into sexual relations.

32. The literature sometimes refers to seductive offers as "undue inducements." I prefer to avoid this phrase because it is unclear whether the inducements are thought to be "undue" because they compromise the rationality of the target's consent or because they are wrongful for other reasons.

33. I set aside the argument that surrogacy harms the children that result from the surrogacy arrangement. Since these children would otherwise not exist, it is difficult to see how they are made worse off as a result of being conceived.

34. See Wertheimer, *supra* note 26, chaps. 5 and 9.

35. As John Rawls puts it, ideal theory "works out the principles that characterize a well-ordered society under favorable circumstances." *A Theory of Justice* (Cambridge, MA: Harvard University Press, 1971), 245.

36. *Id.* at 8–9.

37. In studies of HIV maternal-fetal transmission in Thailand, the placebo group had a higher transmission rate than the treated group but a lower transmission rate than the local background transmission rate. See Christine Grady, "Science in the Service of Healing," *Hastings Center Report* 28 (1998): 34–38, at 36.

38. In slightly different terms, the sponsor would be issuing a warning and not a threat. See the discussion of this distinction in Wertheimer, *supra* note 29, at 96–99.

39. World Medical Association, Declaration of Helsinki, as quoted in Ezekiel J. Emanuel, "A World of Research Subjects," *Hastings Center Report* 28, no. 6 (1998): 25.

40. Needless to say, similar issues arise with respect to the affluent and the poor in developed societies.

41. An old chestnut used by game theorists asks how a rich man and a poor man should agree to share $200. "The rich man could argue for a $150-$50 split in his favor because it would grieve the poor man more to lose $50 than the rich man to lose $150." Howard Raiffa, *The Art and Science of Negotiation* (Cambridge, MA: Harvard University Press, 1982), 52. Raiffa also observes that an arbitrator might suggest the reverse split because the poor person needs the money more and adds that the rich man might also argue for an even split on the grounds that it is wrong to mix business with charity.

42. Even sweatshops may be ethically underrated. As Nicholas Kristof has written, "The American campaign against sweatshops could make [a child's] life much more wretched by inadvertently encouraging mechanization that could cost him his job." "Let Them Sweat," *New York Times*, June 14, 2002, A25.

43. "Among two hundred patients being treated at the University of Pennsylvania Cancer Center, 40 percent did not know the purpose or nature of the procedure they had undergone and 45 percent could not give even one major risk or cite a possible complication resulting from it." David Rothman, "The Shame of Medical Research," *New York Review of Books*, November 30, 2000. Annas and Grodin suggest that "research will almost inevitably be confused with treatment." See Annas and Grodin, *supra* note 1, at 562. A survey of data on the quality of informed consent in developing countries suggests that there is little evidence to support the claim that the quality of consent in underdeveloped societies is significantly less than the quality of consent in developed

societies. See Christine Pace, Christine Grady, and Ezekiel J. Emanuel, "What We Don't Know about Informed Consent," *SciDevNet*, August 28, 2003, www. scidev.net/en/opinions/what-we-dont-know-about-informed-consent.html.

44. See Rothman, *supra* note 43.

45. Charles Weijer, "Protecting Communities in Research: Philosophical and Pragmatic Challenges," *Cambridge Quarterly of Healthcare Ethics* 8 (1999): 501–13, at 503.

46. "Soft paternalism" refers to cases in which we have reason to question B's competence. "Hard paternalism" refers to cases in which we prevent B from doing X even though we have no reason to question the competence of B's decision. Requiring motorcyclists to wear helmets may be a case of hard paternalism.

47. Annas and Grodin, *supra* note 1, at 562.

48. Crouch and Arras, *supra* note 5, at 28.

49. Robert Gilpin, *U.S. Power and the Multinational Corporation* (New York: Basic Books, 1975), 289.

50. Lurie and Wolfe, *supra* note 6, at 855.

51. *Id.*

52. Marcia Angell, "The Ethics of Clinical Research in the Third World," *New England Journal of Medicine* 337 (1997): 849–51, at 849.

53. "Research that is unacceptable in one society because its risks outweigh the risks posed by the disease may have a favorable risk-benefit ratio in another society where the risks posed by the disease are significantly greater. Adapting these requirements to the identities, attachments, and cultural traditions embedded in distinct circumstances neither constitutes moral relativism nor undermines their universality; doing so recognizes that while ethical requirements embody universal values, the manner of specifying these values inherently depends on the particular context." Ezekiel J. Emanuel, David Wendler, and Christine Grady, "What Makes Clinical Research Ethical?" *Journal of the American Medical Association* 283 (2000): 2701–11, at 2708.

54. Peter Lurie and Sidney Wolfe, letter to Tommy Thompson, *Public Citizen*, February 22, 2001.

4

Testing Our Drugs on the Poor Abroad

THOMAS POGGE

Determining whether U.S. companies and some of the persons involved in them are acting ethically when conducting the research described in the Havrix trial and the Surfaxin trial requires reflection on the moral objections that could be raised against what they did. Given the wide range of possible moral objections, it would be folly to try to discuss them all in the space of this chapter. I concentrate, then, on a kind of moral objection that strikes me as especially interesting, plausible, and important. I try to work out whether such objections are valid and, if so, what significance they have for the conduct of the pharmaceutical companies in question—and for the conduct of ourselves as citizens of democratic countries under whose jurisdiction these companies operate.

The moral objections treated in this chapter can be identified, more specifically, as moral *complaints*. These are moral objections that point to some particular person or group as one whom the conduct (here: research) in question should not have treated as it did. A complaint is always presented *in behalf of*, but not necessarily *by*, this person or group. (The victim of a homicide has become unable to formulate a moral complaint against her killer and his act, for instance, but there may nonetheless be a valid such complaint that can be formulated in the victim's behalf.) By focusing on moral complaints, I am not denying, or affirming, that it is possible to act badly without acting badly against anyone. I am merely leaving such possible moral objections aside in order to concentrate on certain moral complaints and questions about their validity.

The contours of the specific kind of moral complaint I am interested in will emerge as the chapter unfolds. It could be discussed in terms of exploitation, but I avoid this label in favor of more accessible language.

Justifying Clinical Trials by Appeal to Benefit

Examining our two clinical trials, it appears that those in whose behalf a moral complaint can most plausibly be advanced are the 325 premature Bolivian infants with acute respiratory distress syndrome (RDS), who were to be given "sham air" in the Surfaxin trial.[1] Some 140 of them were expected to die painfully from their untreated RDS.[2] Did the producer of Surfaxin—Discovery Laboratories Inc., or D-Lab for short—or its agents treat these infants wrongly?

It may seem obvious that they did not. The 325 members of the placebo control group would have received no treatment for their RDS even if D-Lab had not conducted this trial in Bolivia. In that case, the same 140 infants would presumably have died equally painfully. So no one has a valid moral complaint against the trial, since no one is appreciably worse off on account of it. And the trial brings a substantial benefit to the 325 infants receiving Surfaxin, as their survival chances are dramatically improved.

In fact, one might even say that *all* infants enrolled in the study benefit, because they all have their survival prospects boosted by a 50 percent chance of receiving Surfaxin treatment. In this way, the Surfaxin trial is like a compulsory public vaccination program. Even if such a program predictably causes medical complications for a few children each year, it does save thousands of lives by preventing epidemics. Assuming it is not known which children will suffer complications, the program can be justified to all children on the ground that it improves the health prospects of each. Participation in the vaccination program is in each child's best interest *ex ante*. And so is enrollment in the Surfaxin trial.

But the analogy to the described vaccination program is dubious. To see why, consider this analogous story: a rich eccentric is eager to play a paint-bomb prank but wants to make sure it is morally justifiable. So she prepares two gift packages. One contains a paint bomb rigged to open with a loud bang and to splatter the recipient's clothes. The other contains $30,000. She fills in labels with the names of two persons and assigns the labels to the packages by the flip of a coin. This satisfies our eccentric that she is not harming either recipient. In fact, she is benefiting both by giving each a hugely beneficial fifty-fifty chance of $30,000 or splattered clothing.

The paint-splattered recipient, however, is unlikely to be grateful for having been enrolled in the prank. Composing himself, he can point out two important disanalogies between how he has been treated by the eccentric and how children are treated through the compulsory vaccination program. The public vaccination program satisfies the crucial condition that we *cannot* detach the harms it produces from its benefits: We can neither identify vulnerable children in advance nor alter the vaccine so that it provides the same benefits without causing medical complications to anyone. We can then defend the risk of harm to which we expose each child as an undetachable side effect of a program that brings each child an expected net benefit. We can justify this risk *to each child*.

Such a justification fails in the eccentric's case. Her claim that she is probabilistically benefiting both package recipients appeals to an uncertainty that is entirely of her own making and easily avoidable. She could simply detach the harm from the benefit, giving money to people without recoloring anyone.

The analogous justification of the Surfaxin trial fails analogously: the uncertainty about which infants will receive which treatment is entirely of D-Lab's own making and thus easily avoidable. And the harm is detachable from the benefit because D-Lab can give Surfaxin treatment to all or else can use an active-control design rather than a placebo-control design.[3] To be sure, an active-control design might make the study more expensive by requiring D-Lab to dispense more medication and also, perhaps, to enroll a larger number of subjects (in order to ensure statistically significant results). But this point does not invalidate the moral complaint brought in behalf of the sham-air-treated infants; it merely shows how this complaint can perhaps be answered by reference to some other good. While the mandatory vaccination program can be justified as treating each child as best we know how, the Surfaxin trial cannot be so justified to the infants in the placebo control group.

Justifying Clinical Trials by Appeal to Consent

The eccentric is unenthusiastic about the suggestion that she could just give money away to people without watching anyone splattered with paint. So she revises her prank in a way that allows her to appeal to informed consent. She asks persons to volunteer to open one of her gift packages while accurately informing them that, so doing, they have a 50 percent chance of being recolored with a bang and a 50 percent chance of finding $30,000. In this way, half her volunteers end up splattered with paint, to the eccentric's delight, and worse off for having participated. But since they are fully informed beforehand of the risk they are taking, they have no moral complaint against her.

The eccentric's justification of her revised prank has a venerable pedigree in the ancient saying *volenti non fit iniuria*, no injustice is being done to the willing. The idea is that a person, even when he is being harmed, has no moral complaint against those harming him if he consented to the harm or to the risk thereof. This justification is thought to be decisive at least when the consent is rational and fully informed—conditions that can be satisfied in the revised prank. In the Surfaxin trial, of course, consent cannot be given by the infant subjects. But so long as their parents' consent is given and clearly rational from the standpoint of each infant in light of full information, it is hard to object to this substitution.

There is a powerful objection, however, to the underlying idea that a recipient's fully informed rational consent always justifies the treatment he receives as permissible. To illustrate:

Monitoring her radio equipment, a successful U.S. filmmaker staying in a hotel south of Calcutta finally hears what she was waiting for—a distress call from a fishing vessel far out at sea. Having sprung a leak, the tiny boat is sinking in calm waters and, lacking proper flotation devices, its crew of three will try to survive by treading water in hopes of rescue. They are natives of very poor Bangladesh, which will make no effort to save them. Ships rarely pass through those remote waters, and, even if some received the call, they will hardly make large detours to rescue indigent fishermen.[4] The filmmaker radios back with her proposal: she will fly to the scene in her helicopter and will then flip a coin. If it comes up heads, she will rescue the crew and fly them to safety at no charge. If it comes up tails, she will film whatever happens to them "naturally" (their slow deaths, almost certainly). She intends this documentary to be shown in wealthier countries where audiences may gain therefrom useful information about panic behavior and its effect on a person's survival time in ocean water. She also promises that, should the coin come up tails, she will rescue the next crew of fishermen in mortal danger with no strings attached. The crew accept her offer, and quite rationally so: the value of the 50 percent chance of being saved vastly outweighs any despair added to a drowning death by seeing safety so close at hand. So the filmmaker flies to the scene and flips the coin. It comes up tails, and she films their slow deaths for the benefit of her "first world" audience.

We are familiar with conduct such as that of D-Lab, and many are thus not especially shocked by it. The rather unusual conduct of the filmmaker, by contrast, seems much worse and quite horrendous, if not grotesque. She is hovering right above drowning men, whom she could easily save, while recording their desperate struggle for survival.

But consider D-Lab's researchers: they force a tube down an infant's throat and pump sham air into its lungs even while they have Surfaxin (and possibly other advanced medicines for RDS) close at hand. They do this 325 times and then observe how these children struggle for breath and how about 140 of them die painfully while their desperate parents are waiting, hoping, and praying for their survival. To be sure, the researchers have prevented themselves from knowing which of the 650 infants they are treating in this way. But they do fully intend so to treat half of them. And this presumably after having—unlike the filmmaker—taken a Hippocratic oath. It appears, then, that if the filmmaker's conduct is wrong, then so is that of D-Lab and its staff.

The case of the filmmaker shows vividly that a recipient's prior fully informed and rational consent may not justify the treatment he receives as permissible when such consent is exacted as a condition for giving him some chance of being saved from a horrible predicament. The exception clearly extends as well to *hypothetical* consent (the recipient, if fully informed, would rationally consent if he had an opportunity to do so) and *proxy* consent such as the parents are giving to their infants' enrollment in the Surfaxin trial.

The Incentives a Morality Provides

The case of the filmmaker appeals powerfully to our moral intuitions: her conduct as described just cannot be right. The Surfaxin trial seems closely parallel, yet it may initially strike us as comparatively harmless. It may help, then, to work out in some more detail how these cases really are parallel in respects that matter to their moral assessment. One respect is obvious, and we have already highlighted it: the agent in both cases is interacting with the recipients, does nearly all that is necessary to save their lives, but then deliberately fails to take the last little step while knowing that this puts the recipients' survival at great risk. Let me highlight another respect in which the two cases are closely parallel.

Like any normative code, a morality provides incentives of two kinds. *Compliance incentives* guide those committed to a code to act as it commands. For an ideal adherent, compliance incentives are decisive—she never acts in ways that her code (considered as a whole and assumed to be consistent) forbids. Through *reward incentives*, a code, working in conjunction with the interests and circumstances of its adherents, encourages or discourages certain kinds of conduct. The distinction is familiar from the legal realm, and from the tax law in particular: a tax code requiring that one pay taxes on interest income not deriving from municipal bonds provides a compliance incentive to pay taxes on such income, and a reward incentive to invest in municipal bonds. Moralities analogously provide incentives of both kinds. For example, a morality that requires single young adults to volunteer for a stint in the military provides a compliance incentive to enlist and a reward incentive to get married early.[5]

The plausibility of a code depends in large part on how it guides its ideal adherents by means of incentives of both kinds. Many tax codes are marred by absurd reward incentives that encourage savvy taxpayers to take advantage of illogical opportunities for tax avoidance.[6] Insofar as we ordinary taxpayers understand these loopholes, our confidence in the tax code is undermined. We judge a code in part by what it rewards and penalizes.

Now suppose our morality counted fully informed rational consent to some treatment as a sufficient condition of its permissibility. It would then encourage and reward *preying* on other people in hopes that they will be overtaken by some misfortune in the context of which it will be rational for them to consent to the treatment we have in store for them. Remember the successful U.S. filmmaker spending hours monitoring her radio in hopes for a distress call, which would give her the chance permissibly to film an authentic drowning death from her helicopter. Her hopes and plan are inspired by a reward incentive her morality provides. And something similar holds in the Surfaxin trial. In order to test its new medication in a placebo-control trial that is permissible by the lights of its morality, D-Lab must hope for a location where infants in sufficient numbers are born with RDS and where such infants lack access to treatment for their condition. Like the filmmaker scours the airwaves in hopes of finding sailors in distress whose deaths she can permissibly film, so D-Lab's staff are scouring the earth in hopes of finding RDS infants whom they can permissibly infuse with sham air. It is hard to have confidence in a morality that encourages and rewards such predatorial behavior.

The Origin of Emergencies and Its Moral Significance

D-Lab's conduct may in fact be *more* wrong than the filmmaker's, for it may be relevant to the moral assessment of such conduct how the horrible predicament it seeks to take advantage of has come about. The fishermen are not entirely faultless in their emergency. They might perhaps have kept closer to shore, taken better care of their boat, or at least brought along some simple floatation devices. By contrast, infants born with RDS are plainly not even ever so slightly culpable for their condition.

This difference may matter morally. It may be less wrong to take advantage of another's predicament if this person implicitly risked this predicament through his recklessness or negligence. Thus, lending someone money at an excessively high interest rate for an urgent car repair may be more acceptable if the borrower damaged the car while driving drunk than it would be if the car had suffered an accidental breakdown.

While the victim's fault in a predicament may make it *less* wrong to take advantage of this predicament and its victim, such conduct may be rendered *more* wrong by the fact that the predicament is partly due to wrongful conduct on the part of people other than the victim. To see this, we might redescribe the loan case so that the car was vandalized by people hateful of its owner's race or religion. Under these circumstances, it would seem more wrong to take advantage of the owner's urgent need by charging interest at an exorbitant rate. Similarly, we may judge the filmmaker's conduct even more harshly when we imagine that the fishermen's poverty, constraining and influencing their choice of work and equipment, is to some extent due not to the poverty of their country but to the injustice of its social institutions and policies. To the extent that this is so, the lender and the filmmaker are seeking to take advantage not merely of an acute emergency but also of a wrong, namely, of a hate crime and a social injustice, respectively.

Social injustice clearly plays a role in the predicaments D-Lab is seeking to take advantage of. The Latin American countries it has targeted display some of the highest rates of income inequality in the world, and these enormous inequalities—reflected in and reinforced by their economic, legal, and political institutions—account for their high incidence of severe poverty, adult illiteracy, and infant mortality as well as for their poor public health systems.[7] Without this social injustice, D-Lab would not have found in Bolivia what it was looking for: rampant RDS routinely left untreated among the poor.

So D-Lab is taking advantage of social injustice. But we have yet to examine whether and how this should make a difference to our moral assessment of its conduct. Toward answering this question, consider a pair of cases that are quite similar to each other and differ in this one respect only:

> A self-employed U.S. author nearing completion of a major writing project needs secretarial assistance for typing, fact checking, and the like. To save money, she is willing to relocate, for the relevant period, to a place where secretarial wages are low. In scenario 1, she chooses a foreign country that is structured in a just way but also is rather poor, thus taking advantage of the much lower sec-

retarial wages there. In scenario 2, she chooses another foreign country that, considerably richer than the first, has a much despised (racial, ethnic, or religious) minority whose members suffer heavy market discrimination and are therefore generally paid only a fraction of the wages their compatriots receive for the same work. Not harboring any animosity toward this minority, our author hires several of its members at their going market rate.

I would think that the author has moral reason, even in scenario 1, to share some of the net benefit she derives from the temporary relocation with her employees, especially if they do not, in the world as it is, enjoy anything like the international mobility she enjoys. In any case, her moral reason to do this is surely stronger in scenario 2, where some of this net benefit derives from the discrimination rampant in the foreign country. By paying her minority workers only the going market rate, the author would be taking advantage of, even become complicit in, the unjust discriminatory practice. To avoid acting wrongly in these ways, the author must pay her employees at least the going rate for equally skilled members of the majority group.

Transferred to the Surfaxin trial, these thoughts suggest that D-Lab's conduct is rendered more wrong by the fact that social injustice plays a major role in landing Bolivian infants in the desperate situation that then makes them available for the placebo-control trial. To avoid taking advantage of such injustice, D-Lab must treat these children as it would have to treat them if this injustice did not exist. As the author ought to pay her minority employees at least as much as members of the majority can earn for such work, so D-Lab ought to treat Bolivian infants as if they were citizens of a just country and therefore entitled to some basic health care (presumably including some existing RDS treatment) as a matter of course.

Taking Advantage of Wrongs in Conjunction with Contributions to Them

We have found two reasons for judging conduct like D-Lab's more harshly than conduct like the filmmaker's. The victims of the predicament that D-lab is seeking to take advantage of bear not even the slightest fault for this predicament, whereas the fishermen bear some fault at least for negligence. And there is, on the face of it, a much greater element of social injustice manifested in Bolivia's than in Bangladesh's extreme poverty, because the former country has much higher income inequality that could be reduced for the sake of poverty eradication.[8]

There is yet a third aggravating factor likely to be present in the Surfaxin trial and more prominently so than in the cases of the filmmaker and the author. Other things being equal, it would seem morally worse to take advantage of a wrong or (more specifically) an injustice when one shares responsibility for it. The unjust discrimination our author takes advantage of in scenario 2 has presumably evolved independently of herself. It is unlikely, by contrast, that D-Lab played no role in the evolution of the economic injustice manifesting itself in the horrible predicament of RDS infants in Latin America. U.S. pharmaceutical companies are causally involved both in the high level of drug prices and in the persistence of severe poverty in the so-called developing countries.[9] These companies have lobbied very hard for the entitlements to economic rents that were enshrined in the existing Trade-Related Aspects of Intellectual Property Rights (TRIPS) regime and that have since been further strengthened through various bilateral treaties pushed by the United States. Incentivizing pharmaceutical innovation by giving inventor firms monopoly pricing powers, these treaties ensure that new medical treatments are unaffordable to the world's poor until after their patents expire and their inventors' evergreening efforts are finally exhausted (for only then are generic producers allowed to enter the market, thereby lowering prices through competition). These treaties also ensure that pharmaceutical companies have no incentives to fund research on diseases that predominantly affect the poor.[10] Insofar as D-Lab has contributed to these lobbying efforts—either directly or through political action committees or industry associations—it shares responsibility for the unavailability of advanced lifesaving drugs to the world's poor.

Moreover, insofar as the existing global economic order, through its strong centrifugal tendencies, contributes to the persistence of severe poverty in many poor countries, the most powerful states and their corporations and citizens, playing the dominant role in designing and imposing this order, share responsibility for such poverty.[11] Even before entering Latin America, D-Lab is then already both a contributor to, and a beneficiary of, global economic injustice, which effectively excludes most people in poor countries from access to advanced lifesaving drugs. By conducting the proposed Surfaxin trial, the people of D-Lab are taking further advantage of an injustice that they themselves have helped create and sustain.

Is Morality Counterproductive?

Let us take stock. We have found various reasons for believing that conducting the Surfaxin trial does a wrong to the 325 infants to be infused with sham air: the treatment they receive is not essential to the purpose of the trial, which could be conducted with an active-control rather than a placebo-control design. This treatment is inflicted on extremely vulnerable human beings who are unable to give prior consent. The extreme predicament of these 325 infants involves no fault of their own and is due in part to social injustice in whose emergence and persistence D-Lab was and is involved quite independently of the proposed trial. It is not morally permissible for D-Lab to use these infants in this way.

This verdict—though without the arguments and analogies supporting it—is now official policy of the World Medical Association[12] and dominant in the bioethics literature.[13] To be sure, the verdict is not unanimous. The dominant view is actively challenged and its dominance seriously threatened by those who believe that placebo-control trials are permissible in poor countries with patients who, in the absence of the study, would remain untreated.[14] But it is still the dominant view, influential enough to have prompted D-Lab to modify its initial research proposal in favor of an active-control design. This modification apparently removed the reasons for preferring subjects from a poor country: D-Lab conducted Phase II clinical trials of Surfaxin at approximately thirty medical facilities in the United States.[15] Morality has prevailed in the end.

But is this not a hollow victory? Because D-Lab was responsive to the demands of morality, it has shifted the venue of its trial to the United States. As a result, 325 Bolivian infants, initially slated to receive Surfaxin, remained untreated. Some 140 of them are likely to have died as a result—infants who would have lived if the Surfaxin trial had gone ahead as initially conceived. Can we be relieved that D-Lab refrained, in the end, from its unethical trial? Or should we not rather reexamine and revise the morality that blocked D-Lab's initial plan?

The story of the Surfaxin trial poses a difficult challenge to our ethical reflection. The challenge can be formulated in the form of three moral propositions that seem clearly true and yet also difficult to hold together. Because the challenge is general, I give general labels to the three propositions. To make quite clear what is at stake, I do, however, formulate narrow and concrete versions of the propositions themselves:

> *Moral Constraint:* It is wrong to test a new medicine (Surfaxin) for some life-threatening medical condition (RDS) with a placebo-control design when there already exists an effective medicine for this condition against which the new drug could be tested (active-control design).
>
> *Moral Freedom:* A drug company (D-Lab) is under no obligation to test new medicines for life-threatening medical conditions in a poor country rather than in its home country or in another rich country.
>
> *Moral Goodness:* It is morally bad (undesirable, regrettable) that many human beings (infants in Bolivia) should die as a result of a drug company's decision to test a new medicine in its rich home country rather than among the poor abroad.[16]

Each of these moral propositions seems plainly true. What produces the tension among them is an empirical fact: that D-Lab has no good reason to conduct its Surfaxin trial in Bolivia unless it can use a placebo-control design there.

D-Lab has three feasible options for testing Surfaxin, which, in nonmoral, cost-benefit terms, it ranks as follows:

> *Placebo-Poor:* use a placebo-control design and conduct the test in a poor country;
>
> *Active-Rich:* use an active-control design and conduct the test in a rich country;
>
> *Active-Poor:* use an active-control design and conduct the test in a poor country.[17]

We can rank the same three options by comparing the resulting outcomes in terms of their moral goodness, which, in the case at hand, can be expressed simply by the trial's impact on the number of infants who die of RDS. We get the following ranking:

Active-Poor—Surfaxin or alternative treatments save more than 280 infant lives in Bolivia;

Placebo-Poor—Surfaxin treatments save some 140 infant lives in Bolivia;

Active-Rich—Surfaxin and alternative treatments save no lives.

Consider now what happens if *Moral Constraint* closes down the *Placebo-Poor* option. A morality including this constraint provides a compliance incentive to prefer an active-control over a placebo-control design. All agents committed to the morality have this incentive, regardless of their nonmoral motives. But the same morality also provides a reward incentive to prefer doing the test in a rich rather than a poor country. This further incentive presupposes not merely a commitment to the morality but certain nonmoral motives as well. In the Surfaxin case, the relevant additional motive is one of ordinary cost-benefit optimization, which leads D-Lab to rank *Active-Rich* above *Active-Poor*.

Taking both incentives together, the effect of *Moral Constraint* is, then, to *guide* D-Lab not only *away* from its preferred option, *Placebo-Poor*, but also *toward* its next-best option, *Active-Rich*. This latter guidance is, however, profoundly undesirable by the lights of *Moral Goodness:* The imposition of *Moral Constraint* leads to the deaths of some 140 Bolivian infants whom, absent *Moral Constraint*, Surfaxin treatment would have saved.

It would seem, then, that any morality committed to the three moral propositions is flawed and, more specifically, counterproductive. By imposing *Moral Constraint*, such a morality guides agents toward producing outcomes that, *by its own lights* (*Moral Goodness*), are morally worse.

This realization invites the following reasoning: we cannot bring ourselves to believe that avoidable deaths of infants in Bolivia are a matter of moral indifference; so we simply cannot jettison *Moral Goodness*. We also cannot bring ourselves to believe that a pharmaceutical company conducting drug trials is morally required to conduct these trials wherever they will produce the greatest expected benefit. For where would this end? As participants in the global economy, we all affect the lives of many people all over the world, and it would be absurd to demand that our economic decisions be guided by some imperative of moral-benefit maximization. Such a demand would not only be enormously burdensome on corporations and individuals—it would most likely also be counterproductive by greatly reducing the collective benefits produced by markets conceived as morality-free zones.[18] So *Moral Freedom* also looks secure. It would seem, therefore, that *Moral Constraint* should be rejected after all. Given the relatively small additional discomfort inflicted on the infants in the control group of the originally planned *Placebo-Poor* Surfaxin trial (conducted with a placebo-control design in Bolivia), we cannot insist on condemning this trial if this condemnation foreseeably results in some 140 additional infant deaths.

We can appreciate the enormous real importance of this issue by looking briefly beyond clinical trials to note that the reasoning just displayed is often applied to analogous decisions made by corporations and individuals. Firms that produce or sell goods made with sweatshop labor argue that any moral constraints on such activities would be absurd because they would shift production from poor to affluent countries, thereby making poor people even worse off. That so many young women in poor countries are eagerly seeking work at $1 or $2 per day shows clearly that such maquiladoras give these women options that they themselves find superior to the other options they have. Analogous arguments are made with regard to child labor as well, which is claimed to give children in desperately poor countries a better life than they would otherwise have. Consumers in the wealthy countries can employ the same sort of reasoning, pointing out that, if they were legally or morally constrained not to buy imported sweatshop and child-labor products, then less production would be shifted to poor countries, which would deprive the people there of valued employment opportunities. Again, sex tourists and their facilitating enterprises can also argue analogously: if the legal and moral constraints governing the domestic sex trade also applied in poor countries, there would be much less sex tourism into those countries, which in turn would deprive many young women (and boys and men) there of valued income opportunities.

The common refrain of all these arguments is that, if we really care about desperately poor people in the developing world, then we should not put moral roadblocks in the path of any initiative that aims to reach out to these people by building commercial ties that bring them substantial net benefits (relative to the lives they would lead with the moral constraints in place). In fact, we should do our best to facilitate such ties. Instead of criticizing our firms' activities in poor countries, we ought to entice them to commence or intensify such activities: we should inform our entrepreneurs how cheaply labor can be bought in these countries and persuade them to build maquiladoras there as well as unconventional sex tourism resorts and the rest.

The Moral Relevance of Who Is Making the Argument

This line of argument is hard to dismiss. Put yourself in the position of the senior medical researcher at D-Lab, who is asked by her chief executive officer (CEO) to consider the various ways of testing Surfaxin so as to win FDA approval of the drug. She knows that her boss would veto the *Active-Poor* option because an active-control trial could be done more reliably and more cheaply in the United States. (Conducting the trial in Latin America would engender additional expenses for upgrading medical facilities there as well as for travel, lodging, and transportation costs. These additional expenses can be recouped only by doing in Latin America what one cannot do in any affluent country: use the more cost-effective placebo-control design.) She also knows that even a placebo-control trial conducted in Latin America would save some 140 lives. Under these circumstances, should she not suspend her moral qualms and urge her boss to choose *Placebo-Poor*? And, if her boss accepts her proposal, should she not then agree to take charge of D-Lab's placebo-control trial in Latin America—that is, should she not then participate in what she herself regards as wrongful? And, if this is what she should or may do, must she not then revise her belief (*Moral Constraint*) that it would be wrong for D-Lab to proceed with *Placebo-Poor*?

I find most of this argument persuasive. With some 140 lives hanging in the balance, it may indeed be at least permissible for the senior medical researcher to act in the way suggested. But I doubt that the last step of the argument goes through; I do not believe that she has reason to reject *Moral Constraint*. To see why, consider this same argument as presented by the CEO himself: "It is permissible for me to decide in favor of *Placebo-Poor* because it leads to the best available outcome: The outcome of *Active-Rich* is much worse, involving some 140 additional infant deaths, and the outcome of *Active-Poor* is unavailable because I am vetoing this option as too expensive." This argument fails because the unavailability of *Active-Poor* is a fact of his own making. While the senior medical researcher can justify her pushing for *Placebo-Poor* by pointing out that her CEO is firmly (and wrongly) disposed to choose *Active-Rich* over *Active-Poor*, the CEO cannot justify his own choice of *Placebo-Poor* by pointing out that *he himself* is firmly disposed to choose *Active-Rich* over *Active-Poor*.[19] Given that this choice costs more than 280 human lives, the CEO ought not to be so disposed. I conclude, then, that *Moral Freedom* is the proposition we should modify: aware of the facts as we have stipulated them, D-Lab ought not to reject *Active-Poor* in favor of *Active-Rich*.

One might object that the CEO has a fiduciary obligation to his shareholders that does not allow him to honor the moral considerations in favor of *Active-Poor*. However, the CEO can have such a fiduciary obligation only if his principals want him to be unresponsive to moral considerations. If they do, the argument of the preceding paragraph can be rewritten, substituting the CEO for the senior medical researcher and the shareholders for the CEO. The upshot, then, is that the shareholders cannot argue: "It is permissible for our company to decide in favor of *Placebo-Poor* because it leads to the best available outcome: The outcome of *Active-Rich* is much worse, involving some 140 additional infant deaths, and the outcome of *Active-Poor* is unavailable because we are firmly opposed to D-Lab's acting in ways that are not profit-maximizing."

Given that the shareholders have ultimate control over, and hence bear ultimate moral responsibility for, their company's policies, they must inform themselves (and the CEO must inform them) about important policy decisions such as those regarding medical trials. A morality would be perverse if it allowed an agent's fiduciary obligations to cancel any moral responsibilities his principals would otherwise have had. A morality would be perverse if it forbade the owners of a company to inflict certain harms on third parties directly but then allowed the very same harms to be inflicted by an agent (CEO) acting in the owners' behalf. That this would be perverse is easily seen: such a morality would enable, and even encourage, principals to circumvent the constraints it imposes by hiring agents to act on their behalf. And such a morality would implausibly place much tighter restrictions on companies that are run by their owners directly than on companies that are run by hired agents on their owners' behalf.[20]

A Mild Constraint on the Freedom of Economic Agents

The objection invoking fiduciary obligations having failed, let us examine how *Moral Freedom* might plausibly be modified. It was said earlier, in support of *Moral Freedom*, that it would be excessively burdensome and also counterproductive to subject corporations and individuals to a demand of moral-benefit maximization. However, so strong a moral demand is not needed to reach the conclusion that the CEO and the shareholders ought to favor *Active-Poor*. The case at hand is special in that the benefit at stake is huge—more than 280 human lives would be saved by conducting the active-control trial in Bolivia rather than in the United States—and the extra costs involved in securing this benefit are comparatively minor. The case at hand is special also in that a plan for a Surfaxin trial in Bolivia had already been drawn up, so there was no need to scour the earth for a place where the trial might be conducted in a highly beneficial way. All the CEO needed to do was to endorse the existing plan while modifying its design from placebo control to active-control. This is what he ought to have done:

> *Exception to Moral Freedom:* A drug company (D-Lab) should not test a new treatment for a life-threatening medical condition in its home country or in another rich country when it knows that there is a poor country where the test can be performed at reasonable cost and would save many human lives.

Such a narrow modification of *Moral Freedom* suffices to reach a plausible resolution of the case before us. But what will happen if this *Exception*, modifying the three moral propositions, becomes widely accepted? Then the CEOs and shareholders of drug companies will have an incentive not to acquire the requisite information about conducting medical trials in poor countries. They will know that placebo-control trials are impermissible whenever effective alternative drugs are already on hand. And they know that it is often cheaper to conduct active-control trials at home rather than in a poor foreign country. So they will not consider

Active-Poor options and consequently keep their companies outside the scope of the *Exception*.

Once widely recognized as morally binding, the proposed *Exception* thus loses much of its effect. It does not dissolve but merely transforms the tension in our morality, insofar as drug companies, aware of *Moral Constraint* and of the cost advantage of conducting active-control trials in their home country, would adopt policies of testing new treatments for life-threatening medical conditions at home without even considering foreign alternatives. If such a policy remains morally acceptable, then *Moral Constraint* continues to be counterproductive by the lights of *Moral Goodness*, leading to the deaths of many human beings in poor countries who would have been saved if placebo-control trials of new medicines were morally permissible there but not in the drug companies' home countries.

A parallel problem arises in the case of the filmmaker. We may think that morality requires him, once he hears the distress call, to use his helicopter to rescue the fishermen (without foisting his lottery scheme upon them). But, if this were widely accepted, such fishermen would be *more* likely to drown. The filmmaker has no earthly reason to be near Calcutta with his radio equipment and helicopter if this can win him no exciting filming opportunity, but can only slap him with a moral rescue burden.

I believe that morality cannot plausibly be purged of such counterproductivity entirely. When morality places constraints on what an agent may demand from needy people in exchange for improving their situation, many such agents may tend to ignore the plight of needy people. Morality may counteract this tendency by restricting our freedom to ignore the urgent needs of others. But such restrictions cannot plausibly be strong enough fully to counterbalance the effects of the constraints. Morality can hold that the filmmaker is not free to ignore the plight of the fishermen if he can rescue them at little cost and no risk to himself. But morality cannot plausibly restrict his freedom by requiring him to spend his life near the Bay of Bengal monitoring the airwaves for distress signals and holding a helicopter at the ready for rescuing Bangladeshi fishermen in mortal peril. Morality can take away what would entice the filmmaker and D-Lab to venture south. But, having done this, morality cannot plausibly substitute an imperative that would have the same effect. There is a real danger, then, that the very people in whose behalf morality imposes such constraints end up worse off than they would have been without it.

Working on the Empirical Factors That Sustain the Tension in Our Morality

Morality cannot plausibly be revised so as to preclude counterproductivity. Though there is no such theoretical solution, it may still be possible to mitigate the problem practically. As the number of people in severe distress declines, the cost of moral constraints in terms of *Moral Goodness* declines as well. This does not alter the fact that our morality is counterproductive. But it does reduce the impact of this counterproductivity. Moral constraints on taking advantage of people in severe distress may make such people worse off in general than they would be without such constraints. But this problem is more tolerable if severe distress occurs so infrequently and unpredictably that little would be gained by removing the constraints.

This practical solution is thus in the interest, as it were, of morality itself. And morality itself can also foster this solution. The emergencies frequently encountered by poor Bangladeshi fishermen are a predictable result of severe poverty in Bangladesh, which leads to a woefully underequipped Bangladeshi coast guard and compels people to risk their lives in flimsy boats to make a living. Morality can hold that people with ample resources (money, time, etc.) ought to make some effort toward preempting and reducing such root causes of severe distress. If most affluent people, corporations, and governments gave a little of their wealth toward reducing severe poverty or toward beefing up emergency services (hospitals, ambulances, coast guard, fire brigade), then we could avoid and preempt most of the desperate needs and emergencies that agents such as D-Lab and the filmmaker are tempted to take advantage of. Reducing such needs and emergencies is desirable in itself. A further reason for thinking of this task as morally required is that its fulfillment eases the tension within morality itself by reducing the cost in moral goodness entailed by moral constraints.

Though the affluent ought to eradicate severe needs as well as frequent and predictable emergencies, too few will in fact support this effort, and the tension in our morality will therefore remain acute for the foreseeable future. Still, it is worth examining what efforts of this kind can and should be made, and by whom. My examination is focused on achieving basic health care in the poor countries, because this achievement would ease the counterproductivity problem as it arises specifically with regard to clinical trials.

The Practical Solution

The severe needs and emergencies pharmaceutical companies might take advantage of indicate injustices in which these companies are involved. These companies and their owners, like the rest of us privileged citizens of the rich countries, are involved in imposing, and are profiting from, a global institutional order under which the lion's share of global economic growth goes to the more affluent people while billions of human beings continue to live in abject poverty. Global economic inequality has grown relentlessly over the past decades[21]—to the point where the citizens of the high-income economies, only 15.7 percent of the world's population, now have 79 percent of global income,[22] while the world's 2,735 million people living below the World Bank's $2 per day international poverty line, over 40 percent of humankind, share about 1 percent of global income. This poverty line is defined in terms of purchasing power and set at a very low level: to count as poor by the $2 per day standard, the consumption expenditure of a U.S. resident for all of 2007 would have to fall below $1,120.[23] Of course, the global poor live *below* this line—42 percent below it on average[24]—and thus consume about as much per person per year as could be bought for $650 in a typical rich country or for $160 in a typical poor one.

The effects of such severe poverty are staggering. It is estimated that 830 million human beings are chronically undernourished, 1,100 million lack access to safe water, and 2,600 million lack access to basic sanitation.[25] About 2,000 million lack access to essential drugs.[26] Some 1000 million have no adequate shelter, and 2,000 million lack electricity.[27] Some 799 million adults are illiterate,[28] and 250 million children between the ages of five and fourteen do wage work outside their household—often under harsh or cruel conditions: as soldiers, prostitutes, or domestic servants, or in agriculture, construction, or textile or carpet production.[29] Roughly one-third of all human deaths, 18 million annually or 50,000 each day, are due to poverty-related causes, easily preventable through better nutrition, safe drinking water, cheap rehydration packs, vaccines, antibiotics, and other medicines.[30] People of color, females, and the very young are heavily overrepresented among the global poor, and hence also among those suffering the staggering effects of severe poverty.[31]

Although we are deeply implicated in the persistent and severe poverty of half of humankind, our pharmaceutical companies are essentially ignoring the specific medical problems faced by the global poor. In fact, they are aggravating the problem by spending millions on political lobbying efforts in favor of an intellectual property regime that patently encourages such neglect and patently ensures that existing drugs are unaffordable in the poor countries to all but a small "elite" (see discussion in the next section).

Having substantially contributed, in these ways, to the medical emergency conditions avoidably imposed on billions of human beings today, our pharmaceutical companies are not then in a position to adduce the unavailability of drugs to the global poor in defense of placebo-control drug trials. Their moral situation compares to that of a different filmmaker who has, intentionally or otherwise, contributed to the desperate emergency of the fishermen. Such a filmmaker ought to reduce the harms she will have caused these fishermen and must not attach to such efforts any conditions (such as consent to his lottery scheme). Likewise, we and our pharmaceutical companies have been and still are contributing to the ongoing massive catastrophe of global poverty and therefore ought to reduce the harms we will have caused the global poor (without attaching to such efforts any conditions, such as consent to placebo-control tests of drugs to which effective alternative treatments already exist).

Such a moral critique of the conduct of pharmaceutical companies standardly receives the response that these companies simply cannot honor such moral imperatives. If one of them lived up to its moral responsibility—by making a major research effort targeted at poor-country diseases, for example, or through a massive initiative of offering proprietary drugs cheaply to poor people in developing countries—then it would quickly encounter the discipline of the market. It would face declining revenues with which to fund its research, gradually lose ground against its competitors, and eventually end up in bankruptcy.

This response has some truth and shows that none of our pharmaceutical companies can, by itself, undertake a sustainable effort to alleviate the ongoing medical disaster among the global poor. But these pharmaceutical companies can nevertheless make such an effort *together* by lobbying for rules that enable and even encourage them to undertake such a sustainable effort.

Just Rules for Incentivizing Pharmaceutical Research[32]

Bringing new, safe, and effective lifesaving medications to market is hugely expensive, as inventor firms must pay for the research and development of new drugs as well as for elaborate testing and the subsequent approval process.[32] In addition, newly developed medical treatments often turn out to be unsafe or not effective enough, or to have bad side effects, or fail to win government approval for some other reason, which may lead to the loss of the entire investment.

Given such large investment costs and risks, very little innovative pharmaceutical research would take place in a free-market system.[33] The reason is that an innovator would bear the full cost of its failures but would be unable to profit from its successes because competitors would copy or retro-engineer its invention (effectively freeriding on its effort) and then drive down the price close to the marginal cost of production. This is a classic instance of market failure leading to a collectively irrational (Pareto-suboptimal) outcome in which medical innovation is undersupplied by the market.

The classic solution, also enshrined in the TRIPs regime (adopted under World Trade Organization [WTO] auspices in the Uruguay Round), corrects this market failure through patent rules that grant inventor firms a temporary monopoly on their inventions, typically for twenty years from the time of filing a patent application. With competitors barred from copying and selling any newly invented drug during this period, the inventor firm (or its licensees) can sell it at the profit-maximizing monopoly price, typically very far above its marginal cost of production. In this way, the inventor firm can recoup its research and overhead expenses plus some of the cost of its other research efforts that failed to bear fruit.

This solution corrects one market failure (undersupply of medical innovation), but its monopoly feature creates another. During the patent's duration, the profit-maximizing sale price of the invented medicine will be far above its marginal cost of production. This large differential is collectively irrational by impeding many mutually beneficial transactions between the inventor firm and potential buyers who are unwilling or unable to pay the monopoly price but are willing and able to pay substantially more than the marginal cost of production. If modified rules could facilitate these potential transactions, then many patients would benefit— and so would the drug companies because they would book additional profitable sales and typically also, through economies of scale, reduce their marginal cost of production.

One idea for avoiding this second market failure (associated with monopoly pricing powers) involves a *differential-pricing strategy*. One variant would have inventor firms themselves offer their proprietary drugs to different customers at different prices, thereby realizing a large profit margin from sales to the more affluent without renouncing sales to poorer buyers at a lower margin. Another variant is the right of governments, recognized under TRIPs rules, to issue compulsory licenses for inventions that are urgently needed in a public emergency. Exercising this right, a government can force down the price of a patented invention by compelling the patent holder to license it to other producers for a set percentage (typically below 10 percent) of the latters' sales revenues. It is often suggested that poor countries should assert their compulsory licensing rights to cope with their public health crises and with the AIDS pandemic in particular.

Differential-pricing solutions are generally unworkable unless the different categories of buyers can be prevented from knowing about, or from trading with, one another. In the real world, if the drug were sold at a lower price to some, then many buyers who would otherwise be willing and able to pay the higher price would find a way to buy at the lower price. Selling expensive drugs more cheaply in poor countries, for example, would create strong incentives to smuggle this drug back into the more affluent countries, leading to relative losses in the latter markets that outweigh the gains in the former. Anticipating such net losses through diversion, inventor firms typically do not themselves try to overcome the second market failure through differential pricing, resist pressures to do so, and fight attempts to impose compulsory licensing upon them. As a result, differential pricing has not gained much of a foothold, and many poor patients who would be willing and able to purchase the drug at a price well above the marginal cost of production are excluded from this drug because they cannot afford the much higher monopoly price.[34]

Insofar as a government does succeed, against heavy pressure from pharmaceutical companies and often their governments, in exercising its right to issue compulsory licenses, any net losses due to diversion are simply forced upon the patent holders. But, were this to become more common, it would engender the first market failure of undersupply: pharmaceutical companies will tend to spend less on the quest for essential drugs when the uncertainty of success is compounded by the additional unpredictability of whether and to what extent they will be allowed to recoup their investments through undisturbed use of monopoly pricing powers.

Doubtful that the differential-pricing strategy can yield a plan for reform that would constitute a substantial improvement over the present regime, I assume that the *public-good strategy* is more likely to yield a reform plan that would avoid the main defects of the present monopoly-patent regime while preserving most of its important benefits. Let me sketch three components of such a reform plan.

First, the results of any successful effort to develop (research, test, and obtain regulatory approval for) a new essential drug are to be provided as a public good that all pharmaceutical companies may use free of charge. This reform would eliminate the second market failure (associated with monopoly pricing powers) by allowing competition to bring the prices of new essential drugs down close to their marginal cost of production. Implemented in only one or a few countries, this reform would engender problems like those attending differential-pricing solutions: cheaper drugs produced in countries where drug development is treated as a public good would seep back into countries adhering to the monopoly-patent regime, undermining research incentives in the latter. The reform should therefore be global in scope, just like the rules of the current TRIPs regime are.

Implemented in isolation, this first reform component would destroy incentives for pharmaceutical research. This effect is avoided by the second component, which is that, similar to the current regime, inventor firms should be entitled to take out a multiyear patent on any essential medicines they invent, but, during the life of the patent, should be rewarded, out of public funds, in proportion to the impact of their invention on the global disease burden. This reform component would reorient the incentives of such firms in highly desirable ways: any inventor firm would have incentives to sell its innovative treatments cheaply (often even below their marginal cost of production) in order to help get its drugs to even very poor people who need them. It would have incentives also to ensure that patients are fully instructed in the proper use of its drugs (dosage, compliance, etc.) so that, through wide and effective deployment, they have as great an impact on the global disease burden as possible.[35] Rather than ignore poor countries as unlucrative markets, inventor firms would moreover have incentives to work together toward improving the health systems of these countries to enhance the impact of their inventions there. Any inventor firm would have reason to encourage and support efforts by cheap generic producers to copy its drugs, as such copying would further increase the number of users and hence the invention's favorable impact on the global disease burden. In all these ways, the reform would align and harmonize the interests of inventor firms with those of patients and the generic drug producers— interests that currently are diametrically opposed.[36] The reform would also align the moral and prudential interests of the inventor firms who, under the present regime, are forced to choose between recouping their investments in the search for essential drugs and preventing avoidable suffering and deaths.

This second component of the envisioned public-good strategy has yet another tremendous advantage: under the current regime, inventor firms have incentives to try to develop a new medical treatment only if the expected value of the temporary monopoly pricing power they might gain, discounted by the probability of failure, is greater than the full development and patenting costs. They have no incentives, then, to address diseases mainly affecting the poor, for which treatments priced far above the marginal cost of production could be sold only in small quantities. As a result, very few treatments are developed for medical conditions that cause most of the premature deaths and suffering in the world today. Even if common talk of the 10/90 gap[37] is now an over-statement, the problem is certainly real: malaria, pneumonia, diarrhea, and tuberculosis, which together account for 21 percent of the global disease burden, receive 0.31 percent of all public and private funds devoted to health research.[38] And diseases confined to the tropics tend to be the most neglected: of the 1,393 new drugs approved between 1975 and 1999, only 13 were specifically indicated for tropical diseases, and 5 out of these 13 actually emerged from veterinary research and 2 had been commissioned by the military.[39] An additional 3 drugs were indicated for tuberculosis. The next five years brought 163 new drugs, of which 5 were for tropical diseases and none for tuberculosis. Tropical diseases and tuberculosis together account for 12 percent of the total disease burden.[40]

Rewarding pharmaceutical research in proportion to its impact on the global disease burden would attract inventor firms to medical conditions whose adverse effects on humankind can be reduced most cost-effectively. This reorientation would greatly mitigate the problem of neglected diseases that overwhelmingly affect the poor and would afford new profitable research opportunities for pharmaceutical companies.

One may worry that the second component of the reform would also *reduce* incentives to develop treatments for medical conditions that, though they add little to the global disease burden, affluent patients are willing to pay a lot to avoid. This worry can be addressed by limiting the application of the reform plan to *essential* drugs, that is, to medicines for diseases that destroy human lives. Drugs for other medical conditions, such as hair loss, acne, and impotence, for example, can remain under the existing regime with no loss in incentives or rewards.

Incorporating this distinction between essential and nonessential drugs into the reform plan raises the specter of political battles over how this distinction is to be defined and of legal battles over how some particular invention should be classified. These dangers could be averted by allowing inventor firms to classify their inventions as they wish and then designing the rewards in such a way that these firms will themselves choose to register under the reform rules any inventions that stand to make a real difference to the global disease burden. Such freedom of choice would also greatly facilitate a smooth and rapid phasing in of the new rules, as there would be no disappointment of the legitimate expectations of firms that have undertaken research for the sake of gaining a conventional patent. The reform plan should be *attractive* for pharmaceutical companies by winning them new lucrative opportunities for research into currently neglected diseases without significant losses in the lucrative research opportunities they now enjoy—and by restoring their moral stature as benefactors of humankind.

This second reform component requires a way of funding the planned incentives for developing new essential medicines, which might cost some $45 to 90 billion annually on a global scale. (A more precise estimate is impossible because the cost each year would depend on how successful innovative treatments would be in decimating the global disease burden.[41] The reform would cost billions of dollars only if and insofar as it would save millions of lives.) The third component of the reform plan is, then, to develop a fair, feasible, and politically realistic allocation of these costs, as well as compelling arguments in support of this allocation.

While the general approach as outlined may seem plausible enough, the great intellectual challenge is to specify it concretely in a way that shows it to be both feasible and politically realistic. Here one main task concerns the design of the planned incentives. This requires a suitable measure of the global disease burden and ways of assessing the contributions that various new medical treatments are making to its reduction. When several medicines are alternative treatments for the same disease, then the reward corresponding to their aggregate impact must be allocated among their respective inventors on the basis of each medicine's market share and effectiveness. More complex is the case (exemplified in the fight against HIV, tuberculosis, and malaria) of "drug cocktails" that combine several drugs often developed by different companies. Here the reform plan must formulate clear and transparent rules for distributing the reward, proportional to the impact of the drug cocktail, among the inventors of the drugs it contains. It is of crucial importance that all these rules be clear and transparent, lest they add to the inevitable risks and uncertainties that sometimes discourage inventor firms from important research efforts.

Another main task, associated with the third component, concerns the design of rules for allocating the cost of the incentives as well as the formulation of good arguments in favor of this allocation. Effective implementation of the reform requires that much of its cost be borne by the developed countries, which control some 79 percent of the global social product. This is feasible even if these countries, after retargeting existing subsidies to the pharmaceutical industry in accordance with the reformed rules, still had to shoulder around $70 billion in new expenditures. This amount, after all, is only 0.2 percent of the aggregate gross national incomes of the high-income countries, or $70 for each of their residents.[42]

This expense can be supported by prudential considerations. The taxpayers of the wealthier countries gain a substantial benefit for themselves in the form of lower drug prices and/or insurance premiums. Shifting costs, within affluent countries, from patients to taxpayers would benefit less-healthy citizens at the expense of healthier ones. But such a mild mitigation of the effects of luck is actually morally appealing—not least because even those fortunate persons who never or rarely need to avail themselves of recent medical advances still benefit from pharmaceutical research, which affords them the peace of mind derived from knowing that, should they ever become seriously ill, they would have access to cutting-edge medical knowledge and treatments.

A second prudential reason is that, by giving poor populations a free ride on the pharmaceutical research conducted for citizens in the affluent countries, we are building goodwill in the developing countries by demonstrating in a tangible way our concern for their horrendous public health problems. This argument has a moral twin: in light of the extent of avoidable mortality and morbidity in the developing world, the case for funding the reform is morally compelling even on the counterfactual assumption that we bear no responsibility whatever for the persistence of severe poverty abroad. Given that we do, it is far more compelling still.[43]

There are three further prudential reasons. The reform would create top-flight medical-research jobs in the developed countries. It would enable us to respond more effectively to public health emergencies and problems in the future by earning us more rapidly increasing medical knowledge combined with a stronger and more diversified arsenal of medical interventions. And better human health around the world would reduce the threat we face from invasive diseases. The outbreak of severe acute respiratory syndrome (SARS) and the recent avian flu scare illustrate the last two points: dangerous diseases can rapidly transit from poor-country settings into cities in the industrialized world; and the current neglect of the medical needs of poor populations leaves us unprepared to deal with such problems when we are suddenly confronted with them. Bringing enormous reductions in avoidable suffering and deaths worldwide, the reform would furthermore be vastly more cost-effective and also be vastly better received in the poor countries than similarly expensive humanitarian interventions we have undertaken in recent years[44] and the huge, unrepayable loans our governments and their international financial institutions tend to extend to (often corrupt and oppressive) rulers and elites in the developing countries. Last, but not least, there is the important moral and social benefit of working with others, nationally and internationally, toward overcoming the morally preeminent problem of our age, which is the horrendous, poverty-induced, and largely avoidable morbidity and mortality in the developing world.

It is obvious that the proposed reform must be thought through more carefully and then specified in much greater detail than I have done here. This is work to which the pharmaceutical companies, which are to operate under the revised rules, could greatly contribute. The companies are currently subjected to rules that make their perfectly legitimate interest to survive and make a profit collide head-on with their moral interest in alleviating the huge health burdens of the global poor.[45] Clearly, it would be much better for the pharmaceutical industry if its economic and moral interests were aligned. Companies have strong reasons, therefore, to contribute their expertise and their political support to the detailed formulation and political implementation of the proposed reform. They cannot do much, each on its own, toward alleviating the horrendous medical conditions among the global poor. But together, politically, they can do a great deal. In doing so, they would not merely help reduce dramatically the global disease burden, but they would also greatly reduce the moral dilemmas in which, as the Surfaxin trial shows, they and we all are now entangled.

Acknowledgments

This chapter has greatly benefited from the very helpful comments of Ezekiel Emanuel, Jennifer Hawkins, Andy Kuper, Fabienne Peter, Chandrima Roy, Pablo Stafforini, Ling Tong, and Leif Wenar.

Notes

1. The Surfaxin trial was most likely to have taken place in Bolivia—though Mexico, Peru, and Ecuador were also considered as candidate locations. In the text I mostly assume, for simplicity, that Bolivia was the preferred location. The trial was to have involved 650 infants, half of whom would have received Surfaxin and the other half sham air. The trial was canceled but, to avoid an overdose of subjunctives, I discuss it as if it had actually taken place.

2. In a press release on July 18, 2002, Discovery Laboratories Inc. reported the mortality rate for untreated RDS to range from 35 to 50 percent. My figure of 140 deaths reflects the rough midpoint of this range: 43 percent. This press release is no longer available on the Internet.

3. Because Surfaxin is supposed to be marketed in the developed world, where more expensive animal-derived surfactant treatments are already widely available, use of an active-control design would also be superior from a medical standpoint. In deciding whether to license Surfaxin, the FDA, for instance, should want to be assured not merely that the drug works better than no treatment at all, but that it can hold its own against existing treatments. An active-control design is better able than a placebo-control design to provide such assurance.

4. This case is a hypothetical and thus does not purport to reflect accurately the conditions of poor fishermen working in the Bay of Bengal.

5. Giving these two examples, I have assumed that typical code adherents, in the first case, care more about enhancing their own income than the government's and, in the second case, would rather avoid that stint in the military. In the second example, serving in the military is morally required and legally voluntary for unmarried young adults. For a detailed discussion of compliance and reward incentives and their relevance to the analysis of moral codes, see Thomas Pogge, *World Poverty and Human Rights*, 2nd ed. (Cambridge: Polity Press, 2007), chap. 3.

6. Such "loopholes" tend to benefit rich taxpayers the most because only they can generally recoup the cost of finding and exploiting such opportunities. Sometimes loopholes are due to mistakes by legislators or bureaucrats. But all too often they are designed deliberately to benefit specific constituents or political supporters.

7. For detailed statistics on income inequality, poverty rates, adult illiteracy, infant mortality, and the public health system of Bolivia, Mexico, Peru, and Ecuador, see United Nations Development Programme (UNDP), *Human*

Development Report 2006 (Houndsmills: Palgrave Macmillan, 2006), 336–37, 292–93, 324–25, 302–3, 309, 316–17.

8. A plausible rough indicator for the avoidability of severe poverty within a country is its decile inequality ratio, which expresses the collective income of the 10 percent of the population with the highest incomes as a multiple of the collective income of the 10 percent of the population with the lowest incomes. The Latin American countries D-Lab was considering for its Surfaxin trial have some of the highest decile inequality ratios in the world—168.1 for Bolivia, 44.9 for Ecuador, 40.5 for Peru, and 24.6 for Mexico—much above the corresponding ratios for any developed countries. Bangladesh's decile inequality ratio, by contrast, is 6.8—close to Germany's 6.9 and way below that of the United States (15.9). See UNDP, *Human Development Report 2006*, *supra* note 7, at 335-37.

9. "So-called," because many of these countries are not developing at all. Assessed at purchasing power parity (PPP), real per capita income in Peru, for instance, is *lower* today than it was in 1981, and real per capita income in Bolivia is lower than it was in 1977. See UNDP, *Human Development Report 2004*, 332–33.

10. See the next section, and Pogge, *supra* note 5, chap. 9.

11. This claim is more fully elaborated in other work. See Thomas Pogge, *supra* note 5; Pogge, "'Assisting' the Global Poor," in *The Ethics of Assistance: Morality and the Distant Needy*, ed. Deen K. Chatterjee (Cambridge: Cambridge University Press, 2004), 260–88, Pogge, "Reply to the Critics," *Ethics and International Affairs* 19 (2005): 55–84; and Pogge, "Severe Poverty as a Human Rights Violation," in *Freedom from Poverty as a Human Right: Who Owes What to the Very Poor?* ed. Thomas Pogge (Oxford: Oxford University Press, 2007), 11–54.

12. As stated in its Declaration of Helsinki, entitled "Ethical Principles for Medical Research Involving Human Subjects" (www.wma.net/e/policy/b3 .htm): "5. In medical research on human subjects, considerations related to the well-being of the human subject should take precedence over the interests of science and society. . . . 8. . . . Some research populations are vulnerable and need special protection. The particular needs of the economically and medically disadvantaged must be recognized. Special attention is also required for those who cannot give or refuse consent for themselves, for those who may be subject to giving consent under duress, for those who will not benefit personally from the research. . . . 19. Medical research is only justified if there is a reasonable likelihood that the populations in which the research is carried out stand to benefit from the results of the research. . . . 24. For a research subject who is

legally incompetent, physically or mentally incapable of giving consent or is a legally incompetent minor, the investigator must obtain informed consent from the legally authorized representative in accordance with applicable law. . . . 29. The benefits, risks, burdens and effectiveness of a new method should be tested against those of the best current prophylactic, diagnostic, and therapeutic methods. This does not exclude the use of placebo, or no treatment, in studies where no proven prophylactic, diagnostic or therapeutic method exists." (The World Medical Association [WMA] first adopted this declaration in 1964; the last-quoted paragraph 29 was added in 1996.)

13. See, for example, "The Ethics Industry," *Lancet* 350 (1997): 897; Marcia Angell, "The Ethics of Clinical Research in the Third World," *New England Journal of Medicine* 337 (1997): 847–49; Peter Lurie and Sidney Wolfe, "Unethical Trials of Interventions to Reduce Perinatal Transmission of Human Immunodeficiency Virus in Developing Countries," *New England Journal of Medicine* 337 (1997): 853–56; Joe A. Stephens et al., "The Body Hunters," six articles in the *Washington Post*, December 17–23, 2000; Florencia Luna, "Is 'Best Proven' a Useless Criterion?" *Bioethics* 15 (2001): 273–88; Paquita de Zulueta, "Randomized Placebo-Controlled Trials and HIV-Infected Pregnant Women in Developing Countries: Ethical Imperialism or Unethical Exploitation?" *Bioethics* 15 (2001): 289–311.

14. See, for example, David B. Resnick, "The Ethics of HIV Research in Developing Nations," *Bioethics* 12 (1998): 286–306; Robert Levine, "The Need to Revise the Declaration of Helsinki," *New England Journal of Medicine* 341 (1999): 531–34. For discussion, see also Carol Levine, "Placebos and HIV: Lessons Learned," *Hastings Center Report* 28, no. 6 (1998): 43–48; and Troyen A. Brennan, "Proposed Revisions to the Declaration of Helsinki: Will They Weaken the Ethical Principles Underlying Human Research?" *New England Journal of Medicine* 341 (1999): 527–31.

15. Results of these and subsequent Phase III trials (www.drugs.com/NDA/surfaxin_040615.htm) suggest that Surfaxin can be highly effective against RDS. See also Fernando Moya et al., "A Multicenter, Randomized, Masked, Comparison Trial of Lucinactant, Colfosceril Palmitate, and Beractant for the Prevention of Respiratory Distress Syndrome among Very Preterm Infants," *Pediatrics* 115 (2005): 1018–29; and Sunil Sinha et al., "A Multicenter, Randomized, Controlled Trial of Lucinactant versus Poractant Alfa among Very Premature Infants at High Risk for Respiratory Distress Syndrome," *Pediatrics* 115 (2005): 1030–38.

16. I am assuming that the Surfaxin trial is saving no lives in the United States, because participants would be receiving at least equally effective treat-

ment if the trial were canceled or conducted abroad. I am vague about the number of infants who would have survived had the trial been conducted in Bolivia because it depends on the trial's design. Conducting the trial in Bolivia with a placebo-control design would have saved about 140 infants; conducting the trial in Bolivia with an active-control design would have saved at least twice as many—perhaps more. The difference in effectiveness between Surfaxin and the alternative treatment that would be used in an active-control trial is less than the difference in effectiveness between Surfaxin and a placebo. Therefore, an active-control trial of Surfaxin may require more than 650 subjects in order to obtain statistically significant results.

17. The theoretical fourth option, *Placebo-Rich*, is clearly ruled out. It is illegal as well as unethical, if not murderous: it would involve deliberately withholding from 325 RDS infants in the Untied States the existing and lifesaving surfactant treatment that RDS infants in the United States ordinarily receive as a matter of course—giving these infants sham air instead.

18. On this concept, see especially David Gauthier, *Morals by Agreement* (Oxford: Oxford University Press, 1986), chap. 4.

19. The relevance of this difference is interestingly discussed by Jerry Cohen, who sums up the general point as follows: "An argument changes its aspect when its presenter is the person, or one of the people, whose choice, or choices, make one or more of the argument's premises true." See G. A. Cohen, "Incentives, Inequality, and Community," in *The Tanner Lectures on Human Values*, vol. 13, ed. Grethe Peterson (Salt Lake City: University of Utah Press, 1992), 263–329, at 276 and generally sections 3 and 4.

20. See Pogge, *supra* note 5, chap. 3, for a detailed presentation of this argument.

21. The World Bank reports that gross national income (GNI) per capita, PPP (current international $s), in the high-income OECD countries rose 53.5 percent in real terms over the 1990–2001 globalization period (devdata.world bank.org/dataonline). World Bank interactive software (iresearch.worldbank .org/PovcalNet/jsp/index.jsp) can be used to calculate how the poorer half of humankind have fared, in terms of their real (inflation/PPP adjusted) consumption expenditure during this same period. Here are the gains for various percentiles, labeled from the bottom up:

+20.4% for the 50th percentile (median)
+21.1% for the 40th percentile
+18.7% for the 30th percentile
+15.9% for the 20th percentile

+12.9% for the 10th percentile
+10.4% for the 5th percentile
+6.6% for the 3rd percentile
+1.0% for the 2nd percentile
−7.3% for the 1st (bottom) percentile

These data are consistent with Branko Milanovic, *Worlds Apart: Measuring International and Global Inequality* (Princeton, NJ: Princeton University Press, 2005), reporting that real incomes of the poorest 5 percent of world population declined 20 percent in the 1988–93 period and another 23 percent during 1993–98, while real global per capita income increased by 5.2 percent and 4.8 percent, respectively (*Id.* at 108). For the 1988–98 period he finds that the Gini measure of inequality among persons worldwide increased from 62.2 to 64.1, and the Theil from 72.7 to 78.9 (*Id.* at 112). For 1998, Milanovic reports a global decile inequality ratio of 71:1 assessed in PPPs and of 320:1 assessed at market exchange rates (*Id.* at 111–12). Such enormous income inequalities accumulate into even larger inequalities of wealth. A recent WIDER study estimates that in 2000 the wealth decile inequality ratio was over 700:1 assessed in PPPs and over 2800:1 assessed at market exchange rates (Davies et al., *The World Distribution of Household Wealth*. WIDER, December 5, 2006, www. wider.unu.edu, tables 11a and 10a). There is reason to believe that PPPs as calculated by the International Comparison Program tend to overstate the purchasing power that poor-country currencies have specifically in regard to basic necessities. See Sanjay Reddy and Thomas Pogge, "How *Not* to Count the Poor," in *Measuring Global Poverty*, ed. Sudhir Anand and Joseph Stiglitz (Oxford: Oxford University Press, forthcoming), available at www.socialanalysis.org.

22. World Bank, *World Development Report 2007* (New York: Oxford University Press, 2006), 289.

23. The World Bank's $2/day poverty line is defined in terms of monthly consumption expenditure with the same purchasing power as $65.48 had in the United States in 1993. Shaohua Chen and Martin Ravallion, "How Have the World's Poorest Fared since the Early 1980s?" *World Bank Research Observer* 19 (2004): 141–69, at 147. I have multiplied by 12 and adjusted for inflation (www.bls.gov/cpi/home.htm).

24. *Id.* at 152 and 158, dividing the poverty gap index by the headcount index.

25. UNDP, *Human Development Report 2006, supra* note 7, at 33 and 174.

26. See www.fic.nih.gov/about/summary.html.

27. UNDP, *Human Development Report 1998* (New York: Oxford University Press, 1998), 49.

28. See www.uis.unesco.org.

29. The UN International Labor Organization reports that "some 250 million children between the ages of 5 and 14 are working in developing countries—120 million full time, 130 million part time" (www.ilo.org/public/english/standards/ipec/simpoc/stats/4stt.htm). Of these, 170.5 million children are involved in hazardous work and 8.4 million in the "unconditionally worst" forms of child labor, which involve slavery, forced or bonded labor, forced recruitment for use in armed conflict, forced prostitution or pornography, or the production or trafficking of illegal drugs. See ILO, *A Future without Child Labour* (Geneva: ILO, 2002), 9, 11, 17–18, also available at www.ilo.org/public/english/standards/decl/publ/reports/report3.htm.

30. In 2002, there were about 57 million human deaths. The main causes highly correlated with poverty were (with death tolls in thousands): diarrhea (1,798) and malnutrition (485), perinatal (2,462) and maternal conditions (510), childhood diseases (1,124—mainly measles), tuberculosis (1,566), malaria (1,272), meningitis (173), hepatitis (157), tropical diseases (129), respiratory infections (3,963—mainly pneumonia), HIV/AIDS (2,777), and sexually transmitted diseases (180). See World Health Organisation, *The World Health Report 2004* (Geneva: WHO Publications, 2004), 120–25, also available at www.who.int/whr/2004.

31. Children under five account for about 60 percent, or 10.6 million, of the annual death toll from poverty-related causes. See United Nations Children's Fund, *The State of the World's Children 2005* (New York: UNICEF, 2005), inside front cover, also available at www.unicef.org/publications/ files/SOWC_ 2005_ (English).pdf. The overrepresentation of females is documented in UNDP, *Human Development Report 2003* (New York: Oxford University Press 2003), 310–30; in United Nations Research Institute for Social Development, *Gender Equality: Striving for Justice in an Unequal World* (Geneva: UNRISD/UN Publications, 2005), also available at www.unrisd.org; and in Social Watch, *Unkept Promises* (Montevideo: Instituto del Tercer Mundo, 2005), also available at www.mdgender.net/resources/monograph_detail.php?MonographID=38.

32. This point is controversial to some extent. It has been asserted that pharmaceutical companies wildly overstate their financial and intellectual contributions to drug development and that most basic research is funded by governments and universities, with pharmaceutical companies then allowed to reap the benefits by patenting the results. See Marcia Angell, *The Truth about the Drug Companies: How They Deceive Us and What to Do about It* (New York: Random House, 2004); Merrill Goozner, *The $800 Million Pill: The Truth behind the Cost of New Drugs* (Berkeley and Los Angeles: University of California Press, 2004); Consumer Project on Technology (www.cptech.org/ip/health/

econ/rndcosts.html); and UNDP, *Human Development Report 2001* New York: Oxford University Press 2001), chap. 5.

33. The basic idea stated in this section is more elaborately presented in Pogge, *supra* note 5, chap. 9.

34. Panos Kanavos et al., "The Economic Impact of Pharmaceutical Parallel Trade in European Union Member States: A Stakeholder Analysis," LSE Working Paper, 2002, www.lse.ac.uk/collections/LSEHealthAndSocialCare/pdf/Workingpapers/Paper.pdf.

35. The absence of such incentives under the present rules gravely undermines the effectiveness even of donated drugs delivered into poor regions. See UNDP, *supra* note 33, at 101.

36. This opposition was dramatically displayed when a coalition of thirty-one pharmaceutical companies went to court in South Africa to prevent their inventions from being reproduced by local generic producers and sold cheaply to desperate patients whose lives depended on such affordable access to these retroviral drugs. In April 2001, the attempted lawsuit collapsed under a barrage of worldwide public criticism. See David Barnard, "In the High Court of South Africa, Case No. 4138/98: The Global Politics of Access to Low-Cost AIDS Drugs in Poor Countries," *Kennedy Institute of Ethics Journal* 12 (2002): 159–74.

37. "Only 10 percent of global health research is devoted to conditions that account for 90 percent of the global disease burden." See Drugs for Neglected Diseases Working Group, *Fatal Imbalance: The Crisis in Research and Development for Drugs for Neglected Diseases* (Geneva: MSF, 2001), 10; and Global Forum for Health Research, *The 10/90 Report on Health Research 2003-2004* (Geneva: GFHR, 2004).

38. GFHR, *supra* note 37, at 122.

39. Patrice Trouiller et al., "Drugs for Neglected Diseases: A Failure of the Market and a Public Health Failure?" *Tropical Medicine and International Health* 6 (2001), 945–51; and Drugs for Neglected Diseases Working Group, *supra* note 37, at 10–11.

40. Pierre Chirac and Els Toreelle, "Global Framework on Essential Health R&D," *Lancet* 367 (2006): 1560–61, also available at www.cptech.org/ip/health/who/59wha/lancet05132006.pdf.

41. My rough estimate—meant to provide an orientation and thus to illustrate the order of magnitude and hence the degree of realism of the reform—derives from current corporate spending on pharmaceutical research, which is reported to be around $50 billion. Only part of this money is spent toward developing *essential* drugs. But the reformed rules would stimulate substantially greater spending on pharmaceutical research toward developing new essential drugs (especially for heretofore neglected diseases). Such outlays could sub-

stantially increase expenditures on pharmaceutical research. The rewards offered under the reformed rules must not merely match, but substantially exceed these outlays because pharmaceutical companies will brave the risks and uncertainties of an expensive and protracted research effort only if its expected return substantially exceeds its cost.

42. The high-income countries are reported to have had aggregate gross national income of $35,529 billion and an aggregate population of 1,011 million in 2005 (World Bank, *supra* note 22, at 289). The high-end cost estimate of $70 billion for the proposed reform is less than the $106.5 billion (2005) the affluent countries are currently spending on official development assistance (ODA). But the reform would prevent vastly more harm than current ODA, which, understandably, is mostly spent for the benefit of agents capable of reciprocation. A large part of ODA is allocated to support exporters at home or small affluent elites abroad, and only a fraction, approximately $7 billion (2004), goes for "basic social services" (mdgs.un.org/unsd/mdg). (USAID has recently toned down its disarming frankness by removing this passage from its Web site: "The principal beneficiary of America's foreign assistance programs has always been the United States. Close to 80 percent of the U.S. Agency for International Development's [USAID's] contracts and grants go directly to American firms. Foreign assistance programs have helped create major markets for agricultural goods, created new markets for American industrial exports and meant hundreds of thousands of jobs for Americans.") These priorities are evident also when one looks where ODA goes: India, with more poor people than any other country, receives ODA of $0.60 annually per citizen. The corresponding figures are $72.60 for Israel and Cyprus, $102.20 for Estonia, $108.20 for Barbados, $129.40 for the Seychelles, $145.10 for Bahrain (UNDP, *supra* note 7, at 344–46), whose gross national incomes per capita are eleven to twenty-six times that of India (World Bank, *supra* note 22, at 288–89 and 298).

43. The moral significance of our causal involvement in severe poverty abroad is extensively discussed in my works cited in note 11.

44. My estimate of what *all* affluent countries would need to contribute to implement the reform plan—$70 billion annually—is significantly less than what the United States alone is spending on its "humanitarian" intervention in Iraq.

45. See note 36.

5

Broadly Utilitarian Theories of Exploitation and Multinational Clinical Research

RICHARD J. ARNESON

Confronted by fine-grained deontological concepts such as exploitation, the consequentialist is a bull in a china shop. Here are many subtly different varieties of exquisite porcelain dishes, but the distinctions do not matter to the bull, and his hooves smash the plates indiscriminately. For many, this situation exhibits the deep flaws of consequentialism. I disagree, and want to defend the bull's perspective.

The Concept of Exploitation

In the pejorative and morally interesting sense, exploiting a person is using her to one's advantage in a way that is morally wrongful and that specifically wrongs her. In other words, the one who exploits takes advantage of another person unfairly. In this sense, to characterize a person's conduct as exploitive is to mark it either as prima facie wrong or perhaps as wrong all things considered.

This morally charged sense of the term contrasts with another purely descriptive sense, as when one speaks neutrally of traders exploiting market opportunities and athletes exploiting their particular skills by finding situations where these honed traits will give them a competitive advantage.

To call a transaction exploitive is to say that it is wrongful but not why. Exploitation is wrongful use, but which types of use are wrongful? Analysts distinguish the general concept of exploitation from specific conceptions of it.[1] The latter are specifications of what it is that qualifies a transaction as exploitive. Two historically prominent conceptions of exploitation in the realm of voluntary economic transactions are the neoclassical and Marxist theories.[2] The former holds that exploitation occurs when advantages are gained beyond what would occur in perfectly competitive markets where many buyers confront many sellers for each good and no agent can exercise any influence on the price at which transactions occur. The latter holds that any gaining of profit by a property owner when a worker is hired to work this property to produce a commodity for sale is exploitive. These competing conceptions are rival interpretations of the same concept.

The distinction between the concept of exploitation and various conceptions of it is not intended to suggest that anyone who uses the concept must explicitly or implicitly be invoking some conception of it. Ordinary accusations that this or that transaction is exploitive might be based on a gut feeling or hunch that whatever exploitation might turn out to be, this occurrence that one is calling exploitive will turn out to be an instance of the phenomenon.

Exploitation can occur in interactions that are coercively imposed on some participants. Slave masters exploit their slaves. However, the important cases focus on transactions in which all those who are involved voluntarily consent to be involved. Even with this restriction in place, finding a satisfactory conception of exploitation turns out to be searching for something that eludes our nets.

The Consequentialist Perspective on the Notion of Exploitation

Our ordinary commonsense notion of exploitation supposes that if two persons A and B are interacting with one another, whether their interaction is exploitive depends on what each does to the other and the effects of each person's action on the other and nothing else. In particular, effects on third parties have no bearing on the question, whether A is exploiting B or being exploited by B. But this assumption contained in the commonsense idea of exploitation immediately puts this idea in tension with act consequentialist morality.

Here *act consequentialism* is the doctrine that morally one ought always to choose an act among those available that induces an outcome that is no worse than the outcome that would have been induced by anything else one might instead have chosen. An action is morally right just in case it is one of those acts whose outcome is no worse than anything else the agent might have done instead, and morally wrong otherwise. The greater the shortfall between the value of the consequences of the act one chooses and the best one might have done, the "wronger" one's act is.

Whatever two persons A and B are doing to one another, any effects of what (say) A does to B might in principle be overridden by the effects of what A is doing to other people, so wonderful generosity to B might be morally wrong, and heaping evil on B might be morally right. If exploitation is wrongful use of persons, then perhaps the consequentialist should say that the use of persons is wrongful, and so exploitive, just in case the use would violate consequentialist principle.

The words we have just put in the mouth of the consequentialist might sound obviously wrong. The notion of exploitation might seem to belong in the armory of those who believe that some types of action are inherently wrongful and must not be done whatever the consequences. In this spirit a recent report of the National Bioethics Advisory Commission asserts, "The use of human beings as means to the ends of others without their knowledge and freely given permission constitutes exploitation and is therefore unethical."[3]

But consider instances in which one can prevent a grave wrong from occurring but only by acting against someone's moral right. Amartya Sen suggests this example. You can prevent a heinous rape, but only by taking my car without my consent and using it to drive to the scene where the crime is to unfold. One might say that if one identifies the morally best outcome with the outcome in which important human rights are fulfilled to a greater extent, the outcome in which the small wrong of car theft prevents the bigger wrong of rape is better than the outcome in which the car theft does not occur and the rape does. When you take my car, perhaps against my explicit well-informed protest and refusal to give consent, you use me as a means to your ends, but given the moral costs and benefits of various choices, you do not wrongfully use me, so what you do does not exploit me. The same would be true if in similar circumstances I were kept in the dark about what was happening to my car and so had no opportunity to give or refuse consent. In other words, the use of human beings as means to the ends of others without their knowledge and freely given permission does not per se constitute exploitation—at least not exploitation all things considered—and is not always unethical.[4]

Another instance of the same is justifiable paternalistic restriction of a person's liberty. If I am using cocaine freely and voluntarily to my detriment, it might be justifiable, by consequentialist calculation, for you to coerce me for my own good, against my will. Here you would be using me as a means to your altruistic and paternalistic ends, but so what? In this example, I submit that if such paternalism leads to the best outcome, it is not wrongful, hence not exploitive.[5]

However, there is no point in running full speed against the ordinary usage of terms by proposing that exploitation in the consequentialist understanding of it is use of a person that is wrongful in virtue of violating consequentialist principle. After all, an act that uses a person in a way that is overly generous to that person counts as exploitive on this conception if consequentialist principles would condemn the generosity as excessive.

The problem we are encountering is not unique to the problem of linking the concept of exploitation to a consequentialist conception of it. The problem arises whenever we try to link an ordinary concept of wrongful behavior to a consequentialist conception of it.

Just as not all homicides that are morally wrong to commit according to consequentialist principles are murders, not all uses of a person that are morally wrong according to consequentialism are instances of exploitation. Rather, exploitation is the use of a person that is wrong, and a wrong to the victim, the person who is so used. The act consequentialist has a strategy for reconciling her fundamental moral principle and commonsense moral rules. One distinguishes two levels of moral analysis, principles and rules.[6] Principles specify and order the reasons that fix, on each occasion of choice, what one morally ought to do. At the level of principle, the act consequentialist affirms act consequentialism and standards for assessing outcomes. Moral rules as I am going to conceive them are codes of conduct instituted in particular societies. The society is arranged so that its members are trained to accept the code. If the training of a member is successful, she will be disposed to conform her conduct to the code, to expect others to conform, to feel the negative emotions of shame and guilt if she fails to conform, and to punish failures by other members of society to conform their conduct to the code. Let us say a person who has been successfully trained to accept the extant moral code in her society feels obligated to uphold the code in the ways just specified.

Moral rules established in actual societies tend to be fairly simple to learn and to apply to situations to see what the rules tell one to do in various situations. Examples are "Don't tell lies!" and "Keep the promises you make!" Rules of this type tell us to conform our actions to the specified standard, and it is an empirical matter, given the standard, whether or not some action one might choose conforms to it or fails to conform. With the standard understood, one does not need to do any further evaluating in order to know what the standard requires by way of conduct. Moral rules can fail to include a determinate standard such as that contained in the rule against lying. An example is "Be fair in one's dealings with others!" In order to conform one's conduct to this rule in a given situation, one will have to do further evaluation, not laid down by the rule itself, in order to determine whether some action one might choose violates the rule or not. "Don't exploit people!" would be a moral rule of the second type. In order to apply the rule to determine what to do, one needs to do further evaluation beyond the evaluation that is as it were built into the rule.

The moral rules accepted in actual societies run the gamut from reasonably good to horrific, as they would be assessed by a consequentialist. The consequentialist rates moral codes by the consequences of their operation. The degree to which a consequentialist should endorse a prevailing moral code in a particular society will then vary depending on the shortfall between the moral value produced by the operation of the code and the best that might be done in the circumstances.

The act consequentialist position thus implies a certain alienation in thought and allegiance between the reflective member of society who embraces the act consequentialist morality and the moral code actually established in the society and serving, for better or worse, as its moral compass. The reflective member of society, trained in its moral code like anybody else, feels obligated by the code, but also subscribes to the act consequentialist principle, which may instruct the individual to tell a lie, for example, in circumstances when the prevailing code condemns telling the lie.

One should note that there is every reason to think this alienation and split would likely still obtain even if the society's moral code were adjusted to be optimal by consequentialist standards. The hypothetical optimal moral code—one that, if it were in place in given circumstances, could not be improved by the consequentialist standard of assessment—might well tell the individual to do X in circumstances in which the act consequentialist principle correctly applied yields the recommendation that the individual, to produce best consequences, should not do X. In that decision setting, what one morally ought to do conflicts with what one feels obligated to do. Why expect this would occur? Since people tend to be not well informed, not perfectly intelligent, and inclined to be partial to themselves and those near and dear to them in their choices of action, the code of rules the operation of which would yield best consequences in a given social setting will contain fairly simple rules that do not make excessive demands on the decision-making abilities and motivations of the people whose behavior they will guide. These rules will produce generally good consequences as they regulate people's conduct but will often counsel choice of conduct at variance with what act consequentialism would dictate.

What moral rules the act consequentialist should endorse depends not just on the structure of the act consequentialist principle but also on the correct substantive standards for assessing outcomes (states of affairs, consequences) as morally better or worse.

In a very wide array of likely circumstances, act consequentialism favors the inclusion of the rule "Don't exploit people" in the ideal moral code. This rule in effect says to be fair in your dealings with people without specifying what constitutes fairness. The rule is not contentless, however. It combines four broad vague norms:

(1) One should refrain from excessive profit-taking when one has a bargaining edge over others.

(2) One should practice reciprocity, in the sense of returning good for good, in dealing with others.

(3) One should seek the fully informed consent of those with whom one interacts (unless one is in specially understood competitive settings when caveat emptor is the reasonable rule or other familiar scenarios in which impinging on people without first eliciting their fully informed voluntary consent is intuitively fair).

(4) One should be generous to the weak and vulnerable. The rule should be broad and vague, to the point at which trying to render it any more or less precise would make it less productive of good consequences in practice.

But there will be settings in which the rule against exploitation (whether as part of some actual moral code or as part of the best consequentialist code we can devise for the circumstances) will tell an agent to do what the act consequentialist principle says she morally ought not to do. These will include cases like the violation-of-a-little-right-to-maximize-rights-fulfillment-overall cases discussed by Amartya Sen as mentioned earlier. So we should say that an action is all things considered exploitive (truly exploitive, one might say) just in case it both (a) violates the moral rule against exploitation that prevails in the society and (b) is not morally justified, that is, is not morally right to do according to act consequentialist principle (because the act would produce an outcome no worse than the outcome that would be reached by any other action one could do instead).

Exploitation and International Medical Research

Consider medical research studies, like the hepatitis A vaccine study, sponsored by agencies from wealthy industrialized nations, that takes place in impoverished countries in Africa, Asia, and Latin America. The research may be designed to test products that will be sold to treat diseases in the West but that are too expensive or otherwise unsuited for use in the country in which the research was conducted. The research is conducted on poor and illiterate people whose understanding of medical science, medical research procedures, and the import of the enterprise in which they are recruited to participate may be less than rudimentary. In this setting possibilities for exploitation are rife.

One recalls remarks by intellectuals that might appear to be unabashed apologies for exploitation. When Lawrence Summers was head of the World Bank, he was deemed to be responsible for a remark to the effect that it would be desirable for more of the world's toxic waste to be deposited in poor developing nations than is presently the case. This is of a piece with economist Thomas Schelling's observation that there ought to be higher-quality warning lights on airport runways that serve predominantly high-income communities than the warning lights on airport runways that serve predominantly low-income people.[7]

Here the economist's bark is worse than his bite. Neither Summers nor Schelling is asserting that the distribution of wealth and income between rich and poor nations and rich and poor people is just. It may or may not be. The remedy for that would be redistribution of wealth and income. The economists are saying that it is better if people are allowed to use whatever wealth and income they have to satisfy their preferences to a greater, rather than a lesser, extent. In general, with less money, one will tend to prefer less of many goods that one desires, and more of those goods, as one has more money to spend.[8] This applies to consumption of toxic wastes and transportation safety just as it does to consumption of housing, jewelry, and movies. Even if rich and poor people have exactly the same underlying preferences (so that with the same amount of money at their disposal they would purchase identical bundles of goods), being rich and poor, they will prefer to choose different levels of safety and exposure to toxicity. Rather than have the levels of safety and health risks preferred by wealthy people imposed on her, the rational poor person would likely prefer lower safety plus some money that she could spend on higher-valued items other than safety. The remarks rightly interpreted sound unobjectionable to me.[9]

Regarding medical research sponsored by developed countries in poor countries, we need to distinguish the question, what global distribution of wealth and income would be just, from the quite different question, given a global distribution that—whether just or unjust—is for the present not significantly going to alter what policies make sense within this context. If levels of wealth are different in the sponsoring country and the host country, it is ethically wrong to insist on the same level of safety for human subjects in the host country that would be appropriate if the research were conducted within the sponsoring country.

To see this, compare the choices of two rational persons, one with more money than the other, each with the same underlying preferences and values. Whatever level of risk from participation as a subject in a medical experiment the wealthier individual would insist on before willingly participating, the less wealthy person would reasonably prefer a lesser level of safety coupled with a cash payment that she could spend on goods she values more than the extra increment of safety the cash could have purchased. To make the point simply, suppose that people care for nothing except prolonging their expected life span, but that participation in a no-risk medical experiment would be less attractive to the less wealthy individual than participation in a similar medical experiment that imposes some risk on participants along with a cash payment that can be used to purchase extra bread that will do more to increase expected longevity than the forgone increment of medical safety. In this example I am supposing that making the experiment risk-free instead of somewhat risky would be costly for the research sponsor, who would accordingly be willing to pay for participation in the riskier procedure.

One point that immediately follows from this example is that if prohibition of cash payment to induce participation in medical experiments (that have genuine social benefits and are otherwise ethical) is ever appropriate, which I doubt, it is not appropriate for medical research on impoverished subjects.[10] The presumption should be that a fair and nonexploitive transaction may well include substantial payment to participants.

Another immediate implication of the rudimentary analysis to this point is that informed consent, though relevant, may have limited significance in determining what medical research studies in developing nations are morally acceptable.[11] The general point to keep in mind is that for any of us, requiring that others' actions not impinge on us in potentially harmful ways without our consent is a variously adequate safeguard of our basic interests, because we have limited cognitive abilities and decision-making disabilities that prevent us from making sensible and rational decisions. Being selfish, we may not accept impingements that risk harm to our own interests even when we should, all things considered. Being cognitively limited, we may fail to appreciate the likely causal consequences for other people and for ourselves of an impingement when we are deciding whether or not to consent to it.

In the context of a developing nation with widespread illiteracy and limited educational opportunities for many citizens, the general point concerning the limits of informed consent takes on greater salience. Even if information is conscientiously made available to potential research subjects, and strong efforts are made to overcome cultural barriers to understanding, the potential subjects may still have limited grasp of what is at stake and the decision regarding participation may be based on confusion. In these circumstances informed consent may not be attainable. Informed consent is, anyway, surely not sufficient for it to be the case that a particular medical study is morally fair to its research subjects. This claim is not controversial.[12]

More controversially, I would submit that informed consent may also not be necessary for the medical study to be fair to its research subjects. For example, suppose that villagers are very likely to reject participation in a particular experiment for superstitious reasons, if all relevant facts are laid on the table, and suppose further that a responsible village political leader is a good steward and caretaker of her constituents, whose interests and values she knows well. In this case consent by the village political chief might be an adequate safeguard for the villagers' legitimate concerns and a good substitute for informed consent. In no case should obtaining informed consent of potential subjects (or the closest approximation to genuine informed consent that one can gain in the circumstances) obviate the researchers' independent assessment that what they are doing balances costs and benefits for all affected policies in a way that is morally acceptable.

Ethical Problems in the Practice of Medical Clinical Trials in Developing Nations

A stylized description of a clinical medical study sponsored in a developed country and carried out in a less developed country suggests problem areas that, if not adequately addressed, may render the study ethically troubling.

The problem to be investigated may promise significant benefits to inhabitants of wealthier nations but scant benefit to inhabitants of poorer countries such as the one in which the study is conducted. For example, a study might be investigating the efficacy of an expensive malaria remedy, which cannot even if the research outcome is favorable be incorporated into public health programs in poorer countries. In that case the experimental subjects cannot expect to benefit from the clinical trial, even if all goes well and the treatment being tested is proven to be safe and effective, by way of having access to that very remedy, should they or those near and dear to them have need of it.

The study itself may involve significant risk of harm to participants. The harms in question might range from minimal discomfort experienced as research procedures are undergone, to deterioration in health caused by the experimental intervention, to relative deprivation when the experiment ends and temporary positive measures instituted as part of the experiment are withdrawn. The study may fail to gain fully informed consent from all research subjects used in its course.

A clinical trial will involve a group of subjects who receive the treatment that is being tested and another group of subjects who are the experimental control group. In some clinical trials a randomized sequence of treatments is applied to all research subjects, so that each patient is both control and experimental treatment recipient. In this case the control group is not a separate group of research subjects. In some clinical trials, all subjects receive an established effective treatment, and some are chosen randomly to receive an additional experimental treatment in addition, others to receive a placebo as an add-on. In another type of trial, some subjects receive the treatment whose efficacy is being tested, others a placebo. In another type, the control subjects receive an established treatment, others the experimental treatment. The study might aim to compare the effectiveness of the experimental treatment with another type of treatment or with no treatment at all.

If what is being investigated is a new treatment or a medical condition that has an established effective treatment, the new treatment might be tested in a study that uses a placebo as a control or the already established treatment. If the former, the issue arises whether the clinical study is inherently unethical, by violating the norm of nonmaleficence in medical care. The problem is that if one subjects a group of subjects to a placebo instead of giving them an already effective treatment, one is thereby giving them substandard care. To some degree the same issue arises if one gives some research subjects an experimental treatment, which might be ineffective or detrimental or medically efficacious, instead of giving them an already established effective treatment as normally would be done outside the research setting.

Suppose that an established effective treatment for some medical condition exists, but it is expensive, and not standardly available to people in the less developed country, where it is proposed to investigate another mode of treatment for the same condition. If a randomized clinical trial is conducted in which some subjects receive the experimental treatment and some subjects receive a placebo and no treatment for the condition, would this be unethical, a violation of the norm that doctors must do no harm? Some might argue that the subjects receiving a placebo in the clinical trial are no worse off than they would have been if the study had not been conducted, since they would not have been able to get the already established effective treatment for their medical condition in any event. But then one would be in the position of allowing research subjects in the less developed country to be treated in the course of the conduct of research in a way that would be forbidden to researchers conducting a comparable clinical trial in their own more developed country. This should give pause. One might distinguish in this context between suffering reversible harm as a placebo control and suffering death or irreversible harm. At least the latter should be forbidden, some would hold. But there have been actual instances of clinical medical trials sponsored by agencies from developed countries and taking place in less developed countries that imposed just these sorts of risks on placebo controls.

Surfaxin

The Surfaxin trial in Bolivia is a prime example of medical experimentation for profit carried out in poor countries in such a way as to appear to constitute wrongful exploitation of the research subjects.[13] Let us stipulate that the study as planned would have met the standard of informed consent on the part of all research participants. The Bolivian parents who would be enrolling their sick babies in the study would know that their child would have a 50 percent chance of being assigned the possibly effective surfactant Surfaxin and a 50 percent chance of receiving a medically inert placebo. Regarding the latter, worse case, the parents know their children would be receiving treatments for respiratory distress syndrome better than the parents could afford to provide in the absence of the opportunity to enroll in the clinical trial.

Even though each Bolivian parent choosing to participate in the study would have known that her child would reasonably expect to be better off being enrolled than not being enrolled, the proposal is marred by troubling features. A for-profit company is conducting medical research in a poor country with the aim of gaining approval for marketing for a drug that would be too expensive to be available and affordable for the indefinite future in the country in which research is conducted. Some children enrolled in the study, suffering from a life-threatening ailment, would receive a medically inert "treatment" when an effective treatment for the condition is available and standardly prescribed in nonpoor countries, and when for this reason such a study would not be allowed to be carried out in a nonpoor country.

The Consequentialist Response

Whether an action or policy is rightly considered exploitive all things considered and so morally wrong is controlled by consequentialist considerations. Whatever would produce the best outcome in the circumstances is right, not wrong. But what according to consequentialism renders a type of action exploitive in the narrow sense, prima facie unfair use and a wrong to the person used? How finely should we individuate types? Consequentialist considerations should fix the answers to these questions as well.

A type of interaction between persons should be considered unfair use and presumptively wrong (here we are to set aside wider effects on other persons) just in case the consequences of having a social practice of characterizing interaction in this way has better consequences than alternative practices. We should then distinguish the practice of guiding conduct by something in the neighborhood of this moral category in two cases: (1) as it ideally should be and (2) as it actually is in a given society. Both may be relevant in guiding agents' choices.

So, is it exploitation in the moral rule sense to recruit poor people in a poor country to participate in a clinical trial in which they receive a placebo treatment for an ailment when an established effective remedy is available in rich countries for that very ailment? I say, it depends on the answers to the questions posed. Insofar as we are in doubt as to the answers to these questions, we are in a state of perplexity and do not know whether the boundary marker of exploitation has been crossed. My claim is that the questions that the consequentualist poses are the questions to which we need answers if we want to know what morality requires and permits. My hunch is that involvement of people in clinical trials that employ a placebo arm does not mark an ethical bright line and can be permissible provided the overall balance of benefits and burdens between the interacting parties is reasonable. But a hunch is just a hunch.

We can say more. Note that for the act consequentialist, there is not simply one assessment to make of the proposed Surfaxin clinical trial. For the sake of clarity, the assessment should occur at several distinct levels of abstraction. The first-best level postulates that all agents involved in a specified decision problem are willing to do what would bring about the best outcome. Suppose we are considering the agents whose choices will together determine the policy of the firm contemplating international medical research (the officials and shareholders of the firm, roughly). Assuming their willingness to do what is best, I note that the work done by a company that produces health care products for sale mainly to well-off people in Western countries and distributes its profits to already well-off shareholders is undoubtedly not making the best possible use of its resources from the best outcome standpoint. Without entering into detailed analysis, I submit it is clear that the shareholders should agree to liquidate the company's assets and donate them to an organization that will use them effectively to promote long-term improvement in the well-being of poor people. Perhaps donating the money to Doctors without Borders or to a group that will provide small-scale entrepreneurial loans to poor people in some backward area of India or China or southern Africa would be an ideal use of the resources. This suggestion might be thought a recommendation in favor of massive charity, but consequentialism does not sharply distinguish justice and charity in the manner of conventional moral thinking. If readers of this chapter are thinking to themselves that this proposal is crazy, recall that we are not in the business of predicting what will happen but specifying what one ought to do if one is committed to best outcomes. And why be committed to less than best?

With respect to Bolivian children at risk for a life-threatening ailment for which an effective medical treatment already exists, if Discovery Labs is interacting with those children, and the question is what should Discovery Labs do, the naïve and I think morally reasonable answer is that all children at risk should be supplied effective treatment for free (provided there is no more cost-effective alternative use of the money that saves more lives and improves well-being by a greater uptick according to the best outcome standard). Discovery Labs should in effect become Discovery Global Poverty Relief Inc. Call this first-best level of analysis the Peter Singer approach.[14]

It should be noted that according to first-best act consequentialist analysis there is nothing special or unique about the strong obligation of Discovery Labs to aid the distant needy. You and I (assuming the reader of this chapter is affluent) are under the same obligation. For the same reason that it is morally wrong for Discovery Labs to carry on its normal business in its normal fashion, it is morally wrong for an affluent consumer to go to the movies or buy an expensive toy when she could instead put the money to better use by donating it to a worthy cause, a charity organization or protest movement or the like, that would use the money to improve the lives of people who are both very badly off and very capable of benefiting from an infusion of resources. This view offends conventional commonsense morality, but act consequentialists frankly present their doctrine as a criticism and revision of common sense. The issue is not whether it offends common sense but whether it strikes us as reasonable all things considered after careful reflection.

We can pose other questions at different levels of abstraction, assuming different levels of compliance with moral requirements. Here is one question: assume Discovery Labs is constrained by existing contract law and fiduciary obligations to shareholders to maintain the enterprise in its present form and carry on business in a way that earns a reasonable profit (not necessarily the most that any legal market behavior could obtain). The company is then going to test and (if the tests are successful) market a surfactant drug. The drug is to be marketed in the developed world but might be tested in a poor region—a backward area of Bolivia, as it happens. Given these background constraints, how might the company conduct a clinical trial as planned that would satisfy the best outcome standard?

Here act consequentialism yields recommendations very different from what a commonsense morality of constraints and options would recommend. Thomas Pogge develops the latter approach in his chapter in this volume. According to a morality of constraints and options, morality does not require an agent to do whatever would bring about the best outcome, and in many circumstances does not permit this mode of action. An agent has the moral option to live as she chooses provided she does not harm others in certain ways that count as wrongful, and is constrained not to do any of these harmful wrongful acts even when doing so would bring about the best overall outcome. (The view can be qualified by permitting the overriding of moral constraints if the consequences of not overriding them would be extremely bad.) So on this view, the crucial question is whether Discovery Labs would violate any moral constraints in carrying out its proposed Surfaxin clinical trial. The issue is whether harm is done to those affected by its actions, and if so, whether the harm done is wrongful in context.

According to Pogge, whether harm is done is assessed against the baseline of alternative feasible actions that would have left the person better off. (If you come upon an accident victim in a remote location and take the victim to a hospital, you are not permitted to kick the injured person in the shins just for the fun of it on the way to the hospital even though the person is overall better off taken to the hospital and kicked than left untreated. For there is a pertinent alternative, in which you rescue but refrain from kicking.) Interacting with a person triggers a high standard of conduct. So even though there may be some duty to aid distant needy strangers, it does not require Discovery Labs in particular to do anything special for Bolivian children. But given that the firm interacts with these children, acts upon them with a view to its profit, the standards of moral requirement are raised. Given the alternative of conducting a clinical trial in which all those involved in the study receive an established surfactant treatment (an active-controlled trial [ACT]), a placebo-controlled trial (PCT) looks morally objectionable. One-half of the children in the PCT will receive only a treatment with no healing physical effect (air rather than surfactant medicine squirted into their lungs). These children are harmed, made worse off against the baseline of how they would fare with the treatment they would receive under an ACT. So they are wrongly treated, according to the commonsense morality of constraints and options as interpreted by Pogge. He then wrestles with the puzzle that if the Discovery Labs does nothing at all to the Bolivian children, does no study there at all but instead carries out an ACT in a developed country (where costs of such research are less), no wrong is done—even though many of the children who would have been aided by the clinical trial will instead die. But if the Discovery Labs carries out a study in Bolivia—does something to Bolivian children— then it is clearly harmful to some of the children and morally wrong to carry out a PCT when at perhaps greater cost and difficulty for the company an ACT could achieve its research and marketing goal without inflicting harm on one-half of the children enrolled in the study. So if the company is denied permission to carry out a PCT in Bolivia, it then carries out its next-best alternative, an ACT in a developed country. Commonsense morality then seems to demand forbidding the PCT study carried out on Bolivian children even though the effect of the prohibition is to induce the firm to act in a morally permissible way that is worse for the Bolivian children and worse overall for the affected people than the outcome that would have occurred had the PCT trial been permitted.

The consequentialist finds no puzzle here. She can consistently say that it is morally wrong for Discovery Labs to carry out a PCT rather than use its resources in the morally first-best way, and also say that if the controlling officers of the firm like most people are not going to do that, and if forbidding them to carry out the PCT either by law or social norm) would lead to worse consequences than allowing them to carry it out, the firm ought to be allowed to carry out the PCT study. She can also say that if international regulation that requires firms engaged in international medical research to share their profits with people in poor countries would lead to better consequences than no regulation or less stringent regulation, the share-the-wealth regulation should be established and implemented. Different questions, different answers.

It is not clear to me why according to Pogge's version of common-sense morality declining to offer surfactant treatment to at-risk children who would not have had the treatment in any event counts as harming them, but let that pass. The point to note is how what matters crucially for the commonsense moralist is virtually a "don't care" for the act consequentialist. The crucial issue for the commonsense moralist is what one does to the specific persons one causally affects by one's actions and whether this is harmful or unfair to those particular persons. For the act consequentialist, the issue is always overall benefits and losses, compared with alternatives, that accrue to everybody and anybody who might have been affected by any act the agent might choose. ACT versus PCT is a minor factor in this calculation and one that can always be overridden by other factors in the situation. For example, for any ACT Surfaxin clinical trial in Bolivia that commonsense morality à la Pogge approves, the act consequentialist will find morally preferable an alternative company decision that combines a PCT (and failure to offer any effective treatment to children at grave risk who fall in the placebo control group) with more than offsetting aid to other parties—for example, aid in the form of malaria preventives provided for other people in the region. Why should we make a fetish of what we do or do not do to the particular people our actions causally affect, rather than take a wider view and look for the best feasible outcome in the circumstances in which we act?

When we consider whether a practice is exploitive, we often are implicitly approaching the topic at a level of abstraction different from the level of individual choice of particular actions. We might be considering a type of act, or set of acts that fall in a common classification, and considering what policy we should adopt with respect to the class of acts. This is the perspective of a regulator. Considering a class of acts, should the class be condemned? Should it be forbidden by law or international treaty carrying the force of law, if that can be arranged? Should there be a social norm against the practice, if legal prohibition would be counterproductive or for some other reason inadvisable? Conduct that violates no law but violates a social norm will be subject to informal sanction, as occurs when people seeing the norm-violating conduct shun the perpetrator or verbally abuse him or the like.

A broad consequentialist perspective considers the consequences that would flow from legally prohibiting, condemning by social norm, or simply permitting a type of conduct. The act consequentialist insists on a clarification in this regard. For an individual, who might be an official in a position to promulgate an authoritative rule that others will follow, a legislator who has to vote for or against a specific legal prohibition or regulation of the type of act in question, a protester who might join with others to pressure legislators and officials, or simply an individual whose conduct falls under the established rules and who must decide whether to comply with the established rule or not, the question can be asked, what morally ought one to do on this particular occasion of choice? For the act consequentialist, this is another choice to be governed by the act consequentialist standard. One ought morally to choose and carry out an act whose outcome would be no worse than the outcome of any other act one could choose instead.

With this clarification in place, we see that the question, what practice would it produce best consequences to implement, is a different question from the decision problem that an individual official, legislator, social planner, and so on faces. The practice that would produce best consequences if put into place perhaps will not be put in place in one's actual circumstances, whatever one does. What one should do in that scenario is not act as if one could single-handedly produce the best practice but rather act to produce the best outcome in one's actual circumstances, warts and all.

According to consequentialism, correct policy concerning these problematic clinical trials in poor countries depends on a morally sensitive cost-benefit calculation—or, more accurately, on a series of such cost-benefit calculations, carried out at different levels of abstraction from the circumstances of the agent deciding what to do. Consider the issue as it would appear to a social planner setting regulations to govern these proceedings. One ought to set the rules so that one's rule-setting act produces best consequences. One will favor legal prohibition of a practice, however disreputable it appears, only if doing so would produce best consequences in the long term.

This response might seem inherently soft on exploitation. For the consequentialist, no act, even if it is inherently evil, is morally wrong all things considered simply in virtue of its intrinsic nature. The all-things-considered assessment depends on the consequences. This feature of consequentialism attracts criticism from the deontologist, who holds that there are some moral rules that agents should obey even if the consequences of obedience are less than ideal.

From a deontological perspective, consequentialism can appear too demanding in its requirements on individuals as well as too lax. The consequentialist will favor legal prohibition of a practice, however reputable and fair it seems, if doing so would produce best consequences in the long run.

The general consequentialist response to deontological conceptions assumes one of two forms. Some deontological conceptions can reasonably be regarded as means useful for promoting consequentialist goals. The consequentialist embraces deontology to the extent it is instrumentally justified in this way. Faced with rival conceptions of a deontological norm, the consequentialist favors the one that is the best means to promoting consequentialist goals. The alternative consequentialist response to deontological conceptions is that to the extent that they stand alone and claim legitimate authority independently of whether they promote or hinder consequentialist goals, the consequentialist is committed to denying their claim to legitimate authority. We should not accept this position without first investigating thoroughly the nonconsequentialist rival views.

Consequences, Well-Being, and Priority

Act consequentialism (one morally ought always to do an act that leads to an outcome no worse than the outcome that would have been brought about by any other act one might instead have chosen), though controversial, is thin in content. The doctrine becomes thicker, more substantive, with the addition of a standard for assessing outcomes, states of affairs. For the purposes of this chapter, I shall stipulate a broadly utilitarian and prioritarian standard of assessing.[15] A broadly utilitarian standard holds that nothing matters except utility (well-being or the quality of life) of individual persons and the distribution of utility. Utility here is understood as objective: whether something one gets is valuable for its own sake, and how valuable it is, are not determined by one's subjective opinion or attitude on these questions.[16] An individual's life goes better for her (her utility increases), to the extent that she gains goods that are genuinely worthwhile, including friendship, love, and family ties, systematic knowledge and understanding, scientific and cultural achievement, athletic performance, meaningful work, and pleasure. A prioritarian utilitarian holds that the moral value of gaining a benefit (avoiding a loss) for a person is greater, the greater the utility gain it brings, and greater, the lower the person's lifetime utility absent this benefit, and that one should act so as to maximize moral value so construed.[17]

Exploitation, Again

Exploitation is interaction that is stained by wrong. If there is no interaction, there is no exploitation. If a stranded motorist is languishing with a flat tire on his car on a lonely stretch of highway, if I insist on striking a deal that gouges him before I will help fix his tire, I am arguably exploiting him. If I drive by seeing his plight but not bothering to stop to bargain or help, I am not interacting with him at all, not profiting in any way from his plight, hence certainly not exploiting him. Evidently there are worse things than being exploited.

If we imagine ourselves charged with the task of framing social norms for such occasions, we note that the consequentialist must confront a difficult and uncertain trade-off. If people driving by the stranded motorist will stop, then it is better that they offer help without taking advantage of the situation. Perhaps it is better if they do the Good Samaritan deed without any personal profit. But social norms that chip away at profit taking by the person playing the Good Samaritan role raise the cost of stopping and helping and will induce some people not to play the Good Samaritan role at all. The more demanding the role as shaped by social norms, beyond some point, the smaller the number of people who will rise to fill the role. This problem occurs even if we have the option of decreeing that it is obligatory to stop and provide charitable aid. Whatever the social norms stipulate to be obligatory, some people will not be obliged. In principle there will be an optimal trade-off between insisting that those who provide emergency aid to the desperate will not take excessive profit and inducing those who might provide emergency aid but only if there is something in it for them to provide it.

Priority and Exploitation

It might seem that prioritarianism must take a ham-fisted approach to the issue of exploitation. According to the prioritarian, if Rich is gouging Poor, this is bad, other things being equal. But if everything in the situation is the same except that Poor is gouging Rich, this is good, other things being equal. So according to the prioritarian, exploitation is good or bad depending on whether the person doing the exploiting is badly off or well-off. This is tantamount to saying that for the prioritarian, exploitation in and of itself just does not matter, does not register as a significant moral category.[18]

Another discontinuity between priority and ordinary thought is that according to priority the determination of what it is on balance right to do gives no special priority to the quality of interaction between the agent and the specific persons with whom she interacts. The interests of all who would be affected by anything one might do count the same. Thus if Rich, rather than rescue Poor for free, can instead gouge Poor and transfer the gains to Poorer, then that is what she should do, provided the gains do not shrink too much in the course of transfer. (For every proposal that might be made whereby elite private universities pay their unskilled clerical and janitorial workers a decent living wage, a proposal that is superior according to priority can be constructed: let Harvard, Yale, Princeton, et al. pay just the competitive wage rate to their unskilled workers and transfer the difference [assuming it is positive] between the competitive wage and the decent wage to the truly disadvantaged in developing countries.)

I am not shy about defending the Robin Hood quality of prioritarian morality. It is unquestionably better if Robin Hood steals from the rich and gives to the poor rather than the reverse. But of course this point does not settle the issue, what verdict Robin Hood practices should get in the court of prioritarian justice. For this we need a cost-benefit analysis. We need to look at the effects of Robin Hood banditry on the incentives of Rich and Poor to labor productively and to participate in schemes of cooperation that are mutually beneficial. The question is what are the real effects of social banditry on the priority-weighted total of human well-being in the long run. The fact, if it is a fact, that a forced transfer of wealth from Rich to Poor has the immediate effect of taking resources from where they would be deployed to satisfy less important human needs to where they would be deployed to satisfy more urgent and probably greater human needs does not settle the issue.

The perception that others are trustworthy in the sense that they are likely to reciprocate benefits received is a significant influence on people's willingness to cooperate with others especially in ways that involve acceptance of costs that benefit others now in the hope that later those whom one has helped will be willing to accept costs when doing so efficiently secures payback to the initial helper.

That this fragile web of social trust is important in the dealings between advantaged and disadvantaged persons is the theme of the fable Androcles and the Lion. According to the story Androcles the mouse chances upon a lion writhing in pain. The lion has a big thorn embedded in his paw. Androcles responds sympathetically. Upon receiving the assurance that he can approach the lion without being eaten, Androcles skillfully removes the thorn from the lion's paw. The lion, king of the forest, offers payment, and has ample resources to pay, but Androcles declines any compensation, perhaps believing that virtue should be its own reward. Months later, Androcles and his family find themselves sorely menaced by a predatory lynx, but the lion happens to be walking by and sizes up the situation. Recalling Androcles' act of friendship, the lion chases away the lynx and saves the lives of Androcles and his extended family. I believe the story ends with the lion eating dinner with Androcles and his family in their house and toasting their friendship.

The story makes several points that are relevant to the prioritarian analysis of exploitation and reciprocity. At least, this is so if you believe that the mouse in the story is badly off in lifetime well-being prospects and definitely worse off in this regard than the lion king. One lesson is that in the end Androcles is better off being sympathetic and acting sympathetically than he would have been had he worked to extract every drop of gain that could be secured when he had a temporary bargaining advantage over the lion. This result depends of course on the mouse's sympathy being bounded by common sense; an altruistic devotion to the welfare of others come what may would lead Androcles to sacrifice his life if need be to relieve the lion's slightly irritating itch. A second point is that the disposition to reciprocity at least in the world of the story is evidently triggered not just by the objective terms of trade faced in social transactions but by the perception that the individual one is dealing with is sympathetically motivated and is willing to incur costs in order to benefit oneself.

The extent to which the Robin Hood character of prioritarian ethics is inhibited by considerations of incentives is difficult to determine. Reciprocity itself requires terms of trade. One might imagine social norms that condemn exploitive taking of advantage but that interpret unfair taking of advantage according to a sliding scale. This sliding scale specifies that more sacrifice is expected of those who are initially better off prior to the transaction under review, and less sacrifice and more taking advantage is expected and tolerated on the part of those who go into the transaction with low lifetime expectation of well-being. At the limit, reciprocity norms might stretch so far that the norm to refrain from exploitation yields recommendations in particular cases that are for all practical purposes the same as the norm, do whatever maximizes priority-weighted well-being.

Priority versus the Prohibition against Extracting Advantage for Oneself from the Needs of Others

Further light on prioritarian consequentialism is shed by comparing this doctrine to two rival perspectives on exploitation. One holds it to be morally illegitimate to extract any advantage from the vulnerability of others; another identifies exploitation with the taking of advantage that exceeds what one could gain if the transaction in question occurred in a perfectly competitive market. The first view is the subject of this section.

When a transaction is fully voluntary on both sides, what renders the terms of trade unfairly disproportionate, hence exploitive? A stringent partial response would have it that when one party to the transaction is vulnerable, no extraction of advantage from the vulnerability of another is morally acceptable. Allen Wood makes this proposal and ties it to a Kantian norm of respect for persons: "Proper respect for others is violated when we treat their vulnerabilities as opportunities to advance our own interests or projects. It is degrading to have your weaknesses taken advantage of, and dishonorable to use the weaknesses of others for your ends."[19] This position is coherent, but unacceptable, I submit. Call it No-Gain-from-Vulnerability.

Applied to the international medical research issue, No-Gain-from-Vulnerability yields the result that if research subjects in the less developed country are vulnerable, then if any clinical trials occur, no profit or advantage should be extracted. All profit should redound to the vulnerable. This result is close to the first-best prioritarian answer to the question, what is morally best to do (given likely empirical assumptions about the case that I will not try to specify). The shareholders of the pharmaceutical firm that proposes to do research in a less developed country should sell their shares and donate their wealth to the world's truly disadvantaged.

But if we switch from the question, what is best to do, to the question, what rules and norms does it make sense to attempt to establish and enforce, given present actual circumstances, the answer to this second-best question diverges from the austere utopian otherworldliness No-Gain-from-Vulnerability counsels.

Return to the broader issue: Should wrongful exploitation be identified with any taking of advantage from other people's vulnerability?

One reason to reject No-Gain-from-Vulnerability is that sometimes the vulnerable are better off, not worse off persons. In this situation, other things being equal, priority favors transfers from better off to worse off, so long as weighted utility is thereby increased. Even if one rejected maximal extraction of advantage from those who are in a weak bargaining position, insistence on no extraction at all is extreme. If a snowstorm renders Rich in need of a cleared driveway, in principle it is not wrong for Poor to charge some modest fee for the job. (However, in this connection one should recall the complicating lessons of the Androcles story.)

Another type of case to consider involves hard bargaining to extract maximum advantage from a vulnerable person when it is the case that the advantages extracted will be used for a good cause. Priority characterizes good causes as those that advance weighted utility to a greater degree than could otherwise be done. Other things being equal, it would be better to elicit the fully voluntary cooperation of those whom one involves as means to the advancement of one's worthy projects, but things are not always equal. Whether Smith wrongfully exploits Jones in a transaction in which Jones is vulnerable and Smith gouges Jones, using her bargaining advantage to extract maximal advantage, depends on the larger context. In particular, the question to be considered is who benefits and loses from the transaction. Wrongful exploitation all things considered for the prioritarian is a matter that is determined holistically. Gains and losses to one can always in principle be counterbalanced and outweighed by gains and losses to others. Priority rejects No-Gain-from-Vulnerability when the immediate gainer from the transaction passes on the advantages wrested from the vulnerable transaction partner to others who are among the worse off or otherwise placed so that weighted utility is maximized thereby.

Vulnerability can be turned to modest advantage. Refraining from gouging the vulnerable person can be virtuous and is compatible with gaining from the situation. The utility company has me at its mercy, as I face a cold winter and the utility company is the monopoly supplier of power in the region. Suppose the company eschews gouging me by charging me a high price and instead charges a modest price for services rendered that nonetheless brings a profit to the company.

Insistence on No-Gain-from-Vulnerability would leave both parties to a potential transaction worse off in many situations when in fact each party is free to walk away from the negotiation and avoid dealing on any terms.

Even in the ideal prioritarian society in which institutions and practices and social norms are perfectly regulated to achieve prioritarian goals, there will still be advantage taken from vulnerability that happens to arise. (Some vulnerabilities and weaknesses will be turned to profit.) If the person used in this transaction were to complain, the reply would be that given that society is perfectly regulated by prioritarian norms, any further attempt to alter practices and norms to advantage the weaker party to prevent advantage-taking at his expense would result in some other people losing, such that moral value overall would be lessened, not increased.

Against this last point it might be urged that in the ideal world regulated by prioritarian principle, there would have been redistribution of power and resources such that no one is liable to be (seriously) vulnerable and as a result no advantage taking from vulnerability will occur.

But although the world in which no advantage taking is possible might be ideal from some ethical standpoints, it is decidedly not ideal according to the prioritarian outlook.

The world in which resources and power are equally distributed, or distributed to prevent all personal vulnerability, may well be undesirable because power is a scarce resource and like any other resource it should be carefully placed and used so that it yields a maximum of moral value in the form of good consequences. In many circumstances, including empirically likely circumstances, the ideal prioritarian distribution of power and resources would be unequal.[20] If I am mean-spirited and vindictive and my wife is not, the scenario in which she commands the lion's share of the power to determine what we together shall do will predictably generate morally better outcomes than the alternative scenario in which neither of us has any bargaining leverage over the other. Even when agents are identically motivated and none is more morally minded than any other, one agent's having power over the rest may give each agent the right incentive to act in ways that will yield a morally better outcome than any equal power-sharing arrangement would reach.

Exploitation as Gaining Profit above the Baseline of Competitive Market Pricing

Consider next a very different proposal, formulated by the economist A. C. Pigou early in the twentieth century.[21] On this view, exploitation is unfair dealing that is possible in the absence of a perfectly competitive market in which many buyers confront many sellers for each good and no one can influence the prices at which any goods are sold. When perfect competition obtains, prices are fair, not exploitative. When conditions of perfect competition do not obtain, the fair or nonexploitative price mimics the price that would obtain if the market for this and all other goods were competitive.

Here we should distinguish justice in background conditions and justice in transactions. It may be unfair or unjust that an individual commands very few resources and faces a bleak array of options from which to choose in a competitive market. But we should distinguish background injustice from unfair taking of advantage.

Alan Wertheimer articulates this line of thought with exemplary clarity. He flirts with the proposal under review, though so far as I can see does not definitely commit himself to embracing it. He writes, "We may need to distinguish between the claim that the results of a bargain between A and B are unjust and the claim that A acted unjustly toward B. We need to distinguish between the claim that A takes unfair advantage of B and the claim that A takes advantage of an unfairness to B."[22] The suggestion is that only the former is properly speaking exploitation.

Why is perfect competition normatively attractive? A perfectly competitive market has the desirable property of inducing outcomes that are efficient in the economist's sense—Pareto optimal. Efficiency in this sense is a component of fairness, but merely one component, not the entirety of fairness. To my mind one cannot find any deeper sense of fairness in the perfect competition ideal.

Wertheimer notes, quite correctly, that when a market is perfectly competitive no one is able to take "special unfair advantage of particular defects in the other party's decision-making capacity or special vulnerabilities in the other party's situation."[23] Wertheimer adds that when a thin market situation prevails, so particular defects and vulnerabilities can be used to advantage by other parties, the hypothetical market outcome may still define the baseline that fixes what is unfair advantage taking.

The temptation to identify transactions under conditions of perfect competition with transactions that cannot be exploitive should be resisted. The temptation arises because when a market is perfectly competitive, by definition there are many buyers and sellers and perfect information, and no agent can influence the price at which transactions occur. All buyers and sellers are price-takers. But since ought implies can, one might suppose that it follows that when a market is perfectly competitive we cannot say a given transaction ought to have occurred at some other price, so the charge that the transaction is unfair cannot stick.

But in fact this does not follow at all. On a standard model of perfect competition, firms are assumed to aim to maximize profits and individuals aim to maximize their utility from their own consumption and leisure. Given this stipulation, all must take prices as given. But there need be nothing that constrains individuals to have the motives that make the market perfectly competitive. Individuals could choose to act from other motives, and perhaps fairness demands that they do so.

Suppose a perfectly competitive market for doctors' services obtains in some locale. This situation does not prevent Dr. Ann from deciding to work at a medical clinic that serves poor people and pays a below-market price for her services. Of course, if Dr. Ann does not seek to maximize her own utility from consumption and leisure, and the shareholders of the medical clinic serving poor people do not seek maximal profits from their investment, the market is then no longer perfectly competitive. But nothing forces people to have the motives that are stipulated to obtain in models of perfect competition. Moreover, maybe people ought to act from other motives and it would be unfair if they did not do so.

The same holds for the thin market situation in which medical research agencies bargain with potential research subjects in developing nations to determine the terms on which a particular international clinical trial will be conducted. Nothing picks out the terms that would obtain if this market were perfectly competitive as inherently fair and non-exploitive terms. Perhaps the managers of business firms conducting clinical trials abroad ought to accept pay cuts so that their firms can do business in impoverished nations on terms more favorable to their inhabitants than the terms perfect competition would induce. Perhaps the stockholders in such firms have similar responsibilities, and also the medical personnel working in such firms. Or perhaps laws or social norms should press people to give up benefits they would have if the transactions in which they engage had occurred under conditions of perfect competition. According to priority, this will very likely be so.

Conclusion

The wrongful exploiter profits by interacting unfairly with another. So it is said. In response, the consequentialist urges that a norm against exploitation is suitable only as a rough-and-ready guide to decision making, not for inclusion in the set of fundamental moral principles. The norm against exploitation forbids unfair dealing, but so far as I can see, no plausible substantive conception of unfairness that gives determinate content to this norm is in the offing. To this extent there is a hole in the center of the doughnut of any "no exploitation" moral rule. In addition, the norm against exploitation presents itself as transaction-specific. Whether or not my dealings with a person are exploitive depends on the costs and benefits that this person gets from the interaction with me and on what I get from her and nothing else. In contrast, a consequentialist morality is inherently holistic: whether what I do to Smith is right or wrong depends on the total impact of what I do to everybody compared to the total impact on everybody of all of the other things I might have done instead. The impact on Smith, the person I am interacting with, is always just one chip in this larger mosaic. But once this point is stated explicitly, it surely becomes obvious that we should be concerned with the entire pattern, not just the one chip in the mosaic or squiggle in the carpet.

In assessing types of interactions such as medical research conducted in developing countries by agents from more affluent countries, the consequentialist of well-being tells us to choose actions and policies that maximize the well-being of individual persons over the long run, and the prioritarian adds that we should maximize a function of well-being that gives significant extra weight to securing gains for those whose lives would otherwise go badly. If present institutional arrangements perform badly by this standard, we should do the best we can within the existing frameworks while looking for chances to improve them. We should unabashedly seek Robin Hood justice while taking care not to give people perverse incentives that will induce behavior that is counterproductive. For what it is worth, my hunch is that the upshot for international clinical research is that we should seek to put in place regimes of regulation that will alter the terms of trade in favor of poor people in poor countries without tilting so far that the losses stemming from reduction in mutually beneficial cooperation due to the regulation outweigh the gains arising to people from the altered terms of trade. In other words, do not allow exploitation unless the allowing is cost-effective according to the morally appropriate measure of costs and benefits.

Notes

1. An extremely useful overview of the concept of exploitation is in Alan Wertheimer, *Exploitation* (Princeton, NJ: Princeton University Press, 1996). For a helpful application of Wertheimer's analysis to issues concerning the

ethics of international medical research, see the participants in the 2001 Conference on Ethical Aspects of Research in Developing Countries, "Moral Standards for Research in Developing Countries: From 'Reasonable Availability' to 'Fair Benefits,'" *Hastings Center Report* 34, no. 3 (2004): 17–27.

2. On the neoclassical account, see the text of this chapter under the heading, "Exploitation as Gaining Profit above the Baseline of Competitive Market Pricing." On the Marxist account, see John E. Roemer, *Analytical Foundations of Marxian Economic Theory* (New York: Cambridge University Press, 1981); also Roemer, *A General Theory of Exploitation and Class* (Cambridge, MA: Harvard University Press, 1982).

3. National Bioethics Advisory Commission, *Ethical and Policy Issues in International Research: Clinical Trials in Developing Countries* (Bethesda, MD: NBAC, 2001). The quoted statement is focused specifically on the issue of informed consent to participation in clinical trials.

4. See Amartya Sen, "Rights and Agency," in *Consequentialism and Its Critics*, ed. Samuel Scheffler (Oxford: Oxford University Press, 1988), 187–223. For a discussion that accepts consequentialism but rejects the idea that best consequences or outcomes should be identified with most fulfillment of human rights, see Richard Arneson, "Against Rights," *Philosophical Issues* 11 (2001): 172–201.

5. The statement in the text is fully compatible with claiming that using the rational standard for assessing consequences, paternalism almost always will turn out to be unjustifiable on consequentialist grounds. For a nonconsequentialist account that is strongly averse to paternalism as a matter of first principle, see Seana Shiffrin, "Paternalism, Unconscionability Doctrine, and Accommodation," *Philosophy and Public Affairs* 29, no. 3 (2000): 205–50.

6. The analysis to come follows a line of thought proposed in R. M. Hare, *Moral Thinking: Its Levels, Method, and Point* (Oxford: Oxford University Press, 1981), chaps. 1–3.

7. See Thomas C. Schelling, "Economic Reasoning and the Ethics of Policy," in his *Choice and Consequence* (Cambridge, MA: Harvard University Press, 1984), 11.

8. There are complications here. As my wealth decreases, my demand for rice or some other cheap source of calories may increase.

9. The remarks in the text oversimplify to an extent. The economist is appealing to the norm of Pareto efficiency, construed as a requirement of fairness. The idea is that a state of affairs is unacceptable if it can be altered by making someone better off without making anyone else worse off. This idea is variously interpretable, depending on the meaning that is assigned to the idea of making someone better or worse off. One interpretation would have it that an agent's being better off in one situation than another just amounts to the agent's pre-

ferring to be in the one situation rather than the other. This last thought is disputable; in my judgment it is false. Rejecting it is compatible with embracing the Pareto norm along with an alternative construal of what it is to be better off or worse off.

10. For a clear statement of ethical hostility to inducing by an offer of cash an individual's involvement in a medical procedure that is (a) intended to benefit other people and (b) imposes some risk of harm on the individual, see D. Z. Levine's comments in "Kidney Vending: 'Yes!' or 'No!' *American Journal of Kidney Diseases* 35 (2000): 1002–18. See Robert W. Steiner and Bernard Gert, "Ethical Selection of Living Kidney Donors," *American Journal of Kidney Diseases* 36 (2000): 677–86.

11. The reader may be puzzled. A few paragraphs back, I suggested the consequentialist should endorse a nonexploitation norm that incorporates an admonition against interacting with people without securing their fully informed consent to the terms of interaction. Here I seem to be taking back this assertion. Actually I mean to point out that for the consequentialist the nonexploitation norm is a rough-and-ready guide, a rule of thumb, not a principle always to be obeyed.

12. However, it would be disputed by the libertarian at least to this extent: if one does not violate any Lockean rights, and offers any sort of deal to another that does not involve violation or threat of violation of anyone's Lockean rights, free and voluntary acceptance of the deal, whatever its terms, suffices to transfer rights and establish obligations to comply with the terms agreed upon.

13. For details of this case, see chapter 2 of this volume.

14. After Peter Singer's essay, "Famine, Affluence, and Morality," *Philosophy and Public Affairs* 1 (1972): 229–43. Liam Murphy argues that each of the *N* persons who could contribute to solving a large problem is morally required only to do her fair (per capita) share, in "The Demands of Beneficence," *Philosophy and Public Affairs* 22 (1993): 267–92. For Singer's recent thinking on the topic, see his "Outsiders: Our Obligations to Those beyond Our Borders," in *The Ethics of Assistance: Morality and the Distant Needy*, ed. Deen K. Chatterjee (Cambridge: Cambridge University Press, 2004), 11–32. For criticism of Murphy and other critics of Singer, see Richard Arneson, "Moral Limits on the Demands of Beneficence?" in the same volume, 33–58; also Arneson, "What Do We Owe to Distant Needy Strangers?" in *Singer under Fire*, ed. Jeffrey Schaler, forthcoming.

15. On prioritarianism, see Derek Parfit, "Equality or Priority?" (Department of Philosophy, University of Kansas, the Lindley Lecture, 1995).

16. According to an objective or Objective List account of well-being, a person's life goes better for her, the more she gains the items on a correct list of goods. The list fixes what is truly choiceworthy. Candidate lists include such

items as friendship and love, healthy family ties, cultural and scientific achievement, athletic prowess, pleasure, and the absence of pain. See Derek Parfit, *Reasons and Persons* (Oxford: Oxford University Press, 1984), 493. See also Thomas Hurka, *Perfectionism* (Oxford: Oxford University Press, 1993); also Richard Arneson, "Human Flourishing versus Desire Satisfaction," *Social Philosophy and Policy* 16 (1999): 113–42.

17. Prioritarianism as characterized in the text specifies a family of principles. One gets a specific principle only by fixing the relative weight of gaining more well-being versus obtaining gains for the more worse off. At one extreme, prioritarianism yields recommendations for policy barely distinguishable from utilitarianism, and at the other extreme, prioritarianism barely disagrees with leximin, the position that the tiniest gain to a worse-off person always outweighs benefits of any size to any number of better-off persons. By priority I mean to favor a "Goldilocks" version that assigns weights in the middle of the range between these extremes, but I have no precise specification in mind.

18. In other writings I defend a tripartite prioritarian principle that identifies the moral value to be maximized with increasing aggregate well-being, securing gains for the worse off, and channeling benefits to individuals on the basis of an assessment of their exercise of personal responsibility. See my "Desert and Equality," in *Egalitarianism: New Essays on the Nature and Value of Equality*, ed. Nils Holtug and Kasper Lippert-Rasmussen (Oxford: Oxford University Press, 2007), 262–93; also Arneson, "Luck Egalitarianism and Prioritarianism," *Ethics* 110 (2000): 339–49. The responsibility factor makes no difference to the issues discussed in this chapter, so I ignore it.

19. Allen Wood, "Exploitation," reprinted in *Philosophy and the Problems of Work: A Reader*, ed. Kory Schaff (Lanham, MD: Rowman and Littlefield, 2001), 141–56, at 153. Wood also suggests that the key to ending exploitation is to equalize power. See pp. 155–56.

20. On the efficient allocation of bargaining power, see Oliver Hart, *Firms, Contracts, and Financial Structure* (Oxford: Oxford University Press, 1995), chaps. 2–3. Of course, prioritarianism embraces the advancement of values in addition to the Pareto norm.

21. A. C. Pigou, *The Economics of Welfare* (London: Macmillan, 1920).

22. Wertheimer, *supra* note 1, at 70.

23. *Id.* at 23.

Kantian Ethics, Exploitation, and Multinational Clinical Trials

ANDREW W. SIEGEL

Human nature never seems less lovable than in relations among entire peoples.

—IMMANUEL KANT[1]

In the recent profusion of literature on the ethics of multinational clinical trials, exploitation has been cast as the central iniquity that rules and guidelines for international research must address. The fundamental concern is with investigators reaping benefits from conditions of social and economic deprivation in developing countries while disregarding the health needs of persons in those countries. This concern is heightened when private industry conducts clinical trials in developing countries, as the salient feature of deprivation within the corporate *Weltansicht* is the opportunity for profit, not the tragic character of existing and perishing in poverty.

Although there has been little careful analysis of exploitation in the context of clinical research, there is a solidifying orthodoxy within the research ethics community regarding the specific kinds of clinical trials that are exploitative. There is general agreement that a clinical trial is exploitative where (1) it takes advantage of a person's inability to give informed consent, (2) it fails to address the health needs of the host country, or (3) the sponsor of the trial does not offer to provide posttrial benefits to the population.

But while it is uncontroversial that taking advantage of a person's inability to give informed consent for one's own gain is exploitative, it is not obvious that trials in which one of the other circumstances obtains must involve exploitation. A exploits B (in the moralized sense) when A secures a benefit by taking unfair advantage of B. Thus, to maintain that a research sponsor (A) necessarily exploits citizens (B) of a developing country when enrolling them in a clinical trial that fails to address their health needs or when refusing to ensure the provision of posttrial benefits, we have to assume that there are no terms consistent with these under which A could treat B fairly. Yet this assumption appears dubious at best. In trials that do not address B's health needs, it seems implausible to presume that there are no forms of compensation that could underwrite a fair exchange. For instance, it seems one could reasonably hold that, at least where a trial poses relatively minor risks to participants, there is some (perhaps very high) monetary compensation for trial participants and the host country that would make the transaction a fair one. Likewise, trials that do address B's health needs might offer quite substantial—indeed, sometimes lifesaving—benefits for participants in the trial, as well as other benefits to the community, even though the research sponsor fails to provide benefits after the trial ends. In these circumstances, it is not at all clear that B has been the victim of an unfair exchange.[2]

There are, then, grounds to question some of the central dogmas of international research ethics. At the same time, we should not discount the concerns that animate these views. There is good reason to suppose that pharmaceutical companies and others perceive the desperate conditions of the Third World opportunistically, and that many would take unfair advantage of citizens in developing nations if left unfettered. But before condemning certain research practices and instituting rules under the banner of preventing exploitation, we require a more robust account of the conditions under which it is morally impermissible for research sponsors to advance their interests by using citizens of developing countries. Toward this end, we need to understand the precise nature of the moral wrong involved in exploitation and the kinds of actions and practices that manifest this wrong.

In this chapter, I seek to address these issues from a Kantian perspective. Kant's ethics is well suited to capture and give theoretical shape to our concerns about exploitation in international research. Our basic misgivings about clinical trials in developing countries emerge from concerns about investigators unfairly using persons who are weak and vulnerable due to poverty. Kant's ethics is illuminating in this context because it offers an ideal of human relations that delimits permissible uses of persons and specifies our obligations to those who need aid. This chapter both develops a theory of exploitation that is guided by Kant's ethics and describes the implications of the theory for the ethics of multinational clinical trials.

Exploitation and the Categorical Imperative

To assess whether A exploits B, we need to know whether A has taken advantage of B in a manner that is morally wrongful. An act is not exploitative simply by virtue of the fact that one person gains an advantage from another; rather, exploitation occurs when a person obtains a benefit (for herself or a third party) through the unfair or wrongful use of another person. A substantive theory of exploitation must therefore identify the conditions under which it is morally impermissible to take advantage of persons.

Accordingly, a Kantian theory of exploitation will be built on the principles that Kant adduces for assessing moral permissibility. For Kant, the "supreme principle of morality" is the categorical imperative. The categorical imperative determines the moral permissibility of maxims, which are the "subjective principles" that persons act upon. A provisional and very general formulation of a Kantian account of exploitation is thus as follows: A exploits B when A secures a benefit from B by acting toward B on a maxim that violates the categorical imperative. A more precise rendering of the theory of exploitation will be possible after we identify the specific demands of the categorical imperative.

Kant offers several formulations of the categorical imperative, all of which, he claims, are equivalent. The unifying thread that runs through the formulations and allows us to recognize a relation of identity between them is their commitment to the value of rational agency. Our rational nature is the value that delimits permissible maxims. The categorical imperative both articulates the value of rational agency and helps us establish when our maxims fail to reflect the appropriate appreciation of this value. I will briefly discuss the first two formulations of the categorical imperative, which will serve as a sufficient statement of Kant's view for purposes of developing a theory of exploitation.

The Formula of Universal Law

The first formulation of the categorical imperative, the formula of universal law, states: "Act only according to that maxim by which you can at the same time will that it should become a universal law."[3] Kant adds that this is equivalent to acting "as if the maxim of your action were to become by your will a universal law of nature."[4] One can will a maxim as a universal law of nature only if the maxim does not generate a contradiction when all other persons are permitted to adopt it. There are two kinds of contradiction that may arise through willing universalized maxims: conceptual contradictions and volitional contradictions. A conceptual contradiction occurs where actions "are of such a nature that their maxim cannot even be *thought* as a universal law of nature without contradiction."[5] A volitional contradiction occurs when it is "impossible to will that [an action's] maxim should be raised to the universality of a law of nature."[6]

The paradigmatic case of a maxim that gives rise to a conceptual contradiction when willed as a universal law is the deceitful promise. Kant considers the maxim, "When I believe myself to be in need of money, I will borrow money and promise to repay it, although I know I will never do so."[7] If made universal, this maxim would allow anyone who needs money to take a loan and promise to repay it while intending not to keep the promise. Yet, as Kant remarks, "This would make the very promise and the end one had in making it impossible, since no one would believe what was promised him but rather would laugh at such an utterance as vain pretense."[8] Kant appears to suggest here that universal deceitful promising would be both logically and practically impossible. It would make the "very promise" logically impossible because there could be no promises where deceitful promising was a universal law. The universalized maxim would make "the end one had in making [the promise]" practically impossible because one's ability to obtain a loan through a deceitful promise presupposes a world in which such promises are exceptional.[9]

The moral problem with the maxim of deceit is that it violates conventions that persons rely on as agents. As agents, we depend on the convention that persons who make promises do so in good faith. Our reliance on this convention makes us susceptible to being taken advantage of by others. The deceitful promise takes unfair advantage of the promisee because, as Barbara Herman puts it, "deceit manipulates the circumstances of deliberation."[10] The maxim of deceit must be rejected because it "exploits the vulnerability of human agents to manipulative control" and thereby interferes with the conditions of rational agency.[11]

Maxims that generate volitional contradictions when universalized also fail to properly acknowledge the conditions of human agency. This is well illustrated in Kant's case of the person who wills a maxim of nonbeneficence. Consider the person who refuses to help a person he sees in need because he thinks, "What does it matter to me? Let everybody be as happy as Heaven wills or as he can make himself; I shall take nothing from him nor even envy him; but I have no desire to contribute anything to his well-being or to his assistance when in need."[12] While it is possible to conceive of a world in which this maxim is a universal law of nature, it is not, according to Kant, possible to will a world in which the maxim is a universal law. Given that we are finite and dependent beings who cannot guarantee our survival in the absence of aid from others, to will the maxim of nonbeneficence as a universal law of nature would be to relinquish resources that may be required for the preservation of our agency. Willing universal nonbeneficence is never rational because we can never presume that complete self-sufficiency is attainable.[13]

The formal procedure of testing maxims for conceptual and volitional contradictions thus serves to identify the limits on willing that are essential for maintaining the conditions of rational agency. Acting on maxims that give rise to conceptual contradictions when made universal laws—for example, the maxim of deceit—directly interferes with agency. Maxims that generate volitional contradictions when universalized— for example, the maxim of nonbeneficence—fail to acknowledge the conditions that are necessary to preserve or promote rational agency.

The Formula of Humanity

The moral requirements prescribed by the formula of universal law also follow from the second formulation of the categorical imperative, which makes more explicit the value of rational agency. The formula of humanity states, "Act in such a way that you treat humanity, whether in your own person or in the person of another, always at the same time as an end and never simply as a means."[14] Kant develops his argument for the humanity formulation in two general stages. First, he argues that the categorical imperative can be binding on everyone only if there exists an end in itself. Second, he maintains that humanity or "rational nature" must be the end in itself.

Kant shows that the categorical imperative requires an end in itself as its ground by identifying the limits of subjective ends. Subjective ends are reasons persons adopt for acting that are based on empirical desires or "inclinations."[15] Because not all persons have the same inclinations, subjective ends cannot unconditionally require action by all agents. Subjective ends can only ground hypothetical imperatives—that is, imperatives that tell us what to do in order to attain something we want. The categorical imperative can be universally binding only if it is based on a nonrelative end. What is required is an objective end or end in itself, an end that is "given by reason alone" and thus "equally valid for all rational beings."[16]

Kant claims that humanity or rational nature is the end in itself because it is through the rational choice of ends that value comes into existence.[17] Our capacity to set ends according to moral principles has, in Christine Korsgaard's words, a "value-conferring status."[18] It is because rational nature is the source of all value that Kant says we must regard it as absolutely and unconditionally valuable. Of course, one might argue that it does not follow from the fact that the rational will is the source of all objective value that it is itself valuable. But, as Allen Wood plausibly counters, "If rational nature is . . . the prescriptive source of all objective goodness, then it must be the most fundamental object of respect or esteem, since if it is not respected as objectively good, then nothing else can be treated as objectively good."[19]

Kant identifies both a negative and a positive sense in which we are required to treat persons (i.e., rational beings) as ends in themselves. In the negative sense, we must never undermine the conditions of free and rational choice by acting on maxims with which others "cannot possibly concur."[20] For example, acts that employ deceit to achieve their aims violate this requirement, as they deny agents information essential to deliberation.[21] In the positive sense, the duty to treat persons as ends in themselves requires that we sometimes act to support the conditions of agency. This includes a duty to one's self to develop talents that are useful for the pursuit of one's ends, as well as a duty to others to, at minimum, help them preserve their status as agents. Kant calls these latter duties "imperfect," as we have some degree of latitude in choosing when to fulfill them. These are in contrast to "perfect" duties (e.g., the duties not to deceive or coerce), which we must always fulfill. How much latitude we are permitted in the case of imperfect duties is a matter of controversy, one that we will have occasion to return to later.

In addition to the duties to avoid subverting the conditions of agency and to affirmatively support agency, the imperative to treat humanity as an end in itself requires more generally that we not act in any ways that demean or degrade persons. Some acts or attitudes may display a lack of respect for the equal worth of all rational beings without violating duties to preserve the conditions of agency. Among the examples Kant cites are contempt, which involves "*looking down* on some in comparison with others," and arrogance, "in which we demand that others think little of themselves in comparison with us."[22] Such attitudes violate the duty of respect for persons because they issue from the false belief that some persons have greater worth than other persons.

A Kantian Theory of Exploitation

We are now in a position to give a more complete statement of a Kantian theory of exploitation:

> A exploits B when A secures a benefit from B by acting toward B on a maxim that (1) subverts the conditions of B's rational agency, (2) fails to acknowledge needs that are essential to B qua rational agent, or (3) demeans or degrades B despite the fact that preservation of B's agency is not at issue.

What remains is to specify the ways in which clinical trials in developing countries may exploit citizens of those countries. I shall argue that the most profound and pervasive form of exploitation in international research is that which involves the violation of the duty of beneficence. That is, the central problem of exploitation in international research is the problem of indifference toward the needs of persons qua human agents. But before developing this argument, I want to note and comment upon concerns about exploitation in international research that emerge in relation to the other two general modes of exploitation— namely, exploitation involving the subversion of rational agency and exploitation involving the degradation of persons where preservation of agency is not at issue. Concerns about the subversion of agency arise in connection with satisfying the requirements of informed consent; concerns about degradation emerge more generally in connection with the inequalities in wealth and power that characterize the relations between research sponsors and research subjects. I consider each of these concerns in turn.

Agency and Informed Consent

One of the basic principles of research ethics is that investigators must obtain voluntary informed consent from individuals before enrolling them in clinical trials. This requirement is consistent with (if not derivative of) the Kantian imperative that we not act in ways that subvert rational agency. An obvious violation of the informed consent requirement occurs when an investigator (or some other interested party) uses deceit or coercion to get a person to enroll in a clinical trial. Such acts directly interfere with agency by manipulating a person's will. One can also violate the informed consent requirement without directly manipulating a person's will. What is of greatest concern in multinational clinical trials is that persons may have a limited ability to give informed consent because "they are illiterate, unfamiliar with the concepts of medicine held by the investigators, or living in communities in which the procedures typical of informed consent discussions are unfamiliar or alien to the ethos of the community."[23] An investigator who seeks to enroll participants without overcoming these barriers to consent interferes with rational agency by promoting a process of deliberation that cannot yield a properly informed decision.

George Annas and Michael Grodin suggest some additional obstacles to voluntary informed consent in developing countries. One problem is that, "in the absence of health care, virtually any offer of medical assistance (even in the guise of research) will be accepted as 'better than nothing.'"[24] Trials that offer free health care and the hope of dramatically improving one's medical condition will be "irresistible" to those who have no other options. Annas and Grodin further maintain that we should "presume that valid informed consent cannot be obtained from impoverished populations in the absence of a realistic plan to deliver the intervention to the population."[25] This is, they claim, because "it is extremely unlikely that [members of impoverished populations] would knowingly volunteer to participate in research that offered no benefit to their communities . . . and that would only serve to enrich the multinational drug companies and the developed world."[26]

Now, the first thing to note about the putative problems cited here is that they are mutually inconsistent. If a trial is irresistible when it offers a person the hope of receiving a highly beneficial intervention that would otherwise be unavailable to her, then it cannot be the case that she would refuse to enroll in the trial just because the intervention would not be made available to the population. If persons would refuse to participate in research where they understand that the sponsor will not provide posttrial benefits to the community, it would follow that the offer to enter the trial is quite resistible. One of the propositions Annas and Grodin posit must therefore be false.

I think that the truth lies somewhere in the middle, and on terrain that is largely immune to challenges about the validity of consent. It is conceivable that in some cultures persons would choose to forgo potentially lifesaving interventions to prevent their own exploitation. It is also possible that it would be collectively rational for citizens to refuse to agree to participate in clinical trials as part of a strategy for obtaining a commitment from research sponsors to make the intervention available to the community. Persons do have the capacity to make substantial sacrifices of self-interest for the good of the collective and for other values. But there is little reason to presume that citizens of developing countries would or ought to make these sacrifices. Individuals certainly can (and most likely do) believe that preserving their own lives is more important than preventing corporations from becoming unjustly enriched. And there may generally be reason to think that refusing to participate will not serve the collective good (e.g., because companies will simply go elsewhere to conduct the trial). Where strong reasons for self-sacrifice are absent, persons without other health care options will indeed feel compelled to enter potentially lifesaving trials. But this is because entering the trial is the only rational course of action under the circumstances, and not because persons lack the capacity to do otherwise.

The real problem here rests not with the validity of consent but with the tragic circumstances that make the choice to enter clinical trials compelling. It is profoundly disquieting that persons live in conditions where participating in research trials is their best hope for improving their health status. While these persons can in principle make a free and rational decision to enroll in a clinical trial, the fact that they must make this decision in circumstances where their options are so severely limited raises its own set of moral issues. The central question about exploitation that arises is whether it is sometimes morally wrong for research sponsors to take advantage of the circumstances of poverty for their own gain. And assuming it is sometimes morally wrong, what is the precise nature of the wrong?

Inequality and Degradation

Allen Wood argues that the morally objectionable feature of exploitative transactions is that advantages gained through inequalities in bargaining power degrade the weaker party:

> Proper respect for others is violated when we treat their vulnerabilities as opportunities to advance our own interests or projects. It is degrading to have your weaknesses taken advantage of and dishonorable to use the weaknesses of others for your ends, even if the exploitative arrangement is voluntary on both sides and no matter what the resulting distribution of benefits and harms.[27]

This account would clearly implicate clinical trials that private industry conducts in developing countries, as the sponsors of these trials advance their interests by taking advantage of the weaknesses and vulnerabilities of research subjects. These sponsors view the union of illness and impoverishment as an ideal opportunity for efficiently and inexpensively testing pharmaceuticals they wish to take to market. That industry takes advantage of persons in developing countries in this way is sufficient on

Wood's account to support a charge of exploitation: the practice is morally wrongful because it degrades persons in developing countries; and it does so regardless of the benefits pharmaceutical companies provide to research subjects or the population.

To assess this thesis about exploitation, we need to consider whether a person who advances her own interests by taking advantage of another person's weaknesses and vulnerabilities necessarily degrades that person. We should first observe that if one holds an egalitarian view of the worth of rational beings—as Kant and Wood do—an act will not literally degrade a human being unless it undermines her status as a rational agent. From a Kantian perspective, when we speak of an act that does not threaten rational agency as degrading, we can mean only that the act treats a person *as if* she is of lower rank than other persons. On this view, a person acts in a manner that degrades another if and only if her action displays a lack of respect for the equal moral worth of the other.

The question, then, is whether transactions in which persons benefit from inequalities in holdings of wealth and power are compatible with an egalitarian view of moral worth. Wood suggests that they are not compatible because such transactions are degrading. He further claims that "this badness seems to be present even where the exploitation involves no unfairness, injustice, or violation of rights."[28]

But there is good reason to challenge his position. Where inequalities in wealth and power result from distributive principles that reflect a commitment to the moral equality of persons, mutually beneficial transactions that involve disparities in bargaining power need not be degrading. Consider, for example, Rawls's difference principle, which permits inequalities when they work to the advantage of the least well off. This principle reflects an egalitarian view of moral worth because it is arrived at through a hypothetical social contract that models the moral equality of persons. Transactions in which the talented benefit from the (voluntary and fairly compensated) labor of the less talented will not be degrading precisely because the principles that allow such transactions are ones that all of the parties would embrace as free and equal persons.

One can make a similar point by invoking other theories of distributive justice. On egalitarian theories that require an initial equal distribution of resources, inequalities that occur at times subsequent to the initial distribution are compatible with recognizing the equality of persons as long as they result from persons' freely acting on their preferences. It need not be degrading for persons to benefit from vulnerabilities where these inequalities exist. If B has no choice but to work for A because B chose to expend his equal share of resources traveling around the world, A does not exploit or degrade B simply by taking advantage of B's need to work. Again, this is because the inequalities upon which the transactions depend flow from a distributive scheme that treats persons as moral equals. The same general claim is available to some who reject egalitarian views about distributive justice. Indeed, some libertarians consider themselves to be the true descendants of Kant, and suggest that it is because everyone has equal moral worth that everyone has the same entitlement to noninterference with their property rights. While there is some controversy about whether Kant is a proponent of the night watchman state or an advocate of a social welfare state,[29] he certainly believes that transactions flowing from inequalities in wealth and power are compatible with respecting persons as moral equals. One can assume that such transactions are inherently degrading only if one fails to acknowledge the ways in which principles of distributive justice that permit inequalities often reflect a commitment to the equal moral worth of persons.

Of course, one may legitimately challenge whether current distributions of wealth and power are the outcome of principles that manifest respect for the moral equality of persons. One might claim, for example, that the current distribution of holdings is problematic because it is the result of unjust acquisitions and transfers or because the distribution is different than what it would be had there been an initial equal distribution of resources. Arguably, an individual fails to show proper respect for the equal moral worth of persons when she seeks to gain an advantage from vulnerabilities that exist as a consequence of distributive schemes that free and equal persons would reject.

I think there is some merit to this position. But just how powerful an indictment it supports of present social and economic exchanges will depend upon what the correct theory of justice requires, the ways in which the principles of justice have been violated, and the impact of those violations on the distribution of benefits and burdens in society. The implications are even less clear when we consider the international context. For most theories of justice articulate distributive principles that are designed to apply to the structure of a single society, especially where positive duties to provide welfare are concerned.[30] In Kant's case, in the rare moments that he ascribes duties to the state to aid the poor through redistributing wealth, he rather clearly suggests that the state owes these duties only to its own members:

> The general Will of the people has united itself into a society in order to maintain itself continually, and for this purpose it has subjected itself to the internal authority of the state in order to support those members of society who are unable to support themselves. Therefore it follows from the nature of the state that the government is authorized to require the wealthy to provide the means of substance to those who are unable to provide the most necessary needs of nature for themselves.[31]

At the same time, however, Kant's views about the moral duties individuals owe one another are fundamentally cosmopolitan. Kant's "kingdom of ends" does not have geopolitical borders. Whatever limits we place on the obligations of the state, as individuals we have a duty to treat persons as ends in themselves wherever they may be. This idea is reflected in Kant's comments about the duty of beneficence: "[T]he maxim of common interest, of beneficence toward those in need, is a universal duty of human beings, just because they are to be considered fellowmen, that is, rational beings with needs, united by nature in one dwelling place so that they can help one another."[32] Thus, regardless of whether or not principles of distributive justice have a global reach, we can query whether the ways in which affluent persons individually distribute their resources are compatible with the requirements of beneficence. Global inequalities and the exchanges that take place in their foreground may manifest a lack of respect for persons even if it turns out that principles of justice are silent on the matter. A violation of respect for persons occurs where the advantages the affluent gain in their transactions with the poor result from a failure on the part of the affluent to fulfill the duty of beneficence. When one person's gain trades on his indifference to the needs of others, he fails to treat those others as ends in themselves. Consideration of the requirements of beneficence is therefore critical to the examination of exploitation in multinational transactions.

Beneficence and Exploitation

THE SCOPE OF THE DUTY OF BENEFICENCE

There are two issues concerning the general requirements of the duty of beneficence. One issue concerns the range of needs that we have an obligation to help satisfy. The other issue concerns the degree of latitude we have in choosing when to assist persons who have these needs. Kant's texts allow for divergent interpretations of his views on these questions. Though I will set out some of the competing accounts, I will not seek to settle all of the interpretive issues. Instead, my principal aim is to show that serious moral problems about relations between rich and poor arise even when we interpret the duty of beneficence as relatively narrow in scope.

Kant's comments about the range of needs that the duty of beneficence encompasses permit both expansive and restrictive readings. Kant says the duty of beneficence requires that "the ends of any subject who is an end in himself must as far as possible be my ends also."[33] A literal reading of this remark suggests that we are to treat the ends of others as our own to the extent possible, whatever the nature of the ends (assuming, of course, that the ends are permissible). The problem with such a duty is that it would, as Barbara Herman argues, conflict both with the idea that not all ends of others have a claim on us (e.g., the goal of owning a yacht) and with the notion that proper cultivation of "capacities for responsible choice and effective action" generally requires that capable persons take responsibility for the pursuit of their ends.[34]

Kant does elsewhere suggest that the duty of beneficence is concerned with the "true needs" of persons.[35] Although Kant does not specify what counts as a true need, there is good reason to think that he primarily has in mind those needs that are crucial to maintaining our status as rational agents. For the ground of the duty of beneficence as revealed by the categorical imperative is the fact of our finitude and dependency as rational agents. It is because we cannot presume that we are able to sustain our agency in the absence of aid from others that it would be irrational to will a universal law of nonbeneficence. It is also for this reason that principled nonbeneficence is incompatible with treating humanity as an end in itself. Thus, it is reasonable to conclude, as Herman does, that "the needs for which a person may make a claim under the duty of mutual aid are those that cannot be left unmet if he is to continue in his activity as a rational agent."[36]

While this reading narrowly circumscribes the range of needs that we have an obligation to address, it is broad enough to cover the basic conditions of the severely poor. Life for persons in the Third World is characterized by the struggle to survive in the face of rampant starvation and preventable disease. Even for one who survives in extreme poverty, the conditions one subsists in are not "broadly consistent with a sense of oneself as an active agent, capable of taking effective command of the conduct of one's life."[37]

It is clear that the duty of beneficence requires that we recognize the needs of persons in developing countries as strong candidates for our assistance. But the question remains regarding the degree of latitude we have in choosing whether to provide aid. Kant holds that the duty of beneficence is "a *wide* one; the duty has in it a latitude for doing more or less, and no specific limits can be assigned to what should be done."[38] The duty of beneficence requires the adoption of a general maxim to promote the true needs of others. It is a principle that guides actions without determinately prescribing them. While it is always a violation of the duty of beneficence to be indifferent to the true needs of others, Kant allows that there may be occasions when one can choose not to attend to these needs without being indifferent to them. There is, however, some uncertainty about the conditions under which Kant thinks it is permissible to deny aid to those in need.

Kant poses the question, "How far should one expend one's resources in practicing beneficence?"[39] The only direct answer he offers is, "Surely not to the extent he himself would finally come to need the beneficence of others."[40] Thus, we can at least say that one need not help others when doing so would place one's own status as an agent at serious risk. But because Kant's answer does not entail that the preservation of one's agency is the only legitimate reason for refusing to offer aid, it leaves open the question of the full set of conditions under which we may forgo providing aid.

There are passages in which one can interpret Kant as placing very strict limits on when we are permitted to deny assistance to those in need. For example, he writes that "a wide duty is not to be taken as a permission to make exceptions to the maxim of actions, but only as a permission to limit one maxim of duty by another."[41] One might read this as stating that the only permissible ground for refusing aid to someone in need is that one is engaged in another act that is required by a perfect duty (e.g., keeping a promise to someone) or that falls under a principle of imperfect duty (e.g., performing other beneficent acts or developing one's talents). Some reject that Kant holds such a rigid view. Thomas Hill, for example, emphasizes that in the *Groundwork* Kant distinguishes between perfect and imperfect duties on the basis that the latter allow some "exceptions in the interests of inclinations,"[42] while the former permit no such exceptions.[43] It seems to follow that "imperfect duties allow us to do what we please on some occasions even if this is not an act of a kind prescribed by moral principles and even if we could on those occasions do something of a kind that is prescribed."[44]

Assuming we accept that the duty of beneficence allows us to sometimes privilege our purely subjective ends over the true needs of others, how do we determine when a refusal to offer aid violates the duty? We need to know a person's general pattern of behavior and the reasons on which she acts. A person who has sufficient means but never provides aid prima facie acts on a maxim of nonbeneficence. However, a person may fail to provide aid for reasons that defeat the presumption of nonbeneficence. For example, one might not offer aid because one believes that relief organizations invariably mismanage donations and fail in their enterprise. But such cases are exceptional.[45] In general, we can assume with confidence that a person who has the wherewithal but never offers aid is indifferent to the needs of others.

As for the person who does sometimes provide aid, we can determine whether she displays indifference in a particular case of withholding aid by examining her resources and the opportunity costs she would incur in offering assistance. Minimally, assuming A sometimes provides aid to persons, I think we can say that A displays indifference toward B's true needs where:

(a) A chooses not to provide aid to B;
(b) There is no good reason to believe B will receive aid if A
     does not provide it;
(c) A has the means to provide aid to B;

(d) A's providing aid to B would not conflict with A's fulfillment of other duties (that A plans to fulfill) or with his plans or current actions to aid persons other than B; and

(e) A's providing aid to B would not interfere with A's enjoying considerable (but nonextravagant) luxuries.

This is a minimalist account of the duty of beneficence because it allows us to withhold aid whenever doing so is necessary for our remaining well-off. While one might wish to promote a stronger duty, this account is sufficient to ground substantial obligations to provide aid to the poor.

Our current situation is one in which it is possible for most individuals in affluent countries to provide far more aid to the impoverished than they do without significantly forgoing their own interests. Collectively, those in affluent countries are in a position to eliminate the worst consequences of poverty with little sacrifice. As Thomas Pogge writes:

> The figure of 1.5 billion human beings in dire poverty may be daunting. But global inequality has now increased to such an extreme that this poorest quartile of humankind—with annual income of $100 per capita and thus collectively about $150 billion— accounts for merely half a percent of the global product. . . . For the first time in human history it is quite feasible, economically, to wipe out hunger and preventable diseases worldwide without real inconvenience to anyone.[46]

Given these facts, our individual and collective failures to provide aid essential to the eradication of global poverty constitute a violation of the duty of beneficence. Thus, even if we adopt something like the minimalist account of the duty of beneficence, we cannot escape our obligation to radically transform the state of the world.

EXPLOITATION AND INDIFFERENCE: TWO WRONGS

We can now more fully describe the relationship between beneficence and exploitation. There are two kinds of moral transgression that occur when A exploits B by violating the duty of beneficence. The first is the indifference A displays toward B's essential needs as a rational agent. In acting with indifference to B's true needs, A fails to treat B as an end in herself. A may commit this wrong even if she does not succeed in exploiting B.

For exploitation requires that A gain from her interaction with B; and A may be indifferent to B's needs without securing a benefit from B. That A benefits from her indifference to B constitutes a second wrong. This wrong lies in A's gaining from her own failure to fulfill her obligations. To better understand the moral problem here, we must attend to some important subtleties concerning the nature of A's obligations.

The duty of beneficence requires that we not be indifferent to the true needs of others. We display indifference when we withhold aid in the absence of legitimate reasons for doing so (as set forth previously). Persons who are well-off have an obligation to provide some aid to impoverished persons, as there are not sufficiently good reasons for a well-off individual to refuse to provide aid altogether.[47] But the duty of beneficence does not generally entail that a person has an obligation to provide aid to a particular person or population. This is because there are so many suffering individuals in the world that a potential donor can permissibly choose to deny some persons aid in favor of providing it to others. The duty of beneficence does not have a right to aid as a corollary because no individual is in a position to exercise this right against another individual (except, perhaps, in the extraordinary circumstance where there is only one potential donor and one potential recipient— e.g., where there are two castaways on an otherwise deserted island, and one of them needs aid that the other can easily provide). Thus, in ordinary circumstances, when A exploits B, we cannot assert that A gains from violating an obligation to provide aid to B.

Nonetheless, when A exploits B by violating the duty of beneficence, we might legitimately hold that A is complicit in the tragic circumstances from which she gains. This will be the case where B is a member of the class that experiences unnecessary suffering because of the transgressions of the nonbeneficent class to which A belongs. Although no member of the class of persons that violates the duty is directly responsible for the impoverished state of any particular individual, it must be the case that each member of the class is complicit in the suffering of all who live in serious poverty. To deny this, we would have to allow that (1) a group might be involved in a wrong despite the fact that no individual member of the group bears any connection to it, or (2) persons might be complicit in the suffering of a group but not in the suffering of individual members of that group. Both propositions are incoherent because the concepts of group wrongdoing and group harm presuppose that there are individuals who are agents and victims of a wrong. The only coherent thing to say is that all persons who violate the duty of beneficence are complicit in the suffering of all impoverished persons whose lives would be improved if the duty were fulfilled.

Now, when A is able to obtain a benefit from B because of a moral breach in which A is involved, at least part of A's gain constitutes a wrong to B. For A's gain depends in part or whole on B's living in dire circumstances that A is complicit in allowing to persist. If A and all other affluent persons were properly concerned with the plight of the poor, B would either have no need to transact with A or possess the power to set better contractual terms for himself. A wrongs B in gaining from the transaction because the gain trades on a larger moral failing to which A contributes.

Of course, this larger moral failing is one in which most of us are complicit. There are very few among us who can claim in good faith to have satisfied the duty of beneficence. Consequently, almost all of us who are well-off are deeply implicated in the problem of exploitation in developing countries because we fail to satisfy our obligation to eliminate some of the conditions that allow exploitation to thrive.

Beneficence and Multinational Clinical Trials

With the theoretical account of the connections between beneficence and exploitation now in place, I want to show how it illuminates some of the more specific issues concerning exploitation in multinational clinical trials. In particular, I want to examine (1) whether research sponsors or others have an obligation to ensure the provision of posttrial benefits, and (2) whether it is morally permissible for investigators to employ placebo-controlled trials where the use of a known effective treatment as the control is a viable alternative. I will argue that the standard approaches to addressing these issues are inadequate, and that considering the issues in the light of the requirements of beneficence affords greater insight into them.

Posttrial Benefits

The prevailing view in the research ethics community is that clinical trials in developing countries are exploitative when conducted without assurances from research sponsors or others that the intervention being evaluated will be made "reasonably available" to the population of the host country after the trial.[48] The Havrix trial is a paradigmatic case of a clinical trial that would be deemed exploitative on this view. In this trial, an inactivated hepatitis A vaccine developed by SmithKline Beecham (SKB) was tested on 40,000 children in northern Thailand. There are very high transmission rates of hepatitis A infection in Thailand, and there is significant morbidity and mortality associated with the infection among adults. The Thai people thus have a strong interest in receiving the vaccine. However, the Thai government cannot afford to provide it to the population, and SKB has not been willing to make reasonable efforts to ensure that the Thai population receives it.

There are two distinct grounds that research ethicists and others appeal to in support of their view that trials such as this one are exploitative. One claim is that a trial conducted without assurances of posttrial benefits is exploitative because we cannot expect that it will serve the health needs of the population. The other claim is that a pharmaceutical company does not offer fair compensation whenever it fails to ensure the provision of a safe and effective intervention to the population in which the intervention was tested.

As I indicated at the beginning of the chapter, the first claim appears problematic inasmuch as it entails that there are no terms under which a clinical trial that fails to address the health needs of a population might be fair. Suppose that a pharmaceutical company wants to conduct a very low-risk trial in a developing country to test a pill designed to eliminate wrinkles. Further suppose the company offers a very generous package of benefits to participants and to the local community. This trial is exploitative on the consensus view because it fails to address the health needs (or, we can assume, any other needs) of the country. But this seems mistaken. The fact that the wrinkle pill does not address the needs of the population does not appear any more inherently problematic than the fact that high-end athletic shoes do not serve the populations that produce them. In both cases, the relevant consideration is whether the companies offer adequate benefits to their employees and to the communities that welcome them.

The second claim is that a fair distribution of benefits requires that research sponsors make interventions that are of value to the host country reasonably available to the population after the trial. However, it is at least not obvious that the benefits a country receives in the course of a trial will not sometimes constitute fair compensation.[49] In the Havrix case, the trial yielded considerable benefits for participants and other members of the population: the 40,000 participants received the hepatitis A vaccine and the hepatitis B vaccine, which served as the control; the hepatitis B vaccine was provided to thousands of personnel who worked on the trial; Thai researchers received valuable training; and public health stations were furnished with much-needed equipment. To be sure, it would be a good thing for SKB to make Havrix reasonably available to the Thai people. But, given the considerable benefits that the Thai people obtained in the course of the trial, it is not self-evident that the exchange was unfair.

The Kantian theory of exploitation allows for a more nuanced and revealing analysis of the Havrix case. On this account, the morally relevant questions as they relate to the connection between beneficence and exploitation are (1) whether SKB displays indifference in not making Havrix reasonably available to the Thai population, and (2) whether SKB's gain is wrongful.

In principle, a pharmaceutical company can refuse to provide a successful intervention or other posttrial benefits without displaying indifference to the population in which the intervention was tested. There are limits to the aid individuals or corporations can provide consistent with their own flourishing. It is possible that a given company could not guarantee posttrial benefits because it is presently suffering from serious financial woes. It is also conceivable—though quite improbable—that a company would refuse to offer posttrial benefits because the resources it can reasonably allocate for relief aid have already been committed to the pursuit of other beneficent acts. In such instances, the failure to offer posttrial benefits does not evidence indifference.

In the Havrix case, however, there is good reason to think that SKB could do significantly more in making the vaccine available to the Thai population without seriously sacrificing its own interests or the interests of others. In 2001, SKB (now GlaxoSmithKline) had sales (for all products combined) of $29.5 billion, yielding $8.8 billion in profits. It's community investment and charitable donations in 2001 totaled approximately $141 million, or 1.6 percent of their profits for that year.[50] While these donations are not insignificant, SKB could certainly offer much more aid without undermining its status as a highly profitable company. Given these circumstances, it is reasonable to conclude that SKB displays indifference to the Thai people in refusing to make Havrix more readily available to the population.

To address the further issue of whether SKB wrongs the Thai population in profiting from the Havrix trial, we have to pose the following counterfactual question: Would SKB have been able to secure its gains from the trial if everyone fulfilled the duty of beneficence? If SKB's gains depend in part or whole on a transgression in which SKB is complicit, then the Thai people suffer a wrong. It is not clear that we can provide a decisive answer to the counterfactual question. We would need to calculate the total resources for aid that would be available in a beneficent world and determine how these resources would be allocated. One might argue that eliminating hepatitis A would be of relatively low priority, since most infected persons recover completely. On the other hand, since hepatitis A largely results from systemic problems with sanitation, support for important public health measures aimed at improving sanitation more generally would have the effect of greatly reducing the incidence of the disease. I think this latter consideration suggests that it is probable that the level of transmission of hepatitis A in Thailand would be considerably lower in a beneficent world. Indeed, it is possible that in a beneficent world hepatitis A would not be prevalent enough to motivate SKB to develop the vaccine at all, in which case all of the company's gains from the sale of Havrix in our actual, nonbeneficent world would be morally tainted. However, given the empirical uncertainties, the full extent of the wrong SKB commits in exploiting the Thai people remains a matter of speculation.

Placebo-Controlled Trials

There has been much recent debate surrounding the ethics of placebo-controlled trials. The central issue is whether it is ever morally permissible to use a placebo-controlled trial to evaluate a new treatment for a condition when a proven effective treatment exists. Broadly speaking, we can distinguish between three views on the issue:

V1 An investigator who uses placebos when proven effective treatments exist violates the therapeutic obligation to provide trial participants with optimal medical care.[51]

V2 An investigator who uses a placebo control does not violate the therapeutic obligation when a proven effective treatment would not be available to research participants outside of the trial—that is, where the treatment is not the standard of care in the country in which the trial is conducted. Placebo controls are acceptable in these circumstances as long as the experimental treatment will serve the health needs of the population if proven safe and effective (e.g., because it is a treatment that the host country can afford to provide as the standard of care).[52]

V3 An investigator does not have a therapeutic obligation to provide optimal medical care to trial participants. The view that researchers have such a duty "conflates the ethics of clinical research with the ethics of clinical medicine."[53] The obligation of investigators is instead to ensure that participants not be "exposed to excessive risk for the sake of scientific investigation."[54] Placebo controls are permissible where the risks are minimal and the participants understand that the purpose of the trial is scientific rather than therapeutic.[55]

To examine the implications of these views for multinational clinical trials, consider the proposed Surfaxin trial. In 2001, a U.S. biotechnology company proposed conducting a study in Latin America to test a new surfactant drug for the treatment of respiratory distress syndrome (RDS), a common and often fatal disease in premature infants. There is—and was at the time—a safe and effective surfactant treatment for RDS, though the cost of the treatment exceeds what most persons in Latin America can afford. In the proposed study, a control group of premature infants would receive a placebo. The trial could be conducted by comparing the new drug with the existing surfactant, but this would require a larger trial. The drug company preferred the placebo-controlled trial because it would provide the most efficient method of testing the intervention. The new intervention would be marketed primarily in the United States and would be largely inaccessible to Latin American countries because of its cost.

According to V1, this trial is impermissible because there is a proven effective treatment for RDS. On V2, the existence of an effective treatment does not in itself render the use of placebos impermissible, since this is not a treatment that participants in the trial would have access to outside of the trial. Nonetheless, according to this view, the trial would be impermissible on the separate ground that it would not serve the health needs of the population. As to V3, the moral assessment of the trial turns on how one resolves an ambiguity regarding the proposition that placebo controls must not expose participants to excessive risks. There are two ways to understand the proposition:

> V3′ The use of a placebo control must not leave participants exposed to serious risks that are preventable.

> V3″ The use of a placebo control must not create serious risks that participants would not face outside of the trial.

V3′ excludes the use of placebos in all cases where a trial addresses a serious condition for which there is a proven effective treatment. The Surfaxin trial would be impermissible on V3′ because RDS poses life-threatening risks that are preventable. In contrast, V3″ in principle permits placebo-controlled trials where the trial addresses a life-threatening condition for which there is a proven effective treatment. On this view, there is nothing intrinsically wrong with using placebos where the participants who receive them would not receive any care for their condition outside of the trial. Those who embrace V3″ would thus not object to the use of placebo controls per se in the Surfaxin trial, though I gather most would object to the trial on the grounds that it would not ultimately yield sufficient benefits for the host countries.

I think that none of the views cited earlier adequately captures what is at issue with the use of placebos in cases like the proposed Surfaxin trial. On all of these accounts, we are to determine the permissibility of denying trial participants proven effective treatments strictly by assessing the role-specific obligations investigators have to research subjects. According to V1 and V2, the permissibility of employing placebo controls depends upon how we construe an investigator's obligation to provide medical care, while V3′ and V3″ assess the permissibility of placebo controls based on competing accounts of the investigator's obligation to minimize risks to subjects. The problem here is that, in cases in which participants would not receive treatment outside of the trial, the question of whether it is permissible to withhold proven effective treatments is not reducible to the question of the role-specific obligations of investigators. Instead, the issue is whether investigators and research sponsors have duties as members of the global moral community to provide existing treatments. To establish this point, it will be helpful to consider some hypothetical cases.

The first case is a variation on the Surfaxin case:

Case 1: A pharmaceutical company proposes conducting a placebo-controlled trial in a developing country to test a new intervention for a fatal disease. There is a proven effective treatment for the disease produced by one of the company's competitors, but it is too expensive to be the standard of care for the country. The company could conduct the trial just as effectively with the existing treatment as it could with the control, and the overall cost would be the same as the placebo trial (say because of some unusual circumstance that makes it necessary to have a larger group of participants to use the placebo control). However, the company prefers to use the placebo because it has a great deal of animus toward its competitors, and does not want to support them by purchasing their products.

In this case, participants on the placebo control are not deprived of a treatment they would otherwise receive outside of the trial. According to V2 and V3″, investigators do not violate their obligations to participants by employing a placebo control because the use of a placebo neither violates the standard of care of the country nor creates serious risks for those on the placebo. Yet, it seems clear that the use of a placebo control is morally unacceptable. Investigators surely act wrongfully when, as in this case, they withhold a lifesaving treatment from research subjects for patently trivial reasons.[56] And this suggests that investigators do at least sometimes have an obligation to provide proven effective treatments to trial participants even when those treatments would be unavailable to participants outside of the trial.

One might claim that what informs our intuition that it is morally wrong to withhold proven effective treatments in this case is the belief that doing so violates the therapeutic obligation (V1) or the obligation to minimize risks to research participants (V3″). But consideration of a second case creates trouble for this claim:

> Case 2: There is a small nation that has amassed great wealth through the hard work and ingenuity of its citizens. The citizens of this country are strongly committed to alleviating suffering in the Third World and donate very large sums of money to this cause. They are also obsessed with their own health and invest enormous resources in finding ways to lead long and healthy lives. Researchers in the country develop a pill that is highly effective in treating a fatal disease. But the pill is extraordinarily expensive to produce, so much so that this is the only nation in the world in which the pill is considered the standard of care. In the United States, the standard of care is a pill that is only a quarter as effective as this one. Investigators in this small nation believe that they now have an even more effective pill. They want to test the pill in the United States with the U.S. standard of care as the control, because this will serve as the most efficient way to determine the effectiveness of the new intervention.

In this case, the trial would deny participants assigned to the control arm a treatment that is known to be far more effective than the control. Moreover, some participants face a serious and unnecessary risk of dying from the disease. Nonetheless, I do not think most of us would find this trial to be morally troubling. It seems morally acceptable because we do not believe that other countries have an obligation to contribute their wealth to improve our health care. While the research sponsor in this case takes advantage of our relative lack of wealth, our absolute standard of living is too great to allow us to have a legitimate claim on the wealth of other countries. There is no reason to presume that we are the victims of indifference, for we could not reasonably expect to receive this kind of aid in a perfectly beneficent world. Indeed, the philanthropic commitments of the country proposing the trial suggest that this country is appropriately responsive to the needs of persons, and that their providing aid to us might effectively foreclose their providing it to those who have a legitimate claim.

What these cases reveal is that the moral permissibility of denying proven effective treatments to persons who would not otherwise have access to them is not a function of the obligation to provide optimal care or minimize risks. Instead, the morally relevant consideration is whether a research sponsor can refuse to provide effective interventions without violating the duty of beneficence. Withholding effective treatments that research subjects would not receive outside of the trial is morally objectionable if and only if it denies them a kind of aid that investigators have an obligation to provide as members of the global moral community. Placebo-controlled trials in developing countries are exploitative when investigators attempt to benefit from conditions that they have an obligation to improve. But the obligation to improve the lot of the impoverished is one that transcends their role as investigators. It is an obligation that all of us who are in a position to offer aid share by virtue of our humanity.

Perhaps the deepest insight that Kantian ethics affords with respect to clinical trials in developing countries is that the vulnerabilities investigators exploit in conducting these trials exist in large measure because of our collective failure to fulfill the duty of beneficence. We need to show humility in our condemnations of those who exploit the impoverished, as it is our indifference to the true needs of the poor that sows much of the ground of exploitation. We must also exercise caution when legislating against exploitation, for the perverse reality is that the best prospect some persons currently have for improving their lives is to submit to exploitative exchanges. While our indignation at those who exploit the poor is certainly warranted, it is not until the day arrives that our indignation is accompanied by shame that we can hope for real progress.

Acknowledgments

My thanks to the Niarchos Foundation for its generous support of this project and to Richard Dean and Amy Sepinwall for helpful comments.

Notes

1. Immanuel Kant, "On the Proverb: That May Be True in Theory, But Is of No Practical Use," in *Perpetual Peace and Other Essays*, trans. Ted Humphrey (Indianapolis: Hackett, 1992), 89.

2. This point is consistent with the "fair benefits" view, which, in dissent from the general consensus, holds that collateral health benefits from the conduct of research may suffice to prevent exploitation. See "Moral Standards for Research in Developing Countries: From 'Reasonable Availability' to 'Fair Benefits,'" *Hastings Center Report* 34, no. 3 (2004): 17–27.

3. Immanuel Kant, *Groundwork for the Metaphysics of Morals*, trans. J. W. Ellington (Indianapolis: Hackett, 1993), 421.

4. Id.

5. Id. at 424.

6. Id.

7. Id. at 422.

8. Id.

9. Some Kant commentators have argued that we should view his conceptual contradiction test as strictly concerned with logical impossibility, while others have argued that it is practical impossibility that matters. For the former, see A. Wood, "Kant on False Promises," *Proceedings of the Third International Kant Congress*, ed. L. W. Beck (Dordrecht: D. Reidel, 1972); for the latter, see Christine Korsgaard, "Kant's Formula of Universal Law," in *Creating the Kingdom of Ends* (Cambridge: Cambridge University Press, 1996).

10. Barbara Herman, "Murder and Mayhem," in *The Practice of Moral Judgment* (Cambridge, MA: Harvard University Press, 1993).

11. Barbara Herman, "Moral Deliberation and the Derivation of Duties," in *The Practice of Moral Judgment*, 154. This idea is nicely captured in Philip Roth's *Everyman*, in a character's reflections on her husband's lies about an affair: "Lying is cheap, contemptible control over the other person. It's watching the other person acting on incomplete information—in other words, humiliating herself." Philip Roth, *Everyman* (New York: Houghton Mifflin, 2006), 121.

12. *Groundwork, supra* note 3, at 423.

13. See Herman, "Mutual Aid and Respect for Persons," in *The Practice of Moral Judgment*; and Onora O'Neil, "Universal Laws and Ends-in-Themselves," in *Contructions of Reason* (Cambridge: Cambridge University Press, 1989).

14. *Groundwork, supra* note 3, at 429.

15. *Id.* at 427.

16. *Id.* at 428.

17. This is in fundamental opposition to consequentialist and modern decision-theoretic accounts, which view rational choice as serving a merely instrumental role in producing valuable states of affairs.

18. Christine Korsgaard, "Kant's Formula of Humanity," in *Creating the Kingdom of Ends*.

19. Allen Wood, *Kant's Ethical Thought* (Cambridge: Cambridge University Press, 1999), 130.

20. *Groundwork*, *supra* note 3, at 430.

21. As Korsgaard argues, the deceiver treats persons as mere means because he treats an agent's reason "as a mediate rather than a first cause." Korsgaard, "The Right to Lie," in *Creating the Kingdom of Ends*, 141.

22. Immanuel Kant, *The Metaphysics of Morals*, trans. and ed. Mary Gregor (Cambridge: Cambridge University Press, 1996), 463, 465.

23. Council for International Organizations of Medical Sciences (CIOMS), *International Ethical Guidelines for Biomedical Research Involving Human Subjects* (1993), Commentary on Guideline 8, at 25.

24. George Annas and Michael Grodin, "Human Rights and Maternal-Fetal HIV Transmission Prevention Trials in Africa," *American Journal of Public Health* 88 (1998): 560–63, at 562.

25. *Id.*

26. *Id.*

27. Allen Wood, "Exploitation," in *Exploitation*, ed. K. Neilsen and R. Ware (New York: Humanities Press, 1997), 2–26, at 15.

28. *Id.* at 17.

29. The standard view has been that Kant supports only a minimalist state, which is limited to protecting individuals from interferences with their freedom. For some recent challenges to this view, see Alexander Kaufman, *Welfare in the Kantian State* (Oxford: Oxford University Press, 1999); and Allen Rosen, *Kant's Theory of Justice* (Ithaca, NY: Cornell University Press, 1993).

30. Some theorists have made a case for extending the reach of principles of justice beyond our own borders. Thomas Pogge, for example, argues that there is a global economic order, and that this order plays an "important causal role . . . in the reproduction of poverty and inequality." Pogge, "Priorities of Global Justice," in *Global Justice* (Oxford: Blackwell, 2001). While I am sympathetic with this position, I am skeptical about the prospect of demonstrating a causal link between the global economic order and suffering in the Third World that is strong enough to ground obligations to help all the persons who need it. The Kantian account of beneficence that I develop later gets around this problem by providing the moral foundation for aiding all persons with serious needs.

31. *Metaphysics of Morals*, *supra* note 22, at 326.

32. *Id.* at 453.

33. *Groundwork, supra* note 3, at 430.

34. Herman, *supra* note 13, at 70.

35. *Metaphysics of Morals, supra* note 22, at 393.

36. Herman, *supra* note 123, at 67.

37. C. R. Beitz, "Does Global Inequality Matter?" in *Global Justice*, ed. Thomas Pogge (Oxford: Blackwell, 2001), 115.

38. *Metaphysics of Morals, supra* note 22, at 393.

39. *Id.* at 454.

40. *Id.*

41. *Metaphysics of Morals, supra* note 22, at 390.

42. *Groundwork, supra* note 3, at 422.

43. Thomas Hill, "Kant on Imperfect Duty and Supererogation," in *Dignity and Practical Reason in Kant's Moral Philosophy* (Ithaca, NY: Cornell University Press, 1992), 147–73.

44. *Id.* at 152.

45. One might argue that even the person who falsely believes that all relief organizations are ineffective displays indifference. For one who makes an effort at educating oneself about relief organizations would learn that many are quite effective; and a person who adopted the maxim of beneficence would presumably wish to educate herself about such matters.

46. Pogge, *supra* note 30, at 13.

47. The only exception would be in the very rare instance that even the most minimal contribution would undermine one's being well-off.

48. Cf. CIOMS, *supra* note 23; National Bioethics Advisory Commission, *Ethical and Policy Issues in International Research: Clinical Trials in Developing Countries* (Bethesda, MD: NBAC, 2001); Annas and Grodin, *supra* note 24; Robert Crouch and John Arras, "AZT Trials and Tribulations," *Hastings Center Report* 28, no. 6 (1998): 26–34.

49. Again, this point is in line with the "fair benefits" view. See *supra* note 2. However, the "fair benefits" view does not specify the conditions under which benefits offered through the conduct of a trial are sufficient to prevent exploitation. The application of my theoretical account later in the chapter seeks to make progress on this issue.

50. GlaxoSmithKline 2001 Annual Report.

51. See, e.g., Benjamin Freedman, K. C. Glass, and Charles Weijer, "Placebo Orthodoxy in Clinical Research II: Ethical, Legal, and Regulatory Myths," *Journal of Law, Medicine and Ethics* 24 (1996): 252–59, at 253; World Medical Association, "Declaration of Helsinki: Ethical Principles for Medical Research

Involving Human Subjects," *Journal of the American Medical Association* 284 (2000): 3043–45.

52. See, e.g., C. Grady, "Science in the Service of Healing," *Hastings Center Report* 28, no. 6 (1998): 34–38, at 36; S. Salim and K. Abdool, "Placebo Controls in HIV Perinatal Transmission Trials: A South African's Viewpoint," *American Journal of Public Health* 88 (1998): 564–66, at 565.

53. Franklin Miller and Howard Brody, "What Makes Placebo-Controlled Trials Unethical?" *American Journal of Bioethics* 2, no. 2 (2002): 3–9, at 4.

54. *Id.* at 5.

55. *Id.*

56. In the Surfaxin trial, it is possible that considerations of cost were not trivial. The cost for surfactant treatments is $1,100 to $2,400 per newborn. In a trial with several hundred individuals receiving the treatment, the cost could be significant, especially if the biotech company is a small one. This is not to deny that there is an obligation to provide the existing treatment as the control in the Surfaxin case. But it is not as clear-cut a case as Case 1 is.

Exploitation and the Enterprise of Medical Research

ALISA L. CARSE AND MARGARET OLIVIA LITTLE

Introduction

According to some, exploitation is a moral red herring. To be sure, it will be said, we know that coercion is wrong. So, too, manipulation, deception, and fraud: all of these undermine the voluntariness of agreement. But why, it will be asked, is there anything morally amiss when genuine consent has been achieved? A seamstress may agree to modest wages, a person may trade sex for money, but just so long as their agreements are based on an undistorted appreciation of potential burdens and benefits, it is morally permissible to pay the wage and take the sex. One might deplore the background conditions that lead them to make this choice; one might even argue for broad social responsibilities to right these conditions. Given their existence, though, there is no reason further to constrain the permissibility of such voluntary transactions. To do so is needlessly limiting of all parties and, indeed, paternalistic to the weaker party: after all, by that party's own lights, acceptance of the transaction is worthwhile.[1]

For many, though, some of the most vexing moral worries start, rather than end, with voluntary agreement. When a manufacturer pays dressmakers five cents a unit, when a soldier pays a hungry woman a dollar for sex, the voluntariness of the transaction does not seem to render it innocent of wrongdoing: the background conditions in virtue of which the exchange is agreed to, we may worry, can raise the specter of exploitation. For those who share this intuition, the challenge is to articulate what exploitation is and the distinctive form of wrong it constitutes. These sorts of questions about exploitation—concerning both its conceptual bona fides and its application—have long occupied the medical research community. How and when can we justify using a person's body, especially when he or she is ill, to gain knowledge to benefit others? Debate has recently become particularly heated over proposals by researchers in developed countries to test new drugs and procedures in acutely impoverished communities. Some have condemned such research as a paradigmatic example of exploitation: when the drugs tested could be afforded only by the world's most prosperous, or again when the study is designed in a way that withholds interventions already known to improve health and save lives, even genuinely voluntary participants are wronged.[2] Others have rejected the charge of exploitation as misplaced: so long as participants have given informed and rational consent, and especially if their participation yields them net benefits, what is the problem?[3]

In this chapter, we side with those who believe that clinical research trials can be exploitative of participants even if enrollment is voluntary and participation beneficial. Our explanation of such exploitation, though—and what it takes to avoid it—is based on an approach to exploitation that is, in crucial ways, essentially contextualist: on our view, one cannot determine what counts as exploitation without reference to the substantive moral norms governing the kind of enterprise in which one is engaged. On this approach, understanding whether, when, and *why* research on impoverished, often medically needful, communities is exploitative requires reflection on the normative purposes and stakes of clinical research.

In the first half of this chapter, we set out our conception of exploitation. In the second half, we apply this conception to clinical research in developing countries, articulating what we take to be crucial aims and constraints appropriate to that general enterprise. Our hope is that the account of exploitation we offer can help us navigate the defining moral tension confronting research in impoverished communities: the imperative, on the one hand, not to take wrongful advantage of existing conditions of injustice and deprivation while, on the other, remaining responsive to the profound health needs those conditions so often generate.

Fairness, Dignity, and Vulnerability

Often in life, we benefit without burdening others in any way, as when we take advantage of the sunshine to get some warmth, or follow another's taillights to find our way in the fog.[4] Such cases carry no implication that the benefit comes at anyone else's expense—even, indeed, if the benefit is conditional on the existence of another's burden (think of the gratification a Good Samaritan might feel in helping another in need).

But other times, a benefit one party enjoys comes *by way of* a cost or burden to the other. It may be an opportunity cost: the dollar that could have gone to B in the exchange goes instead to A. It may be an added burden: the sexual gratification A enjoys is in fact degrading to B. When A benefits by way of a cost to B, we might call this *exacting a benefit*. One can exact a benefit strategically (as when one actively negotiates the terms of the transaction) or passively (as when one accepts the terms one comes across).

Now, not all exactings are wrongful. When you and I play a clean game of chess and I take your king, I have exacted a win but have not committed a wrong. Or while the customer might prefer to pay even less for the bread the baker sells—to keep ten cents more in her pocket—this hardly entails that the baker is exacting too high a price for his bread. But some exactings are wrongful. Exploitation, in the moralized sense, is meant to refer to a particular subclass of these. The nature of the subclass is most clearly explored by looking at cases in which the wrong of coercion is not in play—by looking, that is, at exactings that are wrongful even though they are entered into by voluntary agreement and even if, in significant ways, they are mutually beneficial.[5] What, then, might make a voluntary and even mutually beneficial exchange nonetheless wrongful and, more specifically, *exploitative*? It is this question we want to address.

Philosophers have looked primarily to two different concepts in giving their answers. For some, exploitation is a species of *unfairness*. Even if a transaction benefits both parties, the *distribution* of those benefits may be unfair. Different criteria of fair distribution are offered. Some, following broadly Marxist lines, argue that transactions are unfair when one party gets a disproportionate amount of the profit relative to the labor or resources each contributes.[6] Others, such as Alan Wertheimer, focus on the division of the "social surplus" generated by the transaction (the division, that is, of the value represented in the overlap of the parties' reserve prices), judging proper distribution often, though not always, by reference to an idealized market price.[7] Still others invoke a favored theory of ideal justice from which to gauge the fairness of an exchange.[8]

For others, exploitation is a species not of unfair distribution but of failure to respect the *dignity* of another. Metaphorically, a transaction is exploitative when one party simply "uses" the other; in exacting benefit from the transaction, one party treats the other as a "mere means" or "instrument" in the service of his or her ends. Working centrally, though not exclusively, from the Kantian tradition, members of this camp once again offer different criteria of their concept's application. Some offer a consent-based criterion: to be treated as a mere means is to be treated in a manner to which one *could* not, or for some, *ought* not, rationally consent.[9] Others connect treating another as a mere means to assaults on his or her subjective sense of dignity. Still others argue that certain *kinds* of exchanges—exacting sex for money, say—are intrinsically degrading, whether or not the exploited party experiences them as such.[10]

Both the fairness- and dignity-based approaches get at something deep; they both characterize morally wrongful exactings. But neither, we believe, successfully locates what would count as the distinctive character of wrongful exactings that are also, and as such, exploitative. To accomplish this, we need to go further. What matters to exploitation is not just *what* is agreed to in an exchange (such that the exchange is unfair, say, or degrading), but also *why* an agreement with such problematic content is accepted by the one for whom it is thusly problematic. Let us explain.

In common parlance, exploitative transactions are thought, most centrally and most deeply, to have something to do with the idea of wrongfully taking advantage of another's *vulnerability*. Such transactions, it is said, wrest benefit from *weaknesses* one should leave be—or alleviate.[11] If Bill Gates cedes all of the social surplus generated in the transaction with his caviar vendor because he cannot be bothered to press for a better deal, we might acknowledge the unfairness of this transaction, but it seems odd to claim that Bill has been *exploited*—at least insofar as it is Bill's riches rather than, say, an irrepressible addiction to caviar, that explain his disinclination to press for a fair price. If there's one thing Bill isn't, it's economically vulnerable. Or, again, consider a sexual exhibitionist who agrees with genuine delight to trade sex for money (he sees this transaction, we will imagine, as doubly good— it presents an opportunity for exhibitionism for which he will even be paid!). Even if one thinks the transaction is inherently degrading, it would seem strange to regard such a transaction as thereby "exploitative." In neither case is the agreement grounded in a genuine vulnerability; whatever other moral concerns these exchanges raise, exploitation is not one of them.

Of course, in the usual case, people do not agree to morally problematic terms *unless* they are in a position of some kind of vulnerability, which is why the point is easy to miss. More deeply, it may well be that the classifications of transactions as "unfair" or "degrading" are built up out of concerns that ultimately trace to what count, within a given realm, as vulnerabilities from which it would, in that realm, be wrong to exact benefit. Consider, for instance, unfairness. Not just any high price counts as unfair: if the unrestricted market price effected by temporary monopolies is often regarded as unfair (the lone snowplow driver who exacts maximum price from stranded motorists), it is not always (the entrepreneur who strikes gold when she introduces her novel invention into the marketplace). Such distinctions may tacitly rely on morally substantive views about which sorts of vulnerabilities, in which kinds of contexts, are *likely* to be present in a given sort of exchange, and which of these, given the broader goals at stake in the context of interaction, we ought to protect. The motorist in question is in dire need of the snowplow's help. He is in this sense acutely vulnerable; and it is his vulnerability that enables the snowplow driver to exact such a high fee—a fee the motorist would, but for his vulnerability in such straits, not agree to.

Or, again, consider the classification "degrading." The judgment that certain transactions compromise others' dignity may tacitly be grounded in assumptions about which forms of dignitary vulnerability are both paradigmatic to and problematic in a given kind of context—in which forms of conduct paradigmatically or predictably cause in the other a sense of shame, humiliation, or diminishment. If the delighted exhibitionist is having fun, he is also unusual: often, publicly traded sex is experienced as, among other things, degrading—a fact that is key to interpreting the meaning of the action more broadly.

Judgments of unfairness and dignitary assault, in short, may well be deeply tied to assumptions about which forms of vulnerability are conceptually central in different kinds of transactional contexts. It is thus no accident that discussions of exploitation often focus on issues of fairness and dignity. Nonetheless, if we focus only on fairness and dignity, we will miss what makes exploitation distinctive. For an essential element of exploitative interactions, we want to argue, is their tie to *actual*, rather than paradigmatic or usual, vulnerabilities. Bill Gates is laughing all the way to the bank; the delighted exhibitionist, "officially" degraded, counts his experience as the highlight of his year: these are not the sorts of transactions that a moralized notion of exploitation is meant to condemn. Even if classifications of fairness and respect are tied to judgments about what kinds of vulnerabilities are paradigmatically present and problematic in certain kinds of cases, then, it is possible for an exchange to count as officially unfair or degrading but not exploitative, if the one who accedes to the exchange is not in fact vulnerable in the ways regarded to be relevantly problematic within this kind of exchange. Exploitation, at its heart, is not just about unfair shares or garden-variety degradation; it is about wrongfully exacting benefit from another's actual vulnerability.

When, then, *is* it wrong to exact benefit from another's actual vulnerability? We believe that the answer is often importantly contextual. Taking advantage of someone's gullibility is problematic when trying to have sex with them, but not when trying to get them to pick a card for the fun magic trick you just learned. Taking advantage of time pressure is improper for the funeral home director making arrangements with a grieving family, but not for the trader on the floor of the stock exchange. Taking advantage of another's susceptibility to distraction is improper when trying to secure their consent to surgery; it is precisely the point, as Alan Wood puts it, when playing chess.[12]

Whether it is wrongful to exact benefit from another's actual vulnerability, we maintain, is often a function of the roles or relationships occupied in a given context, of the practice in which the transaction takes place, of what we will, more broadly, call the *normative enterprise* in which the parties are engaged. What constrains a friend is different from what constrains an economic partner; what constrains a physician is different from what constrains a parent. To be sure, some types of vulnerabilities may ground more global constraints on the benefits it is permissible to take: many will argue that others' dire straits always constrain the benefits we may morally negotiate from them. But many of the most important such constraints are grounded in the morally substantive (and often contested) norms governing a specific enterprise, and even, in some kinds of cases, keyed to the finely grained details of the case at hand as they play out given the actual vulnerabilities present (when one may exact benefit from another's perverse sense of fun may well depend not only on whether one is friend or foe but on what benefit, under what circumstances, is gained).

Sometimes, indeed, the norms identify certain types of vulnerabilities as inappropriate grounds for transaction, even if the terms of the transaction are not worrisome on other grounds. Imagine that you have secured your graduate student's agreement to help you weed your long-neglected garden. If she agrees because she genuinely enjoys your company, or looks forward to the anticipated workout, the agreement might not have been problematic. But if, as may be all too likely, she agrees to help out of deference to your power and authority as her teacher, or out of fear that, were she to decline, you will retaliate with a low grade, then something has gone awry. The benefit you derive here is wrongfully derived, for your student's agreement to render you that benefit is secured in virtue of a vulnerability from which you arguably ought not, as her *teacher*, exact benefit. Here, then, it is the *type* of vulnerability out of which agreement is secured—more specifically, the type of vulnerability given the parties' respective roles—that determines the transaction's nature as exploitative. Of course, the risks of agreement based on problematic grounds may be high: it is precisely because your request is made in the context of a significant power differential that you ought to take care in how you make the request; if the risk is high enough, you should not make it at all. The central point, though, is that transactions can count as exploitative even if their terms look innocuous when abstracted from the relationship or roles of the parties, just in case the transaction is reached by pressing on a type of vulnerability that the relationship or role marks as especially protected.

There are, thus, two basic structures of exchange we characterize as genuinely exploitative:

> *First*, as with someone selling sexual services out of acute impoverishment, a transaction is exploitative if the terms of the exchange both are wrongful in their own right—unfair or degrading (or, for that matter, cruel or obtuse)—and are agreed to out of vulnerability.
>
> *Second*, as with the graduate student, a transaction is exploitative if terms that are not in and of themselves wrongful (e.g., unfair, degrading, or otherwise morally problematic) are agreed to by one party in virtue of a *kind* of vulnerability that the other is especially constrained in benefiting from given the normative enterprise in which the transaction is undertaken.

Particularly worrisome are cases of exploitation in which constraints on terms and types of vulnerability coincide—that is, transactions whose terms are already wrongful to one party are agreed to by that party out of the *very kind* of vulnerability the other is especially constrained in pressing given his role or the enterprise in which the transaction is undertaken. A cosmetic surgeon who charges fees we regard as exorbitant by fair market standards *and* who plays on his patients' low self-esteem and suffering to get them to pay such fees is adding insult to injury, morally speaking: given that one of the defining goals of the physician is to attempt to heal, the vulnerabilities in virtue of which the patient accedes to his fee are precisely those vulnerabilities the surgeon has a role-specific charge to try to alleviate. Many cases of exploitation we find most troubling in the real world take this form. Such exploitation involves, in essence, a double wrong: one party agrees to terms of exchange that would be morally out of bounds even if she herself were not vulnerable, and she agrees out of a vulnerability from which the other party is, in the context at hand, especially constrained in exacting benefit.

Details to one side, exploitation occurs when one party agrees out of vulnerability to let another benefit from them on "the moral cheap." Whether or not it is morally permissible for the exploited party to so agree, note, is its own, complicated question, especially if he or she is in dire straits. We ourselves would argue that in certain conditions, sustaining a core sense of dignity may require participating in exchanges that are even in significant ways dignity-compromising or unfair. (If the only way to feed your children, given exigencies of circumstance, is to stay in a job in which you are, say, sexually harassed, and hence treated disrespectfully, staying in that job may nonetheless be crucial to retaining your more fundamental sense of dignity.) Whatever one thinks about assessments of the exploited party in agreeing to an exploitative exchange, we must distinguish this from assessments of the *exploiter's* engagement in the exchange. It is wrong-making to exploit another, even if that other's decision to participate is rationally and morally defensible. Exploitative transactions are, in this sense, *morally asymmetrical.*

Mere Means Revisited

We have argued that one form of exploitation (type 1 above) involves pressing a vulnerability to get someone to accept terms that are independently morally wrong. We now want to take a closer look at one of the most common ways in which terms can be morally wrongful—namely, when they treat another as an "object of use" or a "mere means." While much ink has been devoted to issues of fairness in the context of exploitation, many of the most important concerns raised by exploitation are not in fact distributive ones—worries about exorbitant prices, profit shares, and the like; they are worries about exchanges in which people's deep vulnerabilities lead them to agree to be treated in *overly instrumental, degrading* ways.

But there is much confusion—and suspicion—surrounding this idea. Unpacking what it means to be treated as an "object of use," or in an overly "instrumental" manner, or improperly as a "mere means" or "tool" in the service of another's agenda, is notoriously difficult. Many have maintained that such notions are so metaphoric that there is no "there" there. Others point to the limits of consent-based criteria, according to which treating others as a "mere instrument" involves treating them in a manner to which they could not, or, again, ought not, rationally consent. Such an approach is of limited use here. After all, on its more empirical version, agents apparently can, and do, consent to even worrisome arrangements; on its more normative version, exploitative transactions turn out to morally censure the exploited: if an exchange counts as exploitative, *both* parties are, on such an account, doing something they ought not.

We propose that there are two key notions of wrongful use that are neither metaphoric nor consent-based; as will become clear, each turns out to be of central importance in the context of human subjects research.

The first conception is a moral psychological one. It concerns, at its core, a subjective *attitude* or mental *construal* one agent has of another, namely, a construal in which the other's usefulness to one's own agenda excessively—and, at the limit, exhaustively—orients one's perceptions, emotional responses, expressive conduct, and treatment of the other. If the toll booth operator drops dead of a heart attack just as you pull your car up and your immediate reaction is one of acute annoyance, you are, in a psychological sense, treating him as a mere object of use.

Such worrisome attitudes are tied to an extremely important subset of worries about exploitation, namely, those concerning actively, strategically, and wrongfully pressing an advantage—what we might call the activity of exploit*ing*. As many have pointed out, it is not necessary that a transaction be intentionally exploitative for it to count as exploitative: exploitation can be unwitting. But actively and strategically exacting benefit does mark a particular wrong, for it precisely involves a psychological attitude toward the other that excessively (or exhaustively) regards him in terms of his usefulness to one's own agenda. Such objectifying attitudes matter, and matter deeply, not only because they bear on issues of virtuous character, but because they inform the "expressivist" import of our conduct—the broader moral *meaning* an action carries. Such meaning can be crucial: it is the expressive character of our conduct that often determines the difference, say, between insult and respect.

Concerns of expressivist import are also broad in scope. Actions, as many have noted, can come to have expressivist meaning independently of the attitudes and intentions lurking in an individual's heart.[13] Calling one's male colleague "boy" has a public or social meaning of denigration, whether or not an insult was literally intended by the speaker. This general point turns out to have particular relevance, as we will see, in enterprises that are governed by regulations and guidelines. For policies and regulations *themselves* can have expressivist import. The regulations we write express the values we hold: what we allow and prohibit, which dangers we note and which we ignore, what rationale we specify and what we leave out. All these factors can contribute to the expressivist import of the actions justified by reference to our policies and regulations.[14]

The first conception of wrongful use we have set out, then, is tied to attitudinal and expressivist notions of objectification. The second conception we would like to mark out is tied to notions of commodification. There is, we want to argue, a helpful functionally specified conception of treating others in an overly instrumental fashion—namely, one that unpacks the metaphors of using another improperly as a "means," "tool," or "instrument" in terms of inappropriately governing one's actions under the positive norms of the marketplace.[15]

According to what we will call "marketplace norms," a transaction is morally permissible just so long as both parties are competent, fully informed, and sufficiently instrumentally rational, and there is no deception, fraud, manipulation, threat, coercion, or force. Within these constraints, the governing regulative ideal is one of *mutual use:* agents should aim to negotiate the highest yield for themselves. Debate exists, of course, over the proper scope of marketplace norms. Marxists will say they are nowhere appropriate; libertarians will say they are appropriate everywhere other than in certain voluntarily assumed roles. Many will at least agree to their propriety in many one-off transactions—say, buying ice cream from a street vendor.

But whatever one's views on these (important) debates, virtually everyone agrees that there are *some* exchanges that ought not be governed by the norms and ideals of the marketplace. There are many types of roles and relationships—parent, physician, teacher—that bring with them a richer array of obligations, ideals, and regulative norms than those constraining marketplace negotiation. Where norms of mutual use are not appropriate, pursuing one's utility or interests in the ways they allow is a form of treating the other in an overly instrumental way. Someone who interprets the reciprocity appropriate to friendship as a matter of quid pro quo exchanges, for instance, has misunderstood the nature of friendship.

The problem, note, is not with the marketplace norms per se. Where they are appropriate, as we think they sometimes are, wresting everything one can within their bounds does not constitute treating the other in a problematically instrumental way (and can, indeed, be a way of expressing respect). What *is* problematic is governing one's behavior by marketplace norms outside of their proper moral scope. Just which constraints we should acknowledge is a question of substantive ethics. While some will point to constraints grounded in the idea of a "person as such," there are also, once again, constraints specific to the goals and aspirations of given enterprises such as family, friendship, or health care. While the basic moral conviction to treat others as having "dignity rather than price" is not itself enterprise or role-specific, that is, many of the ways in which we fill out what more specifically counts as treating another as a "mere means" get fleshed out in enterprise- and role-specific terms.

When we inappropriately downgrade to the marketplace norms, we are improperly maximizing our own utility or interests (broadly construed). We can also, ironically, end up treating others problematically as objects of use in the (often more altruistic) interest of seeking the "greater good." If a firm hires a token woman into a chilly corporate climate to reduce the incidence of sexist jokes, this surely risks treating her in instrumental fashion, even though the motive is improving the corporate culture, and thus the aggregate good of the firm. Once again, it is not utilitarian norms per se that are problematic. There may well be isolated realms or questions for which its terms are exactly right. But where one inappropriately understands another's usefulness in its terms—an issue, again, filled in as a matter of substantive ethics—one has in this sense treated the other in an overly instrumental way.

On this conception of treating others in an overly instrumental way, then, we treat others as mere means, functionally specified, when we ignore certain moral "trade-off" constraints on garnering benefit—more specifically, when we inappropriately govern our behavior and justifications by the norms of the marketplace or, again, of maximizing aggregate utility.

Both conceptions of wrongful use we have highlighted—the one centered on inappropriate objectification and grounded in moral psychology, the other pointing to inappropriate commodification, functionally specified—are key in moral life. On both conceptions, wrongful use turns out to be a *degreed* notion: treating someone as an "instrument," "tool," or market "commodity" can be more or less thoroughgoing (one's attitude may be more or less objectifying, one may ignore one or several trade-off constraints), as well as more or less egregious (the moral import of an attitude expressed, as well as of ignoring a given trade-off constraint, can vary). On both conceptions, too, what counts as degrading is often indexed to the enterprise at hand: expression or conduct that in one context counts as treating another disrespectfully can be fully respectful in another.

Once again, treating others as mere means, in either the moral psychological or the functionally specified sense, does not itself suffice for exploiting them. It is only if another agrees to such terms out of vulnerability that degradation turns into exploitation. And if the vulnerability in virtue of which another agrees to the transaction is of the *very kind* one is especially constrained in pressing, the transaction is doubly wrong. How egregious a case of exploitation is will depend on how morally serious the wrongs involved are and the nature of the vulnerabilities in play; these factors, too, are often indexed to the enterprise at hand.

Clinical Research in the Developing World

With these clarifications in hand, we now want to turn our attention to the exploitative potential of conducting clinical research trials in acutely impoverished, often poorly educated, communities in the developing world. Many different sorts of criticisms have been levied against such research.

One important set centers on the potential *unfairness* of such arrangements.[16] Drug companies stand to amass huge profits from knowledge gained by the research; impoverished communities, lacking basic resources, are in a poor position to bargain for what might be seen as a fair share of compensation. Such trials threaten to be just one more instance of the developed world "raping the resources" of the developing world—here the resource of its citizens' bodies, and of the effort expended in serving as research subjects—for the benefit of those already unjustly privileged.

Important as these worries are, it is a different worry we want to focus on. Depending on their background political theories, people will have very different intuitions on what might count as "fair shares" in such exchanges; more important, considerations of transactional fairness do not adequately capture the special sort of worry many have about exploitation in the present context. When Bolivian infants are used to test a drug designed for sale in the United States, the worry is not just about how much money or how many goods change hands; the worry is that those infants are being somehow wrongfully used—treated as objects in the service of the investigators' agenda. These worries are not assuaged simply by increasing compensation or shares of profits; indeed, doing so can add the specter of undue inducement to the worry of wrongful use.[17] These worries, in short, find their home more squarely in the family of *dignity-based* concerns of exploitation outlined earlier. The worry we want to explore is, in essence, that such trials threaten to use the world's poor and vulnerable as our laboratory.

Some investigators will wonder what the problem is. After all, it is pointed out, those who participate in trials, as well as those in their surrounding communities, stand to garner substantial benefits through the agreements—ancillary medical care for participants, infrastructure built to enable research that stays behind after researchers have gone home. Given the dire straits of potential participants, such benefits should be embraced. Just in case there is no outright fraud, lying, or coercion— just in case the participants' agreement is rational by decision-theory metrics—all is well.

But however we regard this as a framework for thinking about the ethics of widget production (and there are plenty of concerns about it there), it constitutes far too low a standard for *clinical research*. Clinical research is a normative enterprise governed by its own special norms. Familiarly, they are not the norms of health care provision: investigators and institutional review boards(IRBs) are not charged (as would be, say, a hospital board) with a fiduciary responsibility to provide the best treatment for those under their charge. Neither, though, are they bound merely by the minimalist norms of the marketplace: justification for study design looks beyond what participants might agree to under conditions of optimal rationality and information.

While there continues to be significant disagreement about the norms governing clinical research, a core set of regulations have been widely agreed upon as integral to ethical research involving human subjects in both domestic and international arenas: (1) high standards for informed consent (investigators have ambitious positive duties to provide the conditions of understanding, rather than relying on the minimal "buyer beware" standard of the marketplace); (2) imposition of minimal risk, where "minimal" is indexed to the importance of the knowledge gained for the goals of public health; (3) scientific validity: trials must be designed in such a way that they would, if carried out, be capable of providing meaningful, robust, and useful data; (4) equipoise: the investigator can undertake and sustain the study only insofar as he or she (or, alternatively, the "medical community") does not yet know by accepted standards of scientific knowledge which arm of the trial is in fact superior;[18] (5) minima on the standard of care offered in the trial: neither arm of the trial can offer less health benefit than what the participants would have received absent their participation in the trial (one does not take someone about to receive penicillin in a clinic and give him something known to be less effective).[19]

These constraints can be thought of as "core protections" that research participants should be afforded. They serve, for one, as constraints on how much and what kind of personal benefits—profits, knowledge, or professional advancement—investigators may accrue through the research. The norms of ethical research are not equivalent to "whatever the market will bear": even if one did think the minimalist norms of the marketplace were appropriate for negotiating shares of *profits* in clinical research, they are not appropriate for determining the contours of *study design*. The core protections also set constraints on using participants for the benefit of the "greater good." We may not, for example, sanction withholding treatment the participants would have been getting but for their participation in the research, or downgrade standards of informed consent, even if the information gained promises to be greatly valuable to researchers or of tremendous overall health utility. Finally, the core protections present limits on what can otherwise be considered as up for negotiation by those keen on achieving (even ambitious) notions of transactional fairness: we may not allow a community to undertake risks and burdens an IRB would not sanction, or to abandon equipoise or appropriate standards of care, even for much needed water wells or ancillary care.

It is true that, in the broad context of research, exceptions to requirements of equipoise and standards of care are sometimes allowed for participants willing to take additional risks on altruistic grounds (with compensatory increases in the measures needed to achieve informed consent). Crucially, though, such exceptions are resisted for research on vulnerable populations—prisoners, the acutely ill, the homeless, as well as those who are deeply impoverished. This is not because vulnerabilities render genuine altruism impossible; it is, rather, a prophylactic policy to guard against what are here empirically high risks of exploitation. It is very difficult in such circumstances to know when it is unpressured altruism, rather than worrisome commodification or undue inducement, that grounds a given agreement. Given these risks, there may be reasons of public policy to place heavy constraints on such exceptions, especially when the potential beneficiaries are not among participants' "nearest and dearest."

The core protections clearly indicate the existence of widespread agreement that constraints on human subjects research are to be significantly more morally stringent and demanding than marketplace norms. Also agreed upon, if not always adequately emphasized, is the special importance of maintaining high standards of respectful comportment throughout the *conduct* of the research. Given the vulnerabilities that so often characterize participation in research—asymmetries of expertise, tendencies of deference to medical authority, exposure of one's body (or the body of one's child), the well-documented tendency of "therapeutic misconception" on the part of participants (the conviction that the investigative process will in fact offer one therapeutic benefit)—clinical researchers occupy a role marked by heightened responsibility. One key responsibility is to sustain an acute awareness of what we might call *emergent* vulnerabilities, many of which are dignitary ones, generated out of the dynamic of the researcher-participant interaction itself. As a researcher, I may poke, inject, touch, and access parts of your body; I may, in some cases, regard you in your nakedness. But *how* I do this can mark the difference between objectification and respect: researchers have obligations to mitigate such vulnerabilities as much as possible. This will entail respectful communication and engagement, attention to the expressive dimensions of conduct (in the explanations you are offered, the way you are touched, the concern and attentiveness extended you as a person, rather than a mere object of investigation). This may involve seeking explicit permission from you in undertaking invasive, uncomfortable, or risky procedures that are an intrinsic part of the investigative process to which you have already "signed on."[20]

All of these norms—some codified in regulations, others existing as shared recommendations for "best practices"—aim to reduce the risk of exploitation in clinical research trials.

One baseline issue, then, is clear. Studies ought not afford less than the "core protections," even if potential participants could be located who, given their vulnerable conditions, would be willing to enroll in them. Given the incentive structures found in the world economy—the money that stands to be made by pharmaceuticals and the desperation of those in dire straits—those vetting study design do well to police these regulations with vigilance when considering proposals for research in the developing world. So, too, those executing studies must remain keenly aware of participant vulnerability and the implications this has for respectful engagement with them.

Controversies over Standards beyond the Minima

Matters quickly get more complicated, however; for the consensus core protections, it turns out, go only so far. Even though there is wide agreement that core protections constitute minima, there is much disagreement about why the core protections alone are inadequate, let alone what additional constraints and requirements are called for. In this section, we address central worries about the sufficiency of consensus protections. We then argue that responses to these worries have been inadequate in protecting against the exploitation of research participants: while there is a need for above-the-minina constraints, no one has yet generated constraints that draw the right lines. Two issues are central: the standard of care owed trial participants and the assurance of reasonable availability to participants (or morally relevant cohorts) of successful treatment protocols.

Standard of Care

Many have worried that the core consensus standards, as we have called them, do not adequately address concerns about the standards of care trial participants are owed. Consensus standards can be thought of as aimed, in essence, at protecting participants from immediate or direct harm—from worsening their health conditions relative to what they would (or should de jure) be were they not to participate in the study. But for those in dire straits, such standards turn out to require very little. Given how little those in poverty would have gotten by way of health benefits were the trial not to take place, or again, how little they were in a sense directly entitled to by their own deeply constrained public health system, the core protections are consistent with exceedingly low standards of care. Crucial as they are, core protective regulations turn out to be de minima.

Of course, investigators focused narrowly on harm may say there is no problem. It's all very well and good to talk of a trial "withholding" treatments like established surfactants, but that begs the question regarding what standard of care we should use against which to judge an intervention as withholding, rather than not providing, treatment. Once we are above the baseline of core protective regulations, everything is benefit, one might think; even if the benefit is modest rather than ambitious, any is still better than none. We might as a matter of charity choose to do more, but doing so is not morally required.

But this is too weak. The idea that investigators may "cherry-pick" among the world's poor to find those with low levels of baseline health care—levels often themselves the result of deep and systemic injustice—to approximate the cost savings of placebo-controlled trials seems morally suspicious, to put it mildly. To conduct research on suffering populations *because* the de minima standard of care is there so easily met is frankly contrary to the aspirations of clinical research: it exploits a "moral loophole" that meets the letter but violates the spirit of the moral enterprise at issue.

Moved by this concern, the Declaration of Helsinki, reiterated in the guidelines of the Council for International Organizations of Medical Sciences (CIOMS), established a highly restrictive regulation.[21] It requires that "the benefits, risks, burdens and effectiveness of a new method should be tested against those of *the best current prophylactic, diagnostic, and therapeutic methods*."[22] Unrestricted in the scope over which we are to measure "best," this standard, in effect, requires that control arms may not fall below the world's best-known treatment. Administering oxygen to infants in order to study a new surfactant, when we already know that other existing surfactants would save their lives, would, for example, be flatly impermissible.

But these regulations, well intentioned as they are, are too strong. As many have pointed out, the idea that research is unethical unless one can, for example, afford to offer state-of-the-art angioplasty or expensive statins seems exaggerated.[23] More than that, the regulations come at a heavy price: on the requirement set by Helsinki and CIOMS, research that is desperately needed for the benefit of the developing world could not be conducted. If we disallow a trial because it fails to test against the world's best-known interventions, then so, too, we must disallow trials such as the short-course AZT trials in Africa—trials that set out to test whether a short course of AZT administered during the last phases of active labor and delivery could reduce maternal-fetal transmission of HIV, given that the full-course AZT therapy known to drastically reduce such transmission rates is far beyond the financial reach of the public health budgets of sub-Saharan countries.[24] Or, again, we would have to disallow trials proposing to study use of microbicides, which bear promise as an inexpensive and easily disseminated method of providing at least some protection against heterosexual transmission of HIV in communities where gender power relations have made it extremely difficult for women to protect themselves by relying on condom use.[25] These interventions were never thought to be as good as the world's best therapies of full-course AZT regimens, or again condom use; they were, instead, seen as beacons of hope that would help save lives for people in desperately constrained situations.

Considerations of this kind have led some to advocate a "host country relevance" constraint: while the "world's best standard of treatment" should be accepted as a default standard, exception can be made when studying interventions that have potential relevance to the country in which participants live.[26] Such a move, intuitive in one sense, is in fact quite dicey. For one thing, it is not sufficiently fine-grained: it intuitively matters *who* benefits within a country (research conducted on poor South African blacks to help well-to-do South African whites hardly seems like progress). More deeply, why individuate by host country in the first place? Why think that political criteria should be morally decisive in delineating the relevant beneficiaries of research (as opposed to its relevance, understandably, to host governments deciding whether to allow research projects within their borders)? Why should "country" be the community whose individuation matters for pegging the relevant standard of care?

Reasonable Availability

Serious questions also plague what has come to be known as the "reasonable availability" standard. To counter worries that research protocols would allow research on subjects who stood no potential to benefit from the knowledge produced, CIOMS regulations were introduced to require researchers to ensure "reasonable availability" of the drug or intervention studied, if proven effective, to those participating in the study. This requirement, though, has not only proven frustratingly vague (how much, for how many, for how long?), it is also both too strong and too weak. It is too strong because some research entities, such as the National Institutes of Health, are well equipped to conduct research designed for the public good but are not in fact set up to provide drugs or interventions. It is too weak because it does not specify that the target of research be related to the participant community's needs. If the drug being studied would be of little or no use to the participant community, the fact that the regulations require it be made available offers cold comfort at best. This would seem a veiled attempt to engage participants in trials that serve a research agenda essentially benefiting others, given on-the-ground realities.

Most deeply, the rationale for a principle of "reasonable availability" is left unclear. If it is fundamentally aimed at ensuring that participants *benefit fairly* from their participation, why restrict the terms of benefit to those of the intervention being studied? Host communities may have far more pressing needs than esoteric interventions on cholesterol levels; why shouldn't the participant community itself decide how best to benefit? This has led some to argue that "reasonable availability" should be abandoned in favor of a requirement that the host community benefit adequately in the terms it itself set—if diapers and water wells are more useful than the drug at hand, compensation should be made in those terms.[27] This would seem to avoid concerns about treating participants as mere objects of use because participants would, on this proposal, have input into the benefit their participation would provide them.

But such proposals have, once again, raised their own controversies.[28] Given worries of improperly commodifying research and undue incentive (always lurking when we introduce the idea of compensation in medical research), it is not intuitively clear whether the proposal is a step forward or backward. For one thing, in emphasizing fairness per se, such a framework does not explain why we could not measure the adequacy of exchange in terms of television sets rather than water wells, if those are the terms requested; yet there seems something worrisome about the idea of clinical researchers bartering just any sort of good for clinical participation. Second, worries arise about the very real possibility that public authorities might offer up segments of "their" populations as research participants (e.g., women, babies) in exchange for collateral infrastructural resources, multiplying rather than reducing the risk of objectifying individual participants. The realities of political authority and social hierarchies can present heavy risk of merely apparent "consent" on the part of participants (e.g., "consent" given under social or political pressure or in a context in which their group membership renders them without meaningful decisional authority).

In short, real controversy begins when we consider regulations that are concerned not directly with protecting participants from research-related harm—at reducing the risks, opportunity costs, and burdens of participation, but with fundamental justificatory questions about conducting the research in the first place. What is the proper standard of care for those enrolled in a trial: the best available world standard, the local standard, no standard other than not making participants worse off than they literally would have been in the trial's absence (so that the participant who in fact would not have made it the two miles to the clinic in the absence of the trial presents researchers with no baseline constraint other than not to harm)? To *whom* must anticipated medical benefits go to avoid using the trial's participants as mere means? How *much* benefit, of what *kind*, must a study promise if it is to avoid the exploitation of the participants it enrolls?

To make progress on these controversies, we believe we need to take a step back. When current regulations are the source of controversy rather than a consensus on which to draw, we need a better articulation of what sort of normative enterprise we are dealing with in the first place. To understand how regulations should here be fashioned, we need a clearer sense of the moral ends they are meant to serve. A key question must be asked, namely, What are the underlying aims and goods of clinical research?

Public Health and the Investigative Stance

How, broadly put, should we conceive of the norms and purposes governing clinical research? If we take the perspective of those charged with constructing regulations for vetting study design and procedure, what norms should they be looking to? We believe the most cogent answer is one that places the enterprise of clinical research under the umbrella of a broad notion of public health. Public health, most generally conceived, is charged with stewardship for the advancement of human health, where human health is understood not as a commodity but as a fundamental dimension of human flourishing. As such, and as we have seen, justificatory frameworks for decisions falling under its broad purview are not those of the marketplace.[29] Just which norms do govern the enterprise, it turns out, depends on which of the several tasks falling under this broad umbrella is at issue.

One familiar sort of task is the *distribution of public health resources*. Distributive questions are of fundamental importance, faced by agencies both small (public service clinics) and large (the National Institutes of Health, the Department of Health and Human Services, the World Health Organization). Given competing jurisdictions (given, that is, that there is no world government using a whole-budget approach), they are also morally complex questions, requiring agencies to decide how to distribute resources when the assignment of responsibility is unclear or even abnegated. Different proposals have been advanced regarding which substantive ethical standards should properly be adopted by public health agencies for purposes of answering these difficult questions, ranging from purely utilitarian ones, according to which we should spend money where it buys the most health care utility, to justice-based (often egalitarian-based) criteria, such as prioritizing the needs of those already most burdened.

A very different task is the *accumulation of knowledge for public health*—the task of clinical research. Of course, distributive questions arise in the context of this task, too, since funding agencies need to decide which problems to prioritize. (Here important calls have been raised for the "world community" to spend more of its research dollars on medical interventions that would help alleviate more suffering—to move its resources from the diseases of the few and the rich to the diseases of the many and the poor.) But the central normative questions that arise in the context of clinical research as an enterprise, as we have seen, concern the proper attitude toward and treatment of those who would *participate in* research studies. These are not primarily questions about distribution of scarce resources; rather, they are questions about what responsibilities and constraints should be seen as governing what we might call the *investigational stance:* the responsibilities investigators and designers have toward those who participate in their studies.

Animating these questions is a central—indeed, defining—tension of clinical research. The central challenge confronting any clinical research on human subjects—rich or poor, healthy or ill—derives from the fact that one gains benefits, as a researcher, that are not fully justified by the participants' own health benefits. Medical research involving human subjects must justify interacting with participants' bodies—and, if they are sick, with medical needs—in order primarily to gain knowledge rather than to treat them. Such a task is, of course, often laudable, but it introduces special justificatory requirements.

More specifically, there are two things, we believe, that stand in need of special justification, and justification in public health terms, when proposing to conduct medical research on human subjects. First and most familiar are responsibilities entailed by the risks and burdens the research imposes on participants. The protective standards, as we saw, aim to keep them minimal; still, any design has residual burdens and risks—blood draws, intubations, surgeries, intimate examinations, and the like—and many of these, in turn, can affect participant dignity.

Second, put bluntly, clinical research needs to justify why, as agents of public health, we are choosing to investigate rather than treat you. Sometimes, of course, this issue does not arise: issues of treatment are otiose in research on healthy subjects. But when, as is often the case, we are taking a research stance toward subjects' illness or medical need, we need to justify why we are spending our efforts studying rather than treating them: we need to justify, as we might put it, the idealized *differential* between taking a fully *therapeutic stance* and an *investigative stance* toward these participants. That differential is located in the risks and burdens that research participation adds to those encountered in being treated (the incremental risks, invasions, and involvement costs); more deeply, it is located in the resources that researchers, again under the aegis of public health, are taking (this money, this equipment, this personnel, and the like) and committing to the investigative endeavor of a research study rather than to therapeutic intervention to allay the health needs of those studied.

This last is, of course, an idealization: there is no pretense that the very dollars or equipment used in research would actually have gone to treat participants had the research not gone forward (as it is so often pointed out, the clinical entourage usually would not have been geographically proximate to, let alone clinically engaged with, those who are participants were it not for the research project). But the point is not about justifying literal opportunity costs (as though there were some über-agency representing public health deciding when to treat and when to undertake research); it is to articulate a tension, within the norms of the public health enterprise, whose navigation demands justification.

Now with some research, these burdens and again differentials are easily justified by the prospect of direct medical benefit to the very participants to whom they apply. Certain Phase III trials involving advanced cancers, for instance, can rightly be thought of as offering a net (if statistical) benefit to participants, given the dearth of other options and the possibility here of success: in these sorts of cases, the ethical challenge is to ensure fair access to the good of participation. But very often, justification resides far more heavily in the prospective benefit to others. If the study design offers some prospect of direct benefit to participants, it is modest in proportion to the degree of burden and differential implicit in the study design; and many studies, namely, Phase I and Phase II trials, as well as longitudinal Phase III studies, offer no prospect of direct benefit because the potential rewards are many years off. Sometimes, in short, the lion's share of justification for burdening you in this way, and again deciding to study rather than treat you, lies in the benefits to others rather than to "you and yours." All of this adds a third factor relevant to justification—the degree to which the trial's justification is located "on behalf of others."

In summary, then, the justificatory burden of a given clinical research trial is a matter of (1) the absolute burdens undertaken by participants, (2) the differential, implicit in the study design, between taking an investigative rather than therapeutic stance toward participants, all weighted by (3) the degree or proportion to which the benefit is directed at others rather than the participants and those whose welfare matters most to them.

These three factors identify a set of desiderata for guiding clinical research regulations: crudely put, we want to minimize the burdens, soften the differential, and diminish the "on behalf of" proportionality relation—all balanced against the laudable goal of relieving as much disease burden as possible throughout the world. These desiderata, we would argue, generate a series of *benchmarks* or *regulative ideals* concerning both *whom* we may conduct research on, and *how*, morally, we must treat those who do enroll.

Take the first issue first. Whom to study is a question that itself demands justification in public health terms; indeed, part of the expressivist import of research conducted on a given set of participants is set by the criteria that guided us in choosing to approach *them* rather than others. We believe there are four key presumptive guides in choosing whom to study. First, we should choose a given cohort for public health–oriented desiderata—to choose a cohort not because the scenery of their location is lovely or the labor cheap, but because they carry particular scientific relevance to the issue at hand (e.g., the transmission rates of disease make it possible to study effects of proposed preventives, a population has genetic polymorphisms particularly helpful in isolating a virus). Second, among those scientifically relevant, we should try to choose those who are among the least vulnerable (least impoverished, hungry, or disempowered), not just because such conditions make it more difficult to secure genuine and unpressured informed consent but because we should try not to further burden those who are already burdened.

Third, and presumptively, the burdens and again differential implicit in study design should be justified by reference to the health utility of the information gained for those relevantly like the participants to whom the burdens and differential apply—but where "relevantly like" is understood *not* as a political or geographic criterion but as *a public health* measure. There are all sorts of ways of defining a community: political (countries, cities), geographic (regions, neighborhoods), cultural (religious or ethnic affiliation), or psychological (social affiliation or identification). Each is important in its own way. But given that what matters here is justification in public health terms, we propose the criteria need to be grounded in the public health enterprise itself—criteria that, while intuitive and without crisp boundaries, to be sure, derive the terms of relevance from the goals, constraints, and normative focus of public health: which disease is at issue, with what level of risk, against which background susceptibilities and resource constraints—the very sorts of variables, that is, that go into demarcating the contours of public health initiatives themselves.

As Christine Grady puts it, "The value of the research question lies in whether the answer could be used to improve health care and to benefit the people represented by those who participate in the research."[30] "Represented," for again, the mark of research is that justification extends to benefits to those beyond the research participants themselves. Crucially, the terms of representation should not be those designated by drug companies or politicians; they should be made by reference to criteria inherent to public health. Put intuitively, what we are saying to participants is this: "We are imposing burdens and risks on you, and taking an investigative rather than fully therapeutic stance toward you, but it is to help those like you in the terms in which we, as public health professionals, are charged to think—namely, in terms of who suffers with this disease as you do, in background conditions relevantly like yours."

Including, presumptively, the participants and those they care most about. A fourth and final core regulative ideal for clinical research is that those studied should, if the intervention proves successful, be likely to be among those who would subsequently enjoy the future stream of health benefits it offers. Lest we end up using participants as mere instruments to help only distant others suffering from their disease, we should try to locate research among participants who will themselves be able to benefit from its success. Doing so, in essence, displays our commitment to try to minimize the "on behalf of" relation. Where prospective benefits are imminent, we should aim to locate the research among those who would be able so to benefit. And where prospective benefit is more distant, it is better to locate the trial among populations whose descendents would likely be able to benefit from those fruits. If not, we want to know why the research is being located there.

None of these considerations are lexically ordered. We may decide to trade off degrees of scientific potency to gain large decreases in the overall vulnerability of prospective participants, or again to allow research on an incrementally more vulnerable cohort if they are more likely to gain significantly by the future stream of benefits should the trial prove successful. And all must be weighed against real-world considerations of which studies are most likely to help alleviate the world's disease burden (weighted, we would say, by the burdens of those most needy). Nonetheless, the four regulative ideals here named—choosing by scientific relevance; minimizing vulnerability; justifying studies by the health benefits to participants, those they care most about, or those relevantly like the chosen cohort in public health terms; and locating studies among populations likely to participate in the future stream of benefits should the trial prove successful—name key benchmarks that exert moral pressure on our decisions, identifying what stands in need of justification when trade-offs are proposed.[31] And when exceptions to given presumptions are made, as at times they should be, it matters that those decisions are reached through a process in which the health needs of the participants did have weight—namely, presumptive weight—integrally related to the justificatory structure.

Standard of Care and Reasonable Availability

What, then, on the framework we propose, should we say about the controversies surrounding the standard of care offered in a study's control arm, and again the issue of reasonable availability? Let us take standard of care first.

Standard of Care Revisited

Given the preceding discussion, there is good reason to insist on a *presumption* that control arms do not offer interventions less than the world's best. For one thing, those who enjoy the best standards of care are likely to be less vulnerable than those who do not, so looking to those who enjoy such standards when deciding where to locate clinical trials is a helpful proxy for avoiding research on those already burdened. More than that, without such a presumption, the criterion of scientific relevance stands in danger of being co-opted. Given that scientific potency is in part an economic notion (high transmission rates of disease allow us to collect data with fewer enrollees or complicated logistics, hence with less outlay of resources), there is always the danger that investigating entities will propose studying populations whose local standard of care is low because the comparison allows us "efficiently"—that is, inexpensively—to gather useful data. We thus need a broad presumption against studies whose control arms give less than our best-known standards of care.

But only a presumption. For also central to public health's mission is finding out how to abate suffering and decrease mortality in countries that cannot remotely afford that standard of care, and hence may not remotely be able to afford treatments that test as more efficacious over that standard. We also need to develop treatments that can be afforded by those who are impoverished and to develop treatments that deal with the diseases of impoverishment.

To be sure, the suffering and deprivation often trace to injustices. Public health, as a steward of health, has a duty to denounce these injustices. But it also has a duty to then ask how to treat the sick and dying given their existence. Such questions are paradigmatic for public health in the real world: How do we treat dysentery in those who have no access to running water, even though they should? How could we minimize vitamin deficiency among those malnourished, even though they would not be malnourished if the world were just? And, very often, the only way to gain needed knowledge is to study those who suffer the deprivation, and against a control arm of the very baseline conditions whose existence we condemn. Not because doing so is cheaper, but because we cannot ethically study the effects of the proposed intervention among those who would have gotten better treatment outside the context of an investigative trial, and because we need to study the intervention in the context of on-the-ground conditions (patterns of nutrition, breastfeeding habits, and the like) not found elsewhere.

Such research, we believe, can thus be ethically crucial, but only under restricted conditions. More specifically, the last two regulative ideals should turn from presumption to requirement. First, the *only* time we should be conducting clinical research trials among impoverished communities that offer less than the world's best treatment in the control arm is when doing so is needed to help those in similar health circumstances (and not, say, because using this population provides an especially cheap way to collect clean data for those who do not suffer the "useful" deprivation). If others also stand to benefit—if the knowledge gained will help develop treatments for another disease or another population—all well and good; but the potential of benefit to those relevantly like the participants, again measured in public health terms, must itself be sufficient to justify the burdens and differential taken to those participants. For *these* studies, extra benefit to others—such as those in the developed world—must be regarded as justificatory gravy.

Second, the very participants or those they care most about must be among those who would stand to benefit from the fruits of the research should it prove successful. We should, as always, try to locate the study among those who would, in the natural course of events, be most likely able to afford and use the drug if the trial proves successful. If we need to locate the study among those who would not otherwise be able so to afford it, though, the price of justification is negotiating provision of the drug or intervention.

In sum, to justify a protocol that uses less than the world's best standard of care, we want to argue, investigators must be able to point to the reasonable likelihood, given on-the-ground conditions of the world as we find it, of sufficient actual benefit to those relevantly like those being studied, and must ensure that those who participate in the study—or, in studies involving more distant benefit, those they personally care most about—will enjoy those fruits. The potential benefits of such studies, note, must be measured realistically. The probability of benefits accruing is a function not only of abstract scientific potential but of concrete possibilities of implementation. If we have good reason to think the intervention will not be used in the relevant populations—if barriers to implementation are too daunting, the cost too high, local government too corrupt—then justification is not achieved.

On the model we propose, then, a study that offers less than the world's best standard of care is morally permissible *just in case (1) it carries a probability-adjusted stream of future health benefits to those who, in*

public health terms, are relevantly like the participants that is sufficient to jus-
tify both the differential between taking a fully therapeutic stance and an in-
vestigative stance toward participants and the burdens imposed on them, and
(2) the participants or those they care most about would be among those who
would enjoy that future stream, if not in the likely natural course of events,
then by provision made especially to them.

What, though, if pursuing less expensive interventions encourages governments local or otherwise not to provide the better ones they ought already be providing? The worry is a real one. We agree with those who have urged the addition of one last important constraint: neither arm may offer less than the care that participants should be entitled to by the actual agencies de jure responsible for their care if doing so would causally enable wrongful denial (by relieving moral and political pressure, for instance, that might otherwise loosen purse strings). Research should not, for instance, be allowed that will likely divert local government resources, such as clinic space, that ought instead be devoted to discharging basic obligations of health care to participants.[32]

Investigators proposing to study an intervention designed to help the poor must beware the possibility that they are, instead, enabling wrongful deprivation of care to which those studied are entitled.[33] This having been said, it is also important to note that, at some point, pragmatics intervene: if a community is not going to get what it in fact deserves no matter what the investigators do—if, say, local corruption is so entrenched, the world community so callous, the ideal world so far distant, then helping to ameliorate the effects of that deprivation is the right thing to do.

Reasonable Availability Revisited

What, then, about "reasonable availability"? On the framework we are suggesting, the issue is revealed as complex. For those studies using control arms that offer less than the world's standard of treatment, a precondition of justifying the trial is the guarantee that those studied would be among those to enjoy the future stream of benefits should the drug or intervention prove successful. If the population would not itself be able to afford it, then posttrial provision of a successful drug or intervention must be arranged. Provision need not in principle be supplied by the

investigating entity: public health can recognize a division of duties between investigators and other sources of provision, including charities or
the World Health Organization; but plans for provision there must be.

For those studies comparing new interventions against a control arm
that *does* offer the world's best broad standard of treatment, though,
matters are more complicated. As we have seen, study designers already
face a presumptive requirement to try to locate the study among those
who could afford the treatment; but other factors, such as comparative
scientific relevance, may override this. If, where this happens, the intervention itself is something that would be deeply helpful to the host community, its future provision will sometimes, but not always, be required
as a constitutive piece of avoiding objectification. Where the community has important medical need for the treatment, then providing that
treatment posttrial will be a paradigmatic example of meeting—not just
studying—the health needs encountered during research. Again, on
pain of adopting an objectifying stance toward you, your medical need
may not be seen exclusively through the lens of its usefulness to my investigation. While I am here because your medical need is useful to others, I may not regard your need solely in terms of that utility—no matter
how fascinating, promising, or compelling the study of your condition
might be from a public health standpoint. I must also indicate appreciation of the meaning those needs carry for you—namely, as something
to be alleviated. One concrete implication is that, where I encounter
health needs of yours that I can with little effort easily alleviate, given
my expertise and resources—where a small investment on my part would
yield substantial health benefits to you—I must provide ancillary medical treatment: iron for anemia, electrolytes for diarrhea, education about
proper sanitation. Roughly speaking, the more substantial the benefit to
the host community, and the lower the cost of its provision to the pharmaceutical company (including indirect effects on world market price),
the stronger the presumptive demand that provision should be made.

Where these considerations are less pressing, fair and respectful exchange can indeed be measured in terms other than provision of the
drug or intervention studied. Even here, though, not just any terms will
do. We want to urge that, if clinical research as an enterprise falls under
the broad domain of public health, the benefits of exchange must be
measured in public health terms, broadly construed—in water wells or
education, ancillary care, or clinics, not televisions. Further, even within

public health terms, it is not enough that the broad community benefits. However valuable terms of exchange may be to the community from a public health standpoint, research participants and those they most care about must be benefited in a way proportional to the burdens and risks they are asked to undertake through their participation. A cost of not objectifying you through our interactions given the normative context of public health is that the "care" must be health care offered *you* and not simply your community.

Vetting agencies should, then, in certain contexts, make study approval conditional on the investigating entity making the drug available—not because drug companies are being held to some saintly standard of public beneficence but because doing so is sometimes a constitutive piece of justifying studies in public health terms.

Case Applications

To illustrate the framework we propose, we turn to a series of case studies. Consider, first, the Surfaxin study proposal—a proposal to compare a new surfactant in respiratory therapy against old-fashioned positive-pressure oxygen therapy on premature infants in Bolivia. Significant worries were raised about the protocol. Some of the concerns derive from commitment to core consensus protections: worries were raised about the ability of the prospective participants to give genuine informed consent in light of their medical needs and general vulnerability; concern was raised, as well, about whether researchers or the broader medical community was in genuine equipoise about the proposed surfactant in relationship to mere oxygen. But problems went deeper than this. Even if the Surfaxin trial could have achieved full informed consent, and even if we stipulate, as some have argued, that researchers were in equipoise about the surfactant's benefits relative to oxygen (after all, even drugs with high *ex ante* expectations sometimes prove disappointing or even dangerous), something more fundamentally troublesome was at issue.

For one thing, the proposed control arm raised red flags. The pharmacological company proposed testing the new surfactant against positive-pressure oxygen therapy, rather than any of the established surfactants already known to be far superior to oxygen in saving the lives of premature infants. Conducting such a trial would not be permissible in the developed world, where effective surfactants are the standard of care. Furthermore, the surfactant tested was never imagined to benefit those who were enrolled in the study or their surrounding community. If found safe and effective, the therapy would have been far beyond the financial means of those on whom it was studied; the potential market for Surfaxin was exclusive to the developed world.

On our proposed framework, the Surfaxin proposal was rightfully denied. Not, though, just because it proposed to test Surfaxin against an intervention below the world's best standard of care per se: as we have said, this can at times be justified. The Surfaxin proposal was rightfully denied because it was so obviously doubtful that the *public health justification* needed to go beneath the world's best standard of care would be met. Indeed, once we highlight the connection to public health, we can see why the proposal was particularly problematic. The sorts of vulnerabilities that might lead Bolivians to accede to such treatment—poverty and medical suffering—are the *very* sorts of vulnerabilities that clinical researchers working under the aegis of public health are charged with alleviating. Such research would, in essence, commit the sort of double wrong found in particularly egregious exploitation: wresting benefit in ways that treat others in overly instrumental fashion, and doing so in a way that takes advantage of the very vulnerabilities one is charged to alleviate.

While the Surfaxin trial, then, would be denied on our framework, testing the efficacy of microbicides to reduce heterosexual transmission of HIV in sub-Saharan Africa would not. Given the difficulty of ensuring condom use, such an intervention, if successful, would be of enormous benefit to those being studied. True, such a study could not be conducted ethically in the United States, given extant data about the superiority of condom use in reducing transmission; but it is perfectly appropriate in an impoverished community, because it is the community that would be benefited.

The short-course AZT trial to reduce maternal-fetal HIV transmission, in turn, might well pass on this framework, but it would depend. Questions were raised about whether the desperately poor countries in which the study was conducted could actually afford even what the intervention, if successful, would cost;[34] if not, the danger is real that the study, however well intentioned, would in fact have the result of exploiting those women to gain knowledge of use only to richer countries looking to reduce their public health expenditures. If the drugs would otherwise be unaffordable, then, once again, the price of admission to those proposing the study would be finding someone willing to render it available up to the level needed to accrue the relevant justification.

The Havrix trial provides a particularly good example of how contextual the justification of a trial design might be with respect to considerations of both standard of care and reasonable availability. Designed to test a vaccine for hepatitis A, the trial tested 40,000 children in Thailand. Thailand was chosen for scientifically credible reasons: Thailand has one of the highest rates of transmission of the virus; there was no less vulnerable population offering equivalent scientific potency. Further, and crucially, the study involved no compromise in the standard of care offered in the control arm: there is currently no vaccine for hepatitis A; the Thais in this sense are in the same boat as everyone else. On the other hand, the vaccine, if successful, would not be affordable to the Thais; the primary users of the vaccine would be first world travelers and militaries. Because there was no compromise in the control arm's standard of care, posttrial provision of vaccine would not, on our framework, be an immediately necessary precondition of allowing the trial. Whether or not regulators ought to have required subsidized provision depends, instead, on contextual factors—on how expensive the provision would be relative to the benefit it would afford the Thais; on how great the burdens and differential of the trial would be relative to the direct benefits it afforded (in this case, 20,000 children received the vaccine); and on what role, if any, provision would play in the broader expressivist import of the trial.

Conclusion

Clinical research in the developing world has, at its heart, a central tension: how do we gain desperately needed knowledge for the world's poor without thereby objectifying those poor? Navigating this tension, we argue, requires deep appreciation of the public health norms that ought to govern clinical research, as well as understanding the challenge of morality in a nonideal world. Asymmetries of power, need, and voice matter, and matter deeply in the context of medical research. Yet understanding *which* transactions count as truly exploitative is not, as current international standards now insist, simply a matter of invoking the standard of care that would be available in the ideal. The cost of this standard is, in real-world terms, too high; more than that, it is disconnected from the very rubric of public health that ought, we believe, to animate the regulations here fashioned. The enterprise of public health is not governed by the minimalist norms of the marketplace; nor, in the main, is it governed by unfettered pursuit of aggregate utility, indifferent to whom the utility accrues. Fundamentally, though, it is an enterprise that concerns the real world, not the kingdom of ends or a Rawlsian society of ideally just institutions. As such, it balances a dual agenda of trying both to change the conditions that impede health and to work out how best to promote health given the often-stubborn intransigence of those impediments.

Looking to the norms governing the enterprise of clinical research under the aegis of public health helps, then, to explain why we do need a standard of care beyond minima, but not one that would forestall researching help in dire circumstances. It provides us an approach that allows research on some of the most pressing health crises facing the destitute even as it insists that dignity, and not mere aggregate health utility, is a moral constraint.

In the real world, of course, it can be difficult to tell when one's actions risk complicity with existing injustices—when, for example, a study of interventions aimed at alleviating suffering rooted in inadequate health care instead enables those very systems of injustice responsible for the inadequate health care. Actions can have causally diffuse effects, and it is often difficult to predict which direction a confluence of pressures will take. Yet as difficult and important as this issue of application is, the central *conceptual* point is more straightforward: it is not always complicit with injustice to try to decide how to help people in the face of injustice; sometimes, it is an abnegation not to do so.

Acknowledgments

Many thanks to useful conversations with Jon Faust, Jeremy Snyder, and Dave Wendler, and to Jennifer Hawkins and Ezekiel Emanuel for keen, detailed feedback, which greatly improved this chapter. We also wish to thank Jeremy Snyder for excellent assistance with the research for this chapter. Thanks, too, to the members of our graduate seminar on Exploitation, Coercion, and Commodification for lively discussion. Finally, our thanks to Christine Grady, whose insights about the moral aims of clinical research have influenced us deeply.

Notes

1. For representatives of this view, see, e.g., Robert Nozick, *Anarchy, State, and Utopia* (New York: Basic Books, 1974); Milton Friedman, *Capitalism and Freedom* (Chicago: University of Chicago Press, 1962); and Ian Maitland, "The Great Non-debate over International Sweatshops," in *Ethical Theory and Business*, 6th ed., ed. Tom Beauchamp and Norman Bowie (Englewood Cliffs, NJ: Prentice Hall, 2001).

2. See Peter Lurie and Sidney Wolfe, "Unethical Trials of Interventions to Reduce Perinatal Transmission of the Human Immunodeficiency Virus in Developing Countries," *New England Journal of Medicine* 337 (1997): 853–56; Marcia Angell, "The Ethics of Clinical Research in the Third World," *New England Journal of Medicine* 337 (1997): 847–49; Marcia Angell, "Ethical Imperialism? Ethics in International Collaborative Clinical Research," *New England Journal of Medicine* 319 (1988): 1081–83; Kenneth Rothman and Karin Michels, "The Continuing Unethical Use of Placebo Controls," *New England Journal of Medicine* 331 (1994): 394–98; Troyen Brennan, "Proposed Revisions to the Declaration of Helsinki—Will They Weaken the Ethical Principles Underlying Human Research?" *New England Journal of Medicine* 341 (1999): 527–31; George Annas and Michael Grodin, "Human Rights and Maternal-Fetal HIV Transmission Prevention Trials in Africa," *American Journal of Public Health* 88 (1998): 560–63.

3. For a review of the issues, see Harold Varmus and David Satcher, "Ethical Complexities of Conducting Research in Developing Countries," *New England Journal of Medicine* 37 (1997): 1003–5.

4. Joel Feinberg, *Harmless Wrongdoing* (New York: Oxford University Press, 1988), 14.

5. Theorists divide on the relation between coercion and exploitation. Some believe they are fully separate concepts but can be co-instantiated; some believe they are contrasting phenomena that hence cannot be co-instantiated; some believe that coercion is a species of exploitation; some believe that exploitation is sometimes achieved by way of coercion. We believe that the two concepts are

distinct but can be co-instantiated. Coercion is an offer both legs of which leave one worse off by reference to a normatively specified baseline; exploitation is an exchange that involves wresting benefit from a genuine vulnerability in a way or to a degree one ought not. Sometimes, one does the latter by coercion; but not all cases of coercion are cases of exploitation—in particular, "faint threats," which formally coerce, do not threaten appreciable harm; in these cases, the threatened party's response, whatever it may be, will likely not involve any genuine or significant vulnerabilities.

6. Alan Wertheimer calls this the "historical" version; he gives as an example of such a charge the worry that student athletes receive too little of the benefits they accrue to their universities. See Wertheimer, *Exploitation* (Princeton, NJ: Princeton University Press, 1996), chap. 3.

7. *Id.* at 230–36.

8. Denis Arnold and Norman Bowie, "Sweatshops and Respect for Persons," *Business Ethics Quarterly* 13, no. 2 (2003): 221–42.

9. Onora O'Neill, *Constructions of Reason* (New York: Cambridge University Press, 1989), 138.

10. Leon Kass, *Life, Liberty, and the Defense of Dignity: The Challenge for Bioethics* (San Francisco: Encounter Books, 2002).

11. Vulnerabilities, on one broad definition, are susceptibilities to loss. Put this way, the construal is a bit too broad, for it will include factors that are, as it were, vulnerabilities in name only. After all, any time agents agree to a transaction that could have brought them more, or cost them less, there is something in virtue of which they agreed to less than they could have gotten. It is important, then, to distinguish such merely "de facto" vulnerabilities from more genuine ones—those susceptibilities that tend to render precarious one's access to more important goods. Just which vulnerabilities—gullibility, naïveté, fear, say—might thusly count is, again, a point of substance; the crucial issue here is that a commitment to exploitation is, at heart, a commitment to the claim that a genuine vulnerability is being wrongfully taken advantage of. As Robert Goodin reminds us, vulnerabilities in the relevant sense may involve "fears, ignorance, superstitions, gullibility, or naivete, . . . generosity, loyalty, or trust, . . . bad luck, joblessness, homelessness, or illness." Goodin, "Exploiting a Situation and Exploiting a Person," in *Modern Theories of Exploitation*, ed. Andrew Reeve (London: Sage, 1987), 171.

12. Alan Wood, "Exploitation," *Social Philosophy and Policy* 12, no. 2 (1995): 145.

13. See Elizabeth Anderson and Richard Pildes, "Expressive Theories of Law: A General Restatement," *University of Pennsylvania Law Review* 148 (2000): 1503–75, at 1508.

14. Thus, for instance, Tom Hill, in his essay "The Message of Affirmative Action," in *Autonomy and Self-Respect* (Cambridge: Cambridge University Press, 1991), appeals to the expressivist implications of affirmative action regulations and policies—the "message" they send about our moral priorities. Whatever one thinks about affirmative action, the point we are making here is that policies are important in their expressivist meaning, not just in their concrete implications.

15. For more on the concept of commodification, see Margaret Radin, *Contested Commodities* (Cambridge, MA: Harvard University Press, 1996).

16. Questions of transactional fairness are central, for instance, to Wertheimer (chapter 3, this volume) and Participants in the 2001 Conference on Ethical Aspects of Research in Developing Countries, "Fair Benefits for Research in Developing Countries," *Science* 298 (2002): 2133–34.

17. We would define "undue inducement" as positive incentives whose appeal distorts the subjects' practical reasoning in such a way that they trade off future for present goods out of proportion to their own personal future-discount rate.

18. Both clauses—whose knowledge, and the standard of knowledge—are currently heavily contested.

19. These regulations, among others, are set out in National Bioethics Advisory Commission, *Ethical and Policy Issues in International Research: Clinical Trials in Developing Countries*, (Bethesda, MD: NBAC, 2001), available at: http://www.georgetown.edu/research/nrcbl/nbac/pubs.html; and in the Declaration of Helsinki, revised October 2000, available at http://www.wma.net/e/policy/b3.htm. As we are about to see, these regulations go further than the core set of regulations here articulated, taking us into what we regard as contested waters.

20. See Debra DeBruin, "Nurses: Research Integrity in Clinical Trials," supported by the Research on Research Integrity Program, an ORI/NIH collaboration, grant 1R01NR08420-01.

21. CIOMS Guideline 8 requires that "interventions or procedures that hold out the prospect of direct diagnostic, therapeutic or preventive benefit for the individual subject must be justified by the expectation that they will be at least as advantageous to the individual subject, in the light of foreseeable risks and benefits, as any available alternative." Council for International Organizations of Medical Sciences, *International Ethical Guidelines for Biomedical Research Involving Human Subjects* (Geneva: CIOMS, 2002), 47. Note that the NBAC report sets the required standard of care lower, mandating an "established, effective treatment."

22. Par. 29, emphasis added; revised October 2000, www.wma.net/e/home/html.

23. See Barry Bloom, "The Highest Attainable Standard: Ethical Issues in AIDS Vaccines," *Science* 279 (1998): 186–88; and Ruth Faden and Nancy Kass, "HIV Research, Ethics, and the Developing World," *American Journal of Public Health* 88 (1998): 548–50.

24. See Robert Crouch and John Arras, "AZT Trials and Tribulations," *Hastings Center Report* 28, no. 6 (1998): 26–34; Salim Karim, "Placebo Controls in HIV Perinatal Transmission Trials: A South African's Viewpoint," *American Journal of Public Health* 88 (1998): 564–66.

25. See Alex London, "Justice and the Human Development Approach to International Research," *Hastings Center Report* 35, no. 1 (2005): 24–37, at 35.

26. See David Wendler, Ezekiel J. Emanuel, and Reidar Lie, "The Standard of Care Debate: Can Research in Developing Countries Be Ethical and Responsive to These Countries' Health Needs?" *American Journal of Public Health* 94 (2004): 923–28.

27. Participants, "Moral Standards for Research in Developing Countries: From 'Reasonable Availability' to 'Fair Benefits,'" *Hastings Center Report* 34, no. 3 (2004): 17–27.

28. For discussion, see John Arras, "Fair Benefits in International Medical Research," *Hastings Center Report* 34, no. 3 (2004): 3.

29. Which does not, of course, rule out the possibility of allowing suitably regulated profit-seeking agents, such as physicians or pharmaceutical companies, to play a designated role in its tasks.

30. Christine Grady, "Science in the Service of Healing," *Hastings Center Report* 28, no. 6 (1998): 34–38, at 35.

31. The latter two are particularly important: the heavier the absolute burdens, and again the wider the gap between what a therapeutic stance and an investigative stance would have brought those participants (and, we would add, the extent to which injustice is responsible for the needs which are here so scientifically useful), the heavier the presumption should be that benefits be measured by reference to those participants themselves, and, where possible, to those both nearest and dearest to participants and those relevantly like the participants in public health terms.

32. Grady, *supra* note 30.

33. It matters, then, who does the research and, more specifically, the relation between the agent of research and the agent responsible for wrongful deprivation. If one is part of an agency that ought to have been giving a certain level of aid, one cannot apply the above. The Kennedy-Kreiger study of lead abatement in Baltimore-area children living in public housing is particularly fascinating in this regard, pressing as it does questions of how we individuate the

agent of obligation. See Joanne Pollak, "The Lead-Based Paint Abatement Repair and Maintenance Study in Baltimore: Historic Framework and Study Design," *Journal of Health Care, Law and Policy* 6, no. 1 (2002): 89–108.

34. See Leonard Glantz et al., "Research in Developing Countries: Taking 'Benefit' Seriously," *Hastings Center Report* 28, no. 6 (1998): 38–42.

8

Exploitation and Placebo Controls

JENNIFER S. HAWKINS

Nicole is a young, HIV-positive mother in Côte d'Ivoire, where virtually no treatment is available for the deadly disease HIV causes. In the late 1990s, Nicole was one of thousands of HIV-positive pregnant women from developing countries who participated in clinical trials to see if low-dose AZT could reduce the rate of transmission from mother to child.[1] In 1998, when Nicole was interviewed after the trial by a reporter, she still did not know which arm of the trial (AZT or placebo) she had been in, and she did not know the HIV status of her baby.[2]

The reporter asked Nicole how she felt about possibly having received a placebo, given that researchers already knew at the time that AZT could effectively reduce the chance of transmitting the virus. Although Nicole—one of the better-educated subjects who participated—seemed to grasp the concept of a placebo well enough, the fact that AZT was already known to be effective was news for her. She was understandably confused and troubled by this information. Pressed again to say how she would feel if she were now to learn that she had received placebo, she responded, "I would say quite simply that that is an injustice."[3]

Poignant and understandable as her claim is, Nicole does not yet possess *all* of the information relevant to making such a judgment. Certainly if she was unaware that AZT was already in use, she was presumably also unaware of how much the standard treatment with it costs, how difficult it can be to administer, and why some scientists thought they could gain useful information only through placebo-controlled trials. In short, she is unaware of all of the subtleties central to the dispute that raged over the choice of placebo controls.

However, a large number of commentators—people who do have that information and have thought about the case at length—agree with Nicole. More precisely, they have argued that it is unjust to use placebo controls in clinical trials when proven therapies exist and remains so even when local medical scarcity guarantees (as it does in Nicole's case) that placebo controls will not make any participant worse off than she otherwise would have been.[4] Not only do these commentators perceive the use of placebos in these contexts as an injustice—they label it as an injustice of a particular sort. They claim that women like Nicole and their children have been *exploited*.

This chapter is an attempt to determine whether Nicole, her baby, and others like them have really been the victims of injustice, *and* if so, whether this injustice is appropriately labeled "exploitation." To answer such questions is not simple. It requires grappling both with tricky questions about the meaning of "exploitation" and with complex moral questions about certain types of research ethics cases—cases that arise primarily in the developing world.

For ease of discussion, let me stipulate the specific sort of case with which I shall be concerned. These cases satisfy all the following conditions: First, clinical research is undertaken in an effort to develop a new treatment for some condition—call it A—even though other forms of effective treatment already exist for A. Second, the control arm in the trial uses placebo *or some other therapy known to be inferior to the best existing therapies*. Third, no treatment for A is generally available where the trial is to take place. Fourth, the proposed subjects are not healthy volunteers but individuals with condition A. Finally, A is a serious condition, that is, one that if left untreated carries with it a high risk of disability or death or is otherwise quite serious. I shall call these cases *placebo cases**.[5]

With this stipulated definition in hand, the central questions are easier to state: Are all placebo cases* unjust to those who participate as controls? If so, should all placebo cases* be prohibited? Also, if there is injustice here, is it appropriately labeled "exploitation"? In this context, what specific *form* of unfairness is being alleged when such trials are said to be exploitative?

My attempt to answer these questions proceeds in stages. After clarifying certain features of the two cases I use as examples, I turn to the

meaning of "exploitation." I distinguish among the various types of unfairness that may support a claim of "exploitation" and attempt to specify the *particular* type of unfairness that motivates certain critics of
placebo cases*. Both tasks are necessary if there is to be a proper fit between the driving concerns of these critics and the expressed charge of
exploitation. As I see it, criticisms of placebo cases* are best interpreted
as claims that researchers have taken advantage of the situation to get
out of fulfilling certain key moral obligations that they have to their subjects. Such a claim can easily be seen as an exploitation claim. However,
I go on to argue that whether we classify such cases as harmful or nonharmful exploitation depends on our underlying understanding of the
moral obligations of researchers. Thus, in order to determine more precisely the type of exploitation at stake, we must tackle directly the question of what the moral obligations of researchers really are. The rest of
the chapter is devoted to these questions.

Despite their deep divisions over the justice of placebo cases*, the
vast majority of commentators appear to agree that whatever we say
about a case like Nicole's must be said about *all* placebo cases*.[6] They
assume that either all such cases are unjust or none is. I argue that this
pattern of assessment is rooted in certain unexamined assumptions
about the basic nature of a researcher's obligations to her subjects. Traditionally, the moral obligations of researchers have simply been read
off from the familiar obligations of physicians to their patients. I refer
to this as the *medical model* of researcher obligations. While it under-
pins the assumption that all subjects in a trial are automatically owed
the best care the researcher can provide, I believe that the medical
model is incoherent.

However, abandoning the medical model does not lead inexorably to
the conclusion that all placebo cases* are morally permissible, which is
what many theorists fear. There are other significant (albeit *defeasible*)
reasons that, in the developing country context, support requiring researchers to offer treatment to seriously ill control group members. If I
am correct, we simultaneously arrive at a clearer understanding of the
obligations medical researchers have in developing countries and at the
conclusion that *some, but not all*, placebo cases* violate these obligations.
Some, but not all, placebo cases* are exploitative.

Two Placebo Cases*

It is important to have detailed cases before us. However, real-life cases are complex and typically raise not one but several moral questions. Since I cannot hope to do justice to all the moral questions raised by the two cases I have selected, I shall stipulate certain simplifications. I shall refer to the real cases as *AZT* and *Surfaxin* and to my own simplified fictions as *AZT** and *Surfaxin**.[7]

AZT raises two important moral questions. First, were placebo-controlled trials (PCTs) *really necessary* for obtaining useful information?[8] Second, *if* they really were necessary, could that fact justify departing from the usual moral prohibition against PCTs once effective therapy exists? Both questions are incredibly difficult to answer. But I am only interested in the second question here:[9] *If* it really were true that the only way to answer a particular important research question with the degree of rigor needed to make the research worthwhile was to use placebo controls, would it then be permissible to depart from the usual norm (provided that doing so would not make any subject worse off than she otherwise would have been)? Hence, while remaining officially agnostic on the question of whether PCTs were actually necessary in *AZT*, I shall stipulate that they were necessary in my fictional *AZT**.

Now consider *Surfaxin*. Like *AZT*, *Surfaxin* is a placebo case* in my defined sense, since the ventilator therapy offered to control group subjects, while somewhat better than nothing, was still known to be significantly inferior to existing surfactant treatments. In *Surfaxin* a key question is why placebo controls were considered in the first place. Although other synthetic surfactants were on the market and had been used for some time with dramatically positive results in premature infants with respiratory distress syndrome (RDS), the existing data comparing these drugs to placebo were quite variable, making it difficult to determine the *exact degree* to which these drugs were superior to placebo. To license a drug for use in the United States for a particular indication, a manufacturer is required to prove to the Food and Drug Administration (FDA) that the drug is superior to placebo for that indication. In this case, given that Surfaxin was not expected to be greatly superior to existing surfactants, and given the uncertainty about the degree of superiority over placebo of the existing treatments, an ACT comparing Surfaxin to its competitors seemed unlikely to yield useful information. As a result, the FDA told the manufacturer that it must produce data from a PCT. However, both the medical community and the FDA agreed that it would be unethical to run a PCT in the United States, given the widespread use of other surfactants in the United States and the general belief in their vastly superior efficacy.

Again, several questions arise: *First*, was it really scientifically necessary to run a PCT in order to get useful data? Although such a claim was the basis for the FDA's requirement, some critics have argued that not enough other options were explored before concluding that a PCT was the only way to go.[10] Rather than try to settle that issue here, I shall simply stipulate that, in *Surfaxin**, a PCT was indeed the only way to obtain useful information. A *second* question arises about the *value* of the information sought. Surfaxin was being developed as a competitor drug in an area where several effective drugs had already been developed. While it is possible that Surfaxin would turn out to be vastly superior to existing drugs, prospectively that was highly unlikely. Moreover, from a public health perspective, there was no pressing need for another surfactant. To avoid controversy, I shall simply stipulate that, in *Surfaxin** it was reasonable to assume that if Surfaxin proved effective, this would primarily mean profits for the manufacturer. Since every drug variant has a slightly different profile (e.g., of side effects), it would no doubt be true that Surfaxin might be preferred for some patient populations. But the stipulation holds that there would be very little difference in terms of overall lives saved.

I wish to consider the following question in relation to *Surfaxin**: Is the fact that a PCT is scientifically necessary to produce meaningful data enough to justify departure from the usual norm, especially when there is no great need for the drug being developed? In *AZT**, PCTs are necessary for a study that, if successful, could lead to an intervention that would save thousands of lives. In *Surfaxin**, they are also necessary, but for a not-so-valuable result. *If* one thinks that we are sometimes justified in departing from the usual norm, are we justified in both of these cases or only one?

Both *AZT** and *Surfaxin** are placebo cases* in my defined sense. Many would see both as exploitative, while some would deny that either is. In order to sort out these claims, we must first turn our attention to "exploitation."

Exploitation: An Initial Road Map

So what exactly is exploitation? What do the critics mean when they label placebo cases* exploitative? And does the label really fit? Some initial analysis of "exploitation" is crucial, for there are many, distinct moral flaws that this term can legitimately be used to identify.

Most theorists accept the rather simple formulation that A exploits B when A takes unfair advantage of B.[11] In addition, A must *benefit* from her transaction with B. Otherwise, we have at most a case of attempted exploitation.[12] Since, on this account, exploitation involves A using B to A's advantage *in an unfair way*, the key to differentiating exploitative transactions from benign ones is to get clear on the distinction between fair and unfair use. However, we must *not only* distinguish between fair and unfair use, but also between *different species of unfair use*. Having a good map of the varieties of unfairness that are exploitative is key to understanding the real concerns that critics voice when they use the term. It is also key to launching practical responses. Different types of exploitation may require different remedies.

I will begin by reviewing a few highly useful distinctions from Alan Wertheimer's work. First is the distinction between *procedural* and *outcome* unfairness.[13] Second is the distinction—within the category of outcome unfairness—between *harmful* and *nonharmful* (though still unfair) transactions.[14]

Unfairness may enter into A's transaction with B through flawed consent or lack of consent altogether. These types of moral flaws are best thought of as *procedural* flaws—problems with how the transaction comes about. If A benefits from using B without obtaining B's consent, this is unfair, as it would also be if A deceived B, coerced B, or otherwise manipulated B's consent.[15] Alternatively, unfairness may enter in ways not related to consent. These are forms of *outcome* unfairness. Of course, it is also possible for a transaction to be flawed in both ways, though any one form of unfairness is sufficient.

Within the category of outcome unfairness, Wertheimer distinguishes further between outcomes in which B is harmed and outcomes in which B is not harmed, though still treated unfairly.[16] On his account, the form unfairness takes in nonharmful encounters is a *distributive* unfairness. A transaction may be unfair to B, even if B benefits overall from the transaction, if B receives an unfair share of the benefits of transacting. For example, if B is desperately poor, then B may agree to work for excessively low wages because such wages are an improvement over nothing. If the employer's profits are excessively large, then we may feel that B is being treated unfairly, even though both the employer and B gain from the transaction when compared with a no transaction baseline. Indeed, because of the mutual gain, Wertheimer labels this kind of exploitation *mutually advantageous exploitation.*

We can helpfully summarize the account of exploitation given so far with the following diagram:

Exploitation:

---

    1. A transacts with B.
    2. A benefits from the transaction.
    3. The transaction is unfair to B in one of the following ways:

Types of Unfairness
      i. Procedural unfairness
     ii. Outcome unfairness: harm
    iii. Outcome unfairness: no harm: distributive unfairness

---

The question now is: Where in all of this (if anywhere) do placebo cases* fit?

No doubt, there often are genuine procedural concerns in real-life placebo cases*.[17] However, my concern in this chapter is not with consent but with placebo use. If particular study designs are exploitative, this must be because the *outcome* of the transaction is in some way unfair to subjects.[18] If this is correct, then the obvious next question is whether placebo cases* are harmful to participants. If not, then we will have to inquire whether there is any other type of unfairness present.

As a general rule, we respond differently to harm than to other forms of unfair treatment. Harm is that which can uncontroversially be prohibited, even if doing so limits the liberty of others. If no harm is occurring, we are more reluctant to prohibit even morally unsavory activity. Hence, if exploitation comes in harmful and nonharmful varieties, this creates the possibility that some forms of exploitation should be permitted. I emphasize that it creates *the possibility*. It may well turn out that there are good grounds for prohibiting nonharmful exploitative transactions. However, the approach to arguing for prohibition will be quite different in the case of harmful exploitation as opposed to non-harmful. Hence, *if* placebo cases* are exploitative, then before we can say whether they should be prohibited, we will need to know whether they are harmful. As I will now try to show, that is a tricky question.

Harm, Exploitation, and the Claims of the Critics

Harm is whatever has an obviously negative impact on a person's welfare. We generally say that a transaction between two persons, A and B, is harmful for B if the outcome of the transaction lowers B's significant welfare interests or sets them back relative to where they would have been otherwise.

The tricky issues arise when we try to identify the two scenarios to compare to determine whether welfare has improved, declined, or remained steady as a result of the transaction. On the one hand, we need to designate more precisely what we mean by the *outcome* of a research transaction. On the other hand, we need to designate a baseline scenario—one that accurately represents how things would otherwise have been for this individual.

Consider first "outcomes." In the research context, "outcomes" are not identified with the literal outcomes of research participation—with how individual subjects fare posttrial. This is because, while we want to be able to assess the overall package of harms and benefits that research brings a subject, we want to avoid giving undue weight to unforeseeable consequences. In research, it is important to distinguish the potential harms and benefits recognized prospectively and agreed to by both parties from the actual harms and benefits that emerge. Hence, the impact of research on subjects is generally assessed *ex ante*, by considering the *offer* made to subjects and evaluating it in light of reasonable predictions about the probability of various outcomes. As a result, most theorists think about the impact research has on a subject in terms of the expected utility participation offers her at the point when she enrolls.

Consider now the issue of baselines. In the simplest cases, we assess how things "would have been otherwise" by comparing the outcome of the transaction for B with B's welfare condition just prior to the transaction (or by comparing the outcome for B with some other *descriptive* baseline). There is no controversy over whether acts that lower welfare relative to these baselines are harmful. However, there is a controversy over whether this is the only baseline that counts. Sometimes *omissions* seem like harms. The important kind of case is one in which A has a preexisting moral obligation to aid B but fails to do so. I shall refer to these as cases of *positive obligation flouting*. Often, when confronted with such a case, our sense of the relevant baseline shifts to a moralized one; we compare the outcome of the transaction for B with how things *ought* to have gone for B—with what B was owed, but did not receive. If we allow such cases to count as harm, and if A benefits from transacting with B while flouting his obligations to B, then it would seem we have a clear case of harmful exploitation.

Wertheimer allows for this possibility, although he does not analyze such cases in any depth.[19] But elsewhere he offers an example that can illustrate the idea.[20] Imagine a tugboat (A) and a vessel in distress (B). Let us stipulate that tugs have a moral obligation to aid vessels in distress at the usual price (in this case, around $100). Rather than offer to tow B for $100, A demands $1,000 to tow B. Because there are no other tugs around (it is sink or pay up), B agrees and is towed. Is B harmed by this transaction? Clearly, when measured against the baseline of his current distress, B benefits. But given the background moral obligation to help B, it seems that perhaps B has been harmed. Our sense of the relevant "otherwise" scenario is shifted by our knowledge of what A was supposed to do and our sense that B should have been able to count on A. Measured against being saved for $100, paying $1,000 is quite a loss. Against this alternative baseline, B *has* suffered a setback. Since, in addition, A has benefited from using B's dire situation in this way, he has clearly exploited B. Hence, we have a case of harmful exploitation.[21]

These two senses of harm, and the two accompanying ways of understanding harmful exploitation, help to illuminate the conflict over placebo cases*. Defenders of such trials frequently emphasize that subjects are not "harmed." This is true in the narrow sense of harm. After all, by participating, someone like Nicole gains a 50 percent chance of receiving a drug that, in turn, has some chance of blocking the transmission of the HIV virus to her baby. Of course, along with this chance comes the risk of unforeseen side effects. But even so, the overall *ex ante* profile of participation is likely positive—as there is also the prenatal care she will receive either way. Outside the trial, she has no chance at all of receiving AZT and will receive no prenatal care.

However, while all this is true, in speaking this way defenders of placebo cases* tend to talk past the critics, who are deliberately invoking the wider notion of harm. The critics label placebo cases* "harmful" because they view them as instances of positive obligation flouting. They think the researcher has a basic moral obligation to offer effective therapy when such therapy exists. Furthermore, they think this type of obligation flouting should be prohibited.

It is coherent to view instances of positive obligation flouting as exploitative, and this is, I believe, the best interpretation of what certain critics *say*. Moreover, I would argue that placebo cases* are either exploitative in the positive obligation flouting sense or they are not exploitative at all. The question ultimately turns on whether researchers really have obligations that they are flouting in these cases. This follows from our earlier chart. Recall that we already set aside issues of procedural unfairness. If placebo use is unfair, it is not *that form* of unfairness. But if placebo use does not harm in the narrow sense (which seems correct), and is also *not* an instance of positive obligation flouting, then the only remaining way of seeing placebo use as unfair would be to see it as distributively unfair. However, distributive concerns seem out of place here.

The *general* idea that exploitation can sometimes arise simply as a result of distributive unfairness—as, for example, when A gains excessively from the transaction relative to B—is important. Furthermore, I think it sheds significant light on certain *other* concerns that have arisen in connection with developing world research: for example, concerns about making drugs available posttrial. These concerns seem usefully interpreted as concerns about ensuring that subjects and other members of the host community receive a fair share of the posttrial benefits of research.[22] Nor do I wish to deny that, in a particular real-life case, subjects may suffer *both* a distributive unfairness and a second form insofar as they receive placebo. In many cases, the appropriateness of applying the label "exploitation" is overdetermined. My point is simply that the *specific* worry about placebo use is not best understood as distributive. If the special concern that arises here could be reduced to a distributive concern, then the problem could easily be resolved by offering more of other types of benefit to those subjects who receive placebo (benefits other than effective therapy for the illness under study). However, I doubt that this would really seem like an adequate solution to anyone bothered about the use of placebo controls when effective therapy exists. The problem is not that the subjects fail to receive *enough* (though that may also be true). The intuition is that they are failing to receive something *quite specific* that they are owed. If I am right, then the question of whether placebo cases* are exploitative in their design depends on whether researchers have moral obligations to their subjects that are being flouted in placebo cases*.

However, before turning to the question of what researchers' obligations are, I want to return to the question of *harm*. I have so far defended the idea that positive obligation flouting may, in certain cases, constitute exploitation. But I now want to question whether all instances of positive obligation flouting must be viewed as instances of harm. Might not there be cases of positive obligation flouting that represent instances of nonharmful exploitation? Obviously, the answer is significant because, as we have seen, the distinction between harmful and nonharmful exploitation determines the way in which we approach questions about prohibition.

Must Positive Obligation Flouting Always Count as Harm?

In *some* cases, we are clearly willing to label positive obligation flouting as harm. But in other cases this is not so obvious. Furthermore, our intuitions about harm tend to line up with our intuitions about the *kinds* of obligations being flouted and with our sense of whether these obligations are enforceable. To see this, consider two quite different instances of positive obligations to aid.

Consider first the obligations of a doctor qua doctor. A doctor clearly has positive moral obligations to aid, if anyone does. However, these are special, role-related obligations. To a large degree, our intuitions about a doctor's moral obligations are guided by our knowledge of the place this role has in society and by the fact that many of those who occupy the role have publicly promised to act in accordance with certain familiar role-related, moral norms.

A doctor's obligations are internal, however, to a particular relationship: the doctor-patient relationship. The moral obligations are obligations *to one's patients*. In agreeing to be a particular person's physician, a person makes an implicit promise to fill the role to the best of her ability, as it is commonly understood and in relation to *that particular patient*.[23] The promise made when the relationship is entered into need not be explicit or public: the organization of the profession, as well as the professional oath that many doctors swear, serves to give institutional structure to the doctor-patient relationship, and thereby to make it common knowledge what can be morally expected from doctors.[24]

This matters because it shapes our intuitions about the positive obligations in question and their relation to harm. Imagine that someone has agreed to be your doctor. Then one day when you are quite ill, this individual simply decides that she does not want to treat you. Nothing explains her decision, except her dislike of having to be bothered with you. There is no shortage of medical supplies, no other patients in greater need. In this case, if the doctor does not treat you, it seems clear that you have been *harmed*. Intuitively, the relevant baseline here is the one in which the doctor fulfills this positive obligation to you. What supports this intuition, I suggest, is not just that a positive moral obligation has been flouted but that it is a positive moral obligation *of a certain type*. As a result of the institutional structure that supports these obligations, a certain kind of promise has been made and certain expectations established. This makes us more confident that the positive moral obligations belong to enforceable morality.

Contrast this with a different case: what is referred to as a *Good Samaritan obligation*.[25] This is an obligation everyone has simply in virtue of being a moral agent. The classic example is someone walking by a pond who notices a small child drowning. All the person has to do is to scoop the child out of the water. Since no one else is present and so little is required to save a life, the passerby is morally obligated to save the child. In a case like this, it is a difficult question whether failure to help constitutes *harm*.[26] Whereas in the doctor's case the answer is relatively clear, moral theorists have traditionally disagreed about cases like the drowning child. Certainly, if the child drowns, this is very bad. But is it fair to say of the passerby that *he has harmed her*?

While people argue at length about this question, there is little disagreement on the issue of moral condemnation. Everyone grants that letting the child drown is a clear-cut case of morally atrocious omission.[27] What they remain unsure about is whether it is "harm." The distinction between harmful and non-harmful actions tracks the distinction between obviously enforceable morality and moral norms that are not so obviously enforceable. That is why the classification in terms of "harm" seems to matter. Still, it is worth noting that placing an action in the nonharmful category is not yet to concede that is should be permitted. It leaves that question open.

I therefore suggest that we simply grant that flouting Good Samaritan obligations is morally worrisome, but not an instance of *harming*.[28] This leaves the enforceability of Good Samaritan obligations open in a way that the enforceability of a doctor's obligations to her patients is not open. However, if this is correct, it represents a change in the general understanding of exploitation. Amending Wertheimer's view, we arrive at a chart that looks like this:

Exploitation

---

1. A transacts with B.
2. A benefits from the transaction.
3. The transaction is unfair to B in one of the following ways:

Types of Unfairness
   i. Procedural unfairness
   ii. Outcome unfairness: harm
       iia. B is harmed in the sense that B's welfare is lowered relative to simple, descriptive baseline.
       iib. B is harmed in the wider sense. We have a case of positive obligation flouting and the obligation flouted is one that is morally enforceable.
   iii. Outcome unfairness: no harm
       iiia. The transaction is distributively unfair to B.
       iiib. We have a case of positive obligation flouting, but the obligation is not of the sort that can be enforced.

The last category, "iiib," represents a type of exploitation not explicitly recognized by Wertheimer. However, I think it is a real and important category. Indeed, I intend to argue (against many of the critics of placebo cases*) that (iiib) is precisely the category of exploitation that applies to some (though not all) placebo cases*.

One potential problem with recognizing (iiib) as a category of exploitation is that it might seem unclear how we are to describe the type of unfairness present. Where does unfairness enter in? First, we must notice that A has a significant bargaining advantage over B: A can simply refuse to transact with B at all, whereas that would be disastrous for B. By itself a bargaining advantage is not sufficient for exploitation. What matters is what A *does* with his bargaining advantage *in cases where he has moral obligations*. In an ordinary business transaction, it is perhaps permissible for A to push that advantage to the limit. But when A has a preexisting moral obligation to help B, this constrains what A may do with his advantage. Importantly, it is *unfair* for A to use his advantage to get B to release him from his moral obligation. It is also important to consider B's agreement. Normally, if A has an obligation to B, the obligation is unproblematically canceled if B agrees to cancel it. In cases like these, B may appear to cancel A's obligation when B agrees to the less good terms. However, since it is unfair of A to ask for a waiver of moral obligations in such a situation, I would argue that the waiver fails to go through. The obligation remains in play and so is flouted by A if A does not comply with it.

With these distinctions in place, we can reframe the debate about placebo-controlled trials. Most *defenders* of such trials appear not to have seen them as exploitative in any sense. On the other hand, the *critics* have seen them as instances of positive obligation flouting *and* as instances of harm.[29] Furthermore, they view them as harmful precisely because they view a researcher as having all the same obligations to her subjects that a physician has to her patients. In short, they think that a researcher *just is* a doctor first, and a researcher second.[30] Of course, they recognize that researchers have other obligations that stem from their quest for useful, generalizable medical knowledge; and they recognize that this quest may, on occasion, lead to conflicts with the doctor role. But they hold that, whenever such conflicts arise, the moral obligations stemming from the physician role must take precedence. In what follows, I shall call this view *the medical model* of researcher obligations.[31]

If one accepts the medical model, then it makes sense to see placebo cases* as instances of positive obligation flouting. Moreover, even though not all obligation flouting counts as harm, as my previous examples show, it is not odd to label *this kind* of flouting "harm." Nor is it odd to view oneself as having a strong case for prohibiting the practice in question, since it is not odd to place the obligations of doctors within the realm of enforceable morality.

The real issue at the core of the debate, therefore, is whether the medical model is the appropriate vision of researcher obligations. If it is, then placebo cases* are instances of harmful exploitation and ought to be prohibited. However, I shall argue that this vision of researcher obligations is deeply misguided. In what follows, I defend an alternative vision of researcher obligations according to which researchers have (defeasible) obligations that are only *sometimes* flouted in placebo cases*. Furthermore, although it is deeply problematic when these obligations are flouted, it would be misleading on my view to say that subjects are "harmed." Nonetheless, since researchers gain from the unfair flouting of these obligations, I think it does count as a form of exploitation. If I am right, then this will have implications for how we approach the question of prohibition.

First, however, let us consider the more common vision of researcher obligations: the medical model.

Getting beyond the Medical Model

How might the medical model be justified? One problematic answer is that researchers simply *are* physicians, either because they have medical training or because they have sworn a medical oath. While many researchers have medical training and have taken professional medical oaths, this is simply *not* as relevant as it might seem. The argument trades on confusion about what it is to occupy a role. People with medical training do not always occupy the role of physician. They may have decided not to practice, for example. But even practicing physicians do not occupy the role in relation to everyone. They occupy other roles with respect to their spouses, children, friends, and colleagues. In these cases, the special moral obligations physicians have to their patients do not apply. As examples like this reveal, the moral obligations of physicians are internal to a particular relationship. Everything turns on what conditions establish that relationship—what it is that makes one person count as another's patient. Whatever the answer, mere medical training is not sufficient.

Even the medical oath that gives many physicians their sense of moral purpose can be understood in this light. The oath binds the individual conditionally, that is, *insofar as she occupies the role* of being someone's doctor. It tells her that, *when* she occupies that role, she must fulfill it to the best of her ability; and it spells out (to some extent) what is required to fulfill it. But it does not tell her when it is that she is someone's doctor.

The confusion is understandable because, in the past, one individual often not only wore both the doctor hat and the researcher hat *but wore them in relation to the same set of subject-patients.* In such a case, the moral importance of the physician role would indeed have to take precedence. But such concrete instances of role overlap are much less in evidence these days.[32] Some medically trained people are simply career researchers. They do not (at least, not from their point of view) take on patients. Others may be researchers for a while, and then return to medical practice later, or they may occupy both roles at the same time in relation to different nonoverlapping groups of people. Obviously, defenders of the medical model of researcher obligations will want to claim that, even when a medically trained person views herself as occupying *only* the researcher role, she is mistaken. Whether she recognizes it or not, she nonetheless has obligations to her subjects similar to a physician's. However, establishing this conclusion requires more substantive argument.

Having once granted that more argument is necessary, we can see that there are really two strategies a defender of the medical model might pursue to establish obligation overlap between doctor and researcher. The first is to show that whatever rationale supports a doctor's obligations applies with equal force to a researcher. This would be to argue that the *same reasons* apply to both. The second strategy would be to argue for sameness of obligation despite difference in justification. One set of reasons would justify assigning the familiar obligations to doctors, while different reasons would justify assigning researchers *the same* set of moral obligations. Both strategies are ambitious: they aim to establish complete obligation overlap, so that a researcher's obligations to her subjects *in any context whatsoever* include all of those a doctor would have if those individuals were her patients.

The first strategy falls apart as soon as we consider it more closely. This follows from the way in which role obligations are justified.[33] With role obligations, the justification of any particular obligation cannot fully be given apart from consideration both of the value of the role itself and of the importance of that particular obligation for maintaining the role thus conceived. So, for example, if we ask at the ground level why a particular physician whose patient has bacterial pneumonia is obligated to give him antibiotics, the answer initially seems incomplete: *That's just what doctors do under those circumstances.* A deeper justification, however, will appeal to the moral importance in society of the role of healer. It will examine why we have come to understand that role as we have, and why it is important for the role to continue to function in that way. Assuming a good justification at this level is found, we would then consider questions such as: Would it diminish or undermine the role if we altered it so that its occupants were not obligated to give antibiotics to their patients in need? Presumably, the answer would be yes. If that is right, then we would have a satisfactory justification of the specific obligation.

Now consider what reasons might ground the claim that a *researcher* whose subject has developed bacterial pneumonia is obligated to give antibiotics. Even if one believes researchers have such obligations, it should be obvious that the reasons for this *cannot be the very same reasons* appealed to previously. Although treating patients is just what doctors do, it is not obviously just what researchers do. Healing is not internal to the special goals of research. At the more general level, where a doctor's obligations are justified in terms of the societal value of the role, we can also see that this will not require researchers *to adopt* the same role. That justification serves only to explain why it is socially important *for someone* to fill the doctor role. It does not say that this is the job of a researcher.

If the first strategy fails, this leaves us with the second. This is to show that researchers and doctors have completely overlapping obligations, even though different reasons justify these obligations in each case. Most defenses of a medical model take this line. The claim is usually some variant on the following thought: since we already have a well-defined doctor role that has great moral value, and since we assign *greater* moral significance to the smooth functioning of that role (even if we assign due importance to research), the researcher role must be designed, from the outset, so as not to conflict with the doctor role or to undermine its smooth functioning.

These justifications for obligation overlap are quite strong so far as they go. However, they are contextually limited, as I will now try to show. Because they point to possible conflicts between the two roles in society, the justifications rely on particular assumptions about the background functioning of the doctor role. This makes sense historically, for the researcher role was originally defined in settings where certain background facts about medical institutions could be taken for granted and (probably) *were* taken for granted. Against that backdrop, it makes sense to view researchers as having the same (or, at any rate, almost the same) obligations as physicians. Yet as soon as we consider different contexts, where either the doctor role or its supporting institutional framework does not function effectively, the rationale for obligation overlap breaks down.

Consider, for example, the fact that, in developed countries, excellent medical care is available to a sizable majority of people. In that context, to enroll subjects and offer them less than the best care is to *harm* them, in the narrow sense of making them worse off than they would have been relative to a nonparticipation baseline. For here, the nonparticipation scenario is a treatment scenario: we can usually assume that a subject with a serious illness would have sought and received good treatment elsewhere. Since researchers have a strict duty not to harm, failure to treat members of the control group (or refer them to accessible others for such treatment) is morally off-limits in these environments.[34]

Of course, not everyone in developed countries has access to care, but even this does not undermine the general argument. For when a sizable majority has access to care, concerns about avoiding harm can still combine with other moral concerns—such as treating all subjects equally or distributing the benefits and burdens of research fairly—to support the policy of offering the best care to all. Hence, in developed countries, there are excellent reasons why we should view researchers as having obligations similar to a physician's. However, this justification is contextually limited.

It does not apply in most developing countries because, in those contexts, the prohibition against narrow harm is satisfied *even when* placebo controls are used.

Another common argument is what I shall refer to as the "inseparability of hats argument." It claims that it is not so easy to separate the two roles, and that *if* we cannot separate them, we may need to view the obligations as fully overlapping. The argument usually appeals to some aspect of human psychology. The claim might be that no matter how hard one tries to make it clear to people what the two roles are and that exclusive concern for healing can only be expected from doctors, human nature being what it is, some people will inevitably get the two roles confused. Hence, if the roles coexist in society and we allow their moral shape to differ substantially, it is inevitable that numerous individuals seeking treatment, and wanting only to be helped, will end up in the control group of placebo-controlled trials. The only way to prevent this is to ensure that research participation does not carry any prospect of a significant sacrifice of individual welfare. This can be accomplished by obligation overlap, which will require researchers to offer the best-known effective treatment to all subjects.

Assuming that the psychological premises hold, problems still emerge when we press for a clarification of the precise nature of the moral wrong that arises when the roles diverge. There are a couple of candidate clarifications. One invokes the disappointed expectations of people who want treatment and end up with none. This is simply a concern about avoidable psychological distress. A second alleges a moral failure of which the distress is only a sign: people *ought not to be in danger of such disappointment*. That is, the seriously ill are, in some sense, *owed medical care*. So there is a moral problem when institutions are set up in such a confusing way that, predictably, some people will fail to get what they are owed.

The second description seems like a much better interpretation of the moral worry. We may feel sorry for people who do not get what they want, but ensuring that everyone gets what she wants is not a primary moral concern in any society. On the other hand, if what they do not get is something they morally *ought* to get, then the fact that their confusion could have been predicted and avoided seems much more serious.

However, this argument is also contextually limited. For the sake of argument, let us assume that its several premises (psychological and moral) could be made more precise, and let us accept them. *Even so*, the argument still has different implications in different contexts.

Consider the situation in the United States. If there is a general moral obligation to ensure that the seriously ill are always given the best-known treatment, then it is only partially met in this country. Although a sizable majority has access to good care, a shockingly large minority does not. Even so, there is still room to argue that the role of researcher should not be allowed to undermine the delivery of care where it *is* being delivered. It would make an already bad situation worse if some individuals who would otherwise have received care in the United States end up not receiving it. Hence, even against a backdrop of partial moral failure, it can be important for researchers to have the same obligations as physicians.

If we now consider the situation in Côte d'Ivoire or Bolivia, we can see that the moral failure is more widespread. In such resource-poor environments, *most* of the seriously ill do not receive the best treatment. But precisely because the moral failure here is virtually complete, the rationale behind the inseparability of hats argument collapses. In such environments, even if the existence of a distinct researcher role led to some confusion, the confusion itself would be harmless and in some cases positively beneficial.[35] The argument I am criticizing assumes, normatively, that care is owed and, factually, that it is being given. Against this backdrop, it aims to convince us that how we define the researcher role may have an impact on the smooth delivery of that care. In the developing world, however, it is abundantly clear that people are not getting care. So even if we adhere to the moral idea that care is owed, it cannot be that *the way we define the researcher role* keeps them from getting it. Furthermore, no argument we have considered supports the idea that when doctors cannot deliver effective care, *researchers* are the ones who should step in and offer it. Even if everyone is (in some sense) owed care, it remains an open question who exactly is obligated to provide it.

I have tried to show that the medical model—the view that a researcher's obligations *are exactly the same as a physician's obligations in all contexts*—is not easily defended. The accusations of critics to the effect that placebo cases* are exploitative were initially premised on this view. However, as I will now try to argue, we do not need that model to explain what is wrong with certain placebo cases*, nor do we need it to support the idea that some placebo cases* are exploitative.

As I see it, what drives many people's moral intuitions in cases like *Surfaxin* and *AZT* is some combination of the thought that those who are seriously ill are owed care and the thought that the researchers must give it *because they are the only ones who can*. However, if that is correct, then the best explanation of why people focus on researchers has nothing to do with a special normative link between the roles of doctor and researcher. It has, rather, to do with the idea that, in crisis situations, the person best placed to help is (defeasibly) obligated to do so. Thus, even if we abandon all attempts to defend the medical model (as I think we should), we can still point to the contingent fact that, in developing world cases, researchers find themselves in an emergency health situation where they have access to effective forms of therapy.

The Good Samaritan Obligations of Researchers

It is a basic premise of morality, accepted by moral philosophers and ordinary people alike, that everyone has a positive obligation to assist others in need. Admittedly, this is a *limited* obligation. Furthermore, people disagree strongly about what its limits are. It is also generally granted that one has a great deal of discretion in how one fulfills this obligation: over when, where, and whom one helps. So it is often difficult to defend specific claims of the form "X has an obligation to aid Y" because X is usually at liberty to reply that it is up to her to decide whether to help Y or Z or W, and so forth.

In certain circumstances, however, the claim that particular individuals must do something to help particular others is easier to defend. When it is critical, those on the scene who are well placed to help (have the necessary skills, resources, etc.) are the ones who inherit the obligation. As mentioned earlier, such duties to rescue have traditionally been called Good Samaritan obligations.

These obligations are *defeasible*. For the obligation to hold, fulfilling it must not conflict with some other weightier moral aim or require too much in the way of personal sacrifice.[36] To see how other moral concerns might defeat these obligations, consider the drowning child again. Imagine you have just set out to rescue ten people, and on your way to do this, you see the lone drowning child. If stopping to rescue the child will lead to the deaths of the ten, (most people would agree that) your normal obligation to rescue the child is defeated.

It seems to me that a good argument can be made that researchers, just like the rest of us, have Good Samaritan obligations and that what is troubling about their actions in certain placebo cases* is that they are flouting a deeply important obligation to perform easy rescues.[37] Third World poverty and its effects constitute a crisis situation and, by stipulation, we are focusing on cases where this poverty has left the desperately ill without effective treatment. When researchers go to such places, they knowingly enter an environment where people they could easily save are dying all around them. Moreover, they are sometimes the *only ones* in the local environment who could help. (In other cases, they belong to a very small set of individuals who can help.) These cases also satisfy the condition on excessive personal sacrifice: the nonmoral interests at stake here are those of the sponsors who have an interest in running cheap, effective trials. Still, the cost of additional medical supplies is (usually) not too expensive for these sponsors and so would not be a huge sacrifice.[38] The remaining question is whether the Good Samaritan obligations are sometimes defeated by other weightier moral aims. To anticipate the practical conclusions of this chapter, it seems that in *AZT** they are defeated, because by hypothesis a PCT is the only way to prove an intervention that, if successful, would save thousands of lives. In *Surfaxin**, they are not defeated, for although PCTs are necessary for obtaining useful data, the data themselves are not morally significant in the same sense. Here a manufacturer is developing a "me-too" drug that would help the company share in the profits of a lucrative industry.[39]

Focusing on Good Samaritan obligations leads us, I believe, in a more productive direction than focusing on physician duties. However, there are a number of reasons why someone might resist this move. Before trying to answer these worries in detail, I want to anticipate a bit and give the reader a sense of the overall structure of the argument to follow.

I wish to argue for three claims. *First*, Good Samaritan obligations can help us arrive at a better understanding of the real moral worries many people have when they think about these cases. It helps us get a better grip on what is really bothering (most) critics of such trials. This is an *interpretive* claim. As I see it, most critics of placebo use in developing country contexts are deeply bothered by what strikes them as a blatant flouting of an obligation to perform easy rescues.

Second, I want to emphasize that we do in fact have such obligations. I argue that, even on a conservative understanding of what such obligations involve, it is likely that such obligations are flouted in many placebo cases*. This is a *moral* claim. In my experience, many theorists who are initially sympathetic to some such analysis nonetheless shy away from it because Good Samaritan obligations are notoriously difficult to pin down and make precise. This can either lead theorists to avoid discussion of such obligations altogether or lead them to conclude that such obligations, although morally significant, should not be viewed as legally enforceable. However, I hope to show that, in the kinds of developing country research cases that concern me, special structural features of the situation make it possible to give a more precise shape to the obligations in question.

Third, I argue (in §8.0) that such obligations should be enforced. My defense of the idea that we *can* define Good Samaritan obligations in placebo cases* provides *part* (but only part) of the argument for enforcement. The argument relies as well on noting the long-term ill effects for the institution of research of not considering how such trials *morally appear to others*. Good Samaritanism is the key to my *moral* argument. It explains why certain placebo cases* are morally troubling. But enforcement is a distinct issue, since there is deep disagreement about which moral wrongs should be prohibited. Hence, it is the long-term negative effects for the enterprise of research of being *perceived as Bad Samaritans* that is key to the prohibition argument.

Let us now back up and consider in more detail why someone might object to the idea that we can explain the particular moral problem of placebo cases* in Good Samaritan terms. To begin with, someone might point out that researchers are not *always* the *only ones* on the local scene who could help. Even in very poor regions, there may be some wealthy individuals who could fund treatment for others if they so chose. In a typical Good Samaritan scenario, when more than one person is on the scene, it is not so easy to determine who is obligated to help, even if we remain sure that someone is. If two people are on the shore and both can help the child, one of them is surely obligated to do so. But which one? If placebo cases* are like this, then someone might wonder how I can be so confident that the obligation to rescue really does fall to the researchers.

However, this issue is less relevant for placebo cases* than it might seem. Placebo cases* are more analogous to the case where fifty children are drowning and two people are on the shore. Here we no longer need to ask who is obligated to help: clearly *both* are obligated, even if it is not fully clear just how far their joint obligations extend. (Must they work together to save all fifty? Or is each just obligated to save a few? And what are the obligations of one if the other flouts his obligation? Must she do more because the other person flouted or do just the same as she would have been required to do anyway? Answers to these questions seem to depend on more details than we have.)

A second objection is that my interpretation does not fit the way the actual moral criticisms have been made. If I am correct, then researchers are not the only ones flouting obligations.[40] But the criticism has focused on *researchers*, rather than others in the local environment who fail to help. I think this observation can be explained away. It may just be that the omissions of the researchers are much more salient precisely because they interact directly with the sick individuals. They literally have effective treatment in their hands, but then offer it to some individuals and not others. If others on the scene who could help do not, they are *also* guilty of a moral failing. Yet their moral failing does not serve to cancel the moral obligations of researchers.

A third reason to resist is that my interpretation may seem to prove *too much*. It may seem to saddle researchers with extensive obligations to people who are not even in the study and with medical obligations to subjects that far exceed merely offering an effective intervention for the condition being studied. Would not a Good Samaritan faced with an emergency situation try to do as much as she could? For as many people as she could? No, she would not. To borrow a phrase from Judith Thomson, this confuses minimally decent Samaritans with splendid Samaritans.[41] All that Good Samaritan obligations require is minimally decent Samaritanism. By their very nature, they are not supposed to require huge amounts of sacrifice. Hence, assuming researchers have these obligations, it must be possible for them to draw a line between those they will help and those they will not. With respect to individual subjects, researchers must be able to draw a line beyond which no further obligations for medical care are recognized.

The real issue, as I see it, is where to draw the line. Consider first the question of *whom* researchers are obligated to help. In my view, the line must be drawn so as (minimally) to include all subjects in the to-be-helped category. The challenge is to explain why, on the one hand, the line *may permissibly* be drawn so as *not* to extend beyond the subjects in the study; and why, on the other hand, it nonetheless *must* be drawn so as to *include all the subjects* in the study. The trick is to show why it *would* violate Good Samaritan obligations to fail to offer effective treatment to members of the control group, and yet *not* violate Good Samaritan obligations to limit such treatment to trial subjects.

This is not as difficult as it might seem. The fact that Good Samaritan obligations are limited—that only decent Samaritanism is required—ensures in most cases that the obligations do not extend beyond the trial subjects. So it merely remains to show that they extend far enough to cover all the trial subjects.

Good Samaritan obligations are open-ended and indeterminate in scope. However, other moral considerations can often help us to narrow that scope. *Reasons that by themselves would not support any particular line of action can, when considered together, point to a specific solution.* In placebo cases*, several such reasons favor including all the subjects participating in the trial. I shall focus on two mutually reinforcing reasons, reasons of *distress avoidance* and reasons of *gratitude.* By themselves, neither uniquely supports the policy of offering the best-known effective treatment to members of the control group. But taken together, and in conjunction with Good Samaritan obligations, they *do.*

Take distress avoidance first. Consider the situation of the infants in *Surfaxin**who are in the control group (along with the situation of their parents). Contrast this with the situation of other local RDS infants who were not in the trial (along with the situation of *their* parents). Those associated with the control group differ both from those associated with the experimental arm and from those outside the trial. Over and above whatever physical and mental suffering the control group infants and their parents encounter simply as a result of the illness, the parents of infants in the control group *also* experience an additional layer of psychological suffering. This comes from knowing (after the fact) that there was something that might have helped their infant, that they had a chance at it, and that they nevertheless did not get it. Presumably, outside of this trial, parents in Bolivia are largely ignorant of the existence elsewhere of surfactant therapies that can save RDS infants. But even if they do know this, they have no reason to hope they will get it. But parents who enroll in the trial learn more about such drugs, simply in virtue of going through the process of informed consent. For those parents whose infants end up in the control group, the information they gain becomes an extra psychic burden later on, even though it is not recognized as such prospectively.[42] Just as the consent process enables them to form a more definite picture of what they do not have, so the blindness of the randomization process offers them hope that is later dashed.

In placebo cases*, therefore, members of the control group inherit an extra layer of mental distress that sets them apart both from those who receive better treatment in the trial and from those outside the trial who receive nothing at all. Insofar as we have a moral reason to avoid causing gratuitous distress, this reason picks out *just this group*. I think we clearly have moral reasons to avoid causing gratuitous distress. In many cases, these reasons are outweighed by other considerations—particularly if the distress created is not, in itself, sufficient to count as harm. Indeed, even in placebo cases*, if Good Samaritan obligations turn out to be defeated, then this distress might be viewed as a regrettable but unavoidable facet of research.

But now consider the role such reasons play in a placebo case* where Good Samaritan obligations have *not* been defeated. Here reasons of distress avoidance appear to be reinforced: the researchers are independently obligated to offer some aid and are simply trying to decide how *far* this obligation extends. The fact that extending aid to members of the control group would eliminate this kind of mental distress supports drawing the line to include them. Indeed, not to include them would be odd. Allowing gratuitous negatives to be introduced, even while seeking to eliminate other negatives, seems at odds with the beneficent aims that lie behind Good Samaritan obligations.

This brings us to another unique fact about control group members: because they are contributing to medical knowledge, we owe them a debt of *gratitude*. Now gratitude *by itself* does not give us reason to offer members of the control group the best-known effective therapy. Gratitude simply requires us to offer the subjects *something* (perhaps money, perhaps other goods) to recognize their contribution to the project. But *in combination with Good Samaritan duties*, gratitude does seem to support effective treatment for the control. Reflection on the gratitude owed reveals that researchers stand in a special relationship to these people unlike the one they have with any other members of the community. If a Good Samaritan obligation is already in play and the only question is where to draw the line, it would actually seem to flout any sense of what subjects have contributed if the line is not drawn to include them. They need something the researchers can offer, and they are already owed gratitude for their help in furthering medical knowledge. If their needs are ignored, this would undermine any attempt to express gratitude by other means.

Someone might still worry that the Good Samaritan paradigm will require researchers to offer too much even to subjects—for example, that it will require extensive care for health problems unrelated to the research. Once again, however, the key is to recognize that Good Samaritan obligations are limited obligations. Some medical complaints of subjects will be minor, and hence will not constitute a serious health threat. Others may pose such a threat, but if what is required to help with them is very costly or labor intensive, it may just be that this exceeds the limits of the duty. Getting effective treatment for the study condition (by hypothesis, a serious illness) is already a big boon to the subjects. Some additional types of non-research-related care may be required, but this is not problematic. Many research ethicists have already recognized limited duties to offer ancillary care. I doubt that adopting the Good Samaritan paradigm would force us to acknowledge anything beyond what has already been recognized as required.[43]

If I am right, then we can view certain placebo cases* (such as *Surfaxin**) as instances of positive obligation flouting. In virtue of the unfairness present in such situations, we can also label them exploitative. But given that the obligations in question are Good Samaritan obligations, we should *not* say that subjects are *harmed* in these instances. Rather, these are cases of nonharmful exploitation. In *AZT**, by contrast, no obligations are flouted, since the obligations are defeated. Hence there is nothing exploitative about *AZT**.

When Are Good Samaritan Obligations Defeated?

Good Samaritan obligations come into play in all sorts of crisis situations. But here I am concerned only with clinical research conducted in developing countries. When (if ever) may researchers depart from the Good Samaritan obligation to offer effective treatment to all seriously ill subjects? Three conditions are necessary and jointly sufficient to cancel this Good Samaritan obligation. First, the aim of the research must be morally weighty—there must be great need for the information to be gained from the study. Second, a *placebo*-controlled trial must be the *only way* to obtain the information in question.[44] Third, the community from which the subjects will be drawn must be one that could greatly benefit, and is also reasonably likely to benefit, from the research. When these three conditions are met, placebo controls are morally justifiable *even though subjects are seriously ill and effective therapy exists elsewhere.*[45]

The first two conditions are straightforward. Although new scientific knowledge is always valuable, some knowledge is not worth obtaining if the price is ignoring people in desperate need. Our obligations to people in desperate need remain in force if the aim of the research is not terribly important or if an alternative trial design will produce the same useful knowledge. *AZT** satisfies these first two conditions, whereas *Surfaxin** fails the moral weight requirement.

What may seem puzzling is why these two conditions are not sufficient in themselves. The third condition is important for reasons that have little to do with obligations to individual subjects. If the first two conditions are satisfied, it is permissible to conduct a PCT *somewhere*. By hypothesis, this will be a trial on seriously ill subjects, and members of the control group will fail to receive a known effective treatment. However, there may still be a choice about where to conduct the trial. If there is a choice between two different populations of desperately sick subjects, and it is known in advance both that this project involves ignoring desperate need in a particularly harsh way and that one population stands to benefit from the results, whereas another is not likely to—then there is a moral reason to conduct the trial where the population stands to benefit. That reason has to do with avoiding unnecessary resentment, as I will now try to explain.

I have compared placebo cases* to cases of failure to rescue, while arguing that sometimes failure to rescue is justified. Granted that failure to rescue is sometimes justified, we should think about how we could justify it *to* the people involved. In our cases, that means justifying it to the subjects, but also to their immediate families and local communities. They are the ones who perhaps will not be rescued or will perhaps watch as someone they love is not rescued. Even if we could expect them rationally to understand the moral case for placebo controls, they might still feel alienated from the purpose if they do not care about the people who will ultimately be helped. It is fair to assume that most people have at best a limited altruistic concern. I envision them asking: Why did you come *here*, specifically to fail to rescue us? It's true you needed this information for a great moral purpose, but why must you use *our* suffering for that end, when (by hypothesis) you could have gathered this information elsewhere, from people with more of a stake in the project?

If we adopt my third condition, it is more likely that the subjects and those in their community will have a stake in the success of the project. They will share, to a limited extent, the end at which the trial aims. Of course, I do not mean that these aims will line up with the *dominant wishes or needs* of the subjects, nor is this morally necessary. Presumably, Nicole's dominant wish is simply the best care for herself and her baby. While she probably *also* cares about other mothers and other children in her community who are HIV-positive, her own illness and its effects on her child are likely to overshadow her concerns for others. Still, if these are her concerns, then *something Nicole cares about* will come to pass if a treatment is developed that helps other HIV-positive women in her community.

Even if the project in which we engage subjects does not satisfy their deepest desires, we can still show a kind of respect for them and avoid generating unnecessary resentment if the project answers real concerns they have. *AZT** satisfies this third condition because its aim is to develop an intervention for women in Côte d'Ivoire (as well as other developing countries). But *Surfaxin** fails the condition because it is clear from the outset that the trial drug will not become available to poor residents in Bolivia any time soon.

It is vital to emphasize that these conditions are *not general conditions for the ethical conduct of research.* Confusion could easily arise because they are similar to conditions various theorists have suggested as general rules for the ethical conduct of research in developing countries. However, used in that way, my conditions would be far too restrictive. My claim is much more modest: that these three conditions must be satisfied *if researchers are to deviate from the usual norm that requires offering the best-known effective therapy to (seriously ill) members of the control group in placebo cases*.* This allows for deviation from the norm in cases where, for example, the illness being studied is not all that serious. But it also allows for trials in developing countries when the illness being studied *is* serious and when there is no expectation that any products developed will be made available later on—as long as the trial is *not a PCT* (and all other standard ethical requirements are met).

Enforcing Good Samaritanism in Research?

Researchers have Good Samaritan obligations. They apply only in certain limited contexts, but when they do, they have deep moral significance. When they are flouted, this is a form of exploitation. Ought they to be enforced? In cases like *Surfaxin**—dire situations where Good Samaritan obligations have *not* been defeated—should placebo-controlled trials be banned?

It is easy to explain why practices that harm individual subjects should be banned. But it is usually harder to defend enforcement of positive obligations to aid. Outside the research ethics context, there is division on whether duties to rescue should be legally enforced. In the case of clinical research, additional reasons speak against enforcement. After all, many subjects in the experimental arm of PCTs benefit from participating. If morally troubling PCTs like *Surfaxin** were ruled out, many research sponsors would simply do their research at home.[46] In that case, a number of individuals in poor countries who might have benefited will not benefit.[47] Since some subjects really do benefit and no subjects are harmed, why should we prohibit the troubling placebo cases*? Why not allow exploitation that is nonharmful?

Such arguments must certainly be taken seriously. But they do not present the entire picture. There are other—I believe, weightier—reasons for prohibiting exploitative placebo cases*. I will explore only one argument here, but it is one that anyone who sees research as a great public good should take seriously. The claim is that *other people*, beyond the actual subjects, are harmed when we allow exploitative trials like *Surfaxin** to go forward.

It is helpful to begin by reflecting on the type of moral wrong occurring in troubling placebo cases*. When Good Samaritan obligations have not been defeated, but are nonetheless flouted, the moral problem combines an *instance of failure to rescue* with the additional attempt to gain from the failure. There is something particularly distasteful about this kind of behavior. People wrong one another in many ways, but next to direct harming, failures of easy rescue may be among the most troubling types of wrong.

Now insofar as this is a widely shared view, that fact itself turns out to be significant. Should failures of easy rescue be viewed as serious moral offenses across many cultures, the emotional reactions people have to such omissions will be deeply felt and strong. If that is right, then cases like *Surfaxin** will evoke strong emotional reactions not only in subjects but also in others who know about the trial and know how it is being conducted. Although no one likes being unfairly used or seeing members of their community being unfairly used, it is plausible that the emotional fallout from observing particularly egregious moral failings will be greater. If failure of easy rescue lies at the severe end of the spectrum of offenses, then cases like *Surfaxin** will plausibly generate a particularly acute form of moral outrage.

Failure to engage in easy rescue communicates a deep disrespect for the humanity of those one fails to rescue. This message of disrespect may itself be quite damaging to many individuals and through them damaging to the fabric of society and to relations between that society and other societies. However, while I think the negative experiences of those so affected are morally significant, my argument also emphasizes their consequences down the line.

Of course, it is not possible to say exactly what these would be, but they might include reinforcing deeply negative stereotypes of Westerners, adding to anti-Western sentiment, and making the work of other groups that aim to be helpful more difficult. In particular, it could lead to a deep distrust of Western medicine and Western research, and an unwillingness to contribute to future trials (even morally innocent research that aims at developing useful interventions for the community in question). As a result of this distrust, subjects may themselves be harmed in the future if interventions later become available that they refuse to use or if trials need to be conducted that would benefit their community.

While it is difficult, of course, to quantify such harms, it would be foolish to reject them out of hand. Nor should we reject them because they seem in the abstract to point to "irrational" reactions on the part of individuals. Rational or not, such reactions have been known to occur. There is much of importance that medical researchers have yet to learn, and the future success of research is highly dependent on public goodwill.

In his excellent study of the Tuskeegee syphilis study, James Jones records the fact that, after Tuskeegee, many African Americans no longer trusted the American Public Health Service *or the white medical establishment generally*. Thus they refused to pay attention (to their own detriment) to warnings about a new deadly virus (AIDS) in the 1980s.[48] Jones's discussion of the African American case not only shows that such reactions are possible but also highlights the consequential importance of trust. If we grant that (1) it is not irrational to distrust people who have harmed you *or used you unfairly* in the past, and that (2) the effects of distrust (whether rational or not) are real and serious, we cannot afford to overlook this argument. Trust is central to the success of medicine, research, and public health endeavors, and trust can be undermined in more ways than simply by harming people. The ordinary person's trust may be undermined by the perception of motivated failures of easy rescue. Hence, whether theorists want to call that particular type of omission a "harm" (or recognize a "right" to easy rescue) turns out to be beside the point. Since clinical research is highly dependent on the goodwill and trust of the public, failures of easy rescue in cases like *Surfaxin** should be forbidden.

Conclusion

I have argued that *some* but not all placebo cases* are morally problematic. Some but not all placebo cases* are exploitative.

To reach this conclusion, we had to first consider what exploitation really is. The model of exploitation most applicable to these cases is the following: A exploits B when A has a preexisting moral obligation to aid B but, instead of helping, uses his bargaining advantage to try to obtain a waiver of this moral obligation from B. In such a case, the waiver fails and A flouts his obligation to B. Critics of placebo cases* have viewed them through this lens because they think about the obligations of researchers in a particular way. They adopt the *medical model* of researcher obligations, and hence see researchers as physicians, with all the obligations that implies. Therefore, it makes sense that these critics would view the subjects of placebo cases* as victims of harm, since we typically allow that you have been harmed when your physician offers you less than the best possible care.

However, I have argued that we must replace the medical model that has shaped so much of the thinking about research ethics. As an alternative, I suggested that researchers have Good Samaritan obligations, just like the rest of us. When these are defeated, as they sometimes are, then subjects cannot claim to be exploited. This view allows us to see why, given the claims of scientific necessity stipulated in *AZT**, cases like *AZT* would be permissible. If that is correct, then although Nicole's distress remains understandable, she may not have suffered an injustice at the hands of researchers simply because the trial she was in had placebo controls.

Recognizing the Good Samaritan obligations of researchers also allows us to see why admitting that *AZT** was justified does not necessarily lead to endorsing all placebo cases*. Good Samaritan obligations are not always defeated. When they are not defeated, placebo cases* flout the obligation to perform easy rescues. Although many theorists resist the idea of a right to easy rescue and with it the idea that a person who is not rescued is harmed, we can nonetheless see the flouting of such an important obligation, for no good reason, as deeply *unfair*. Since researchers in such cases benefit from this unfair flouting, such cases are exploitative. This helps to explain why it is so important to limit the troubling kinds of placebo cases*. Research depends on trust and support from the public, and this is incompatible with a view of researchers as those who stand by watching while people needlessly drown.

Acknowledgments

Thanks to Ezekiel Emanuel, Frank Miller, Alan Wertheimer, Dan Wikler, Dan Brock, Connie Rosati, Angelo Volandes, Simon Keller, and the members of the Edmund J. Safra Faculty Fellows Seminar at Harvard University, 2004–2005.

Parts of this chapter appeared earlier under the title "Justice and Placebo Controls," *Social Theory and Practice* 32 (2006): 467–96. Reprinted here with permission of the publisher.

Notes

1. AZT is the brand name for the antiretroviral drug zidovudine. A more detailed description of the case appears in the introduction to this volume.

2. H. French, "AIDS Research in Africa: Juggling Risks and Hopes," *New York Times*, October 9, 1997.

3. *Id.*

4. Marcia Angell, "The Ethics of Clinical Research in the Third World," *New England Journal of Medicine* 337 (1997): 847–49; Peter Lurie and Sidney Wolfe, "Unethical Trials of Interventions to Reduce Perinatal Transmission of the Human Immunodeficiency Virus in Developing Countries," *New England Journal of Medicine* 337 (1997): 853–55. These two pieces sparked the debate over the AZT trials. While many other articles have been critical of these trials, they are too numerous to list here.

5. The asterisk is there to remind the reader that "placebo case," as I am using it, only refers to a subset of trials that employ placebo controls. There is a huge general literature on the ethics of placebo-controlled trials, but I am not aiming to engage that entire debate.

6. See, e.g., Angell, *supra* note 4; Lurie and Wolfe, *supra* note 4; Ruth Macklin, *Double Standards in Medical Research in Developing Countries* (Cambridge: Cambridge University Press, 2004).

7. For detailed descriptions of *AZT* and *Surfaxin*, see chapter 2 of this volume.

8. See chapter 1 of this volume for a more in-depth explanation of these trial designs and their typical uses.

9. It is important to emphasize that the first question—whether PCTs are really necessary in a given case—is not a simple one. The question opens up a bitter, on-going methodological dispute that has an important normative component, since in clinical research the degree of methodological rigor we insist upon has real human effects. In real life, many people find it difficult to separate the two questions I outline here. Nonetheless, it is conceptually possible to separate them and morally beneficial to do so.

10. See the discussion of the case by Lurie and Wolfe in *Ethical Issues in International Biomedical Research: A Casebook*, ed. James V. Lavery, Christine Grady, Elizabeth R. Wahl, and Ezekiel J. Emanuel (New York: Oxford University Press, 2007), 159–70.

11. Alan Wertheimer, *Exploitation* (Princeton, NJ: Princeton University Press, 1996), 10. All further references to Wertheimer are to this book unless stated otherwise. See also Richard Arneson, "Exploitation," in *The Encyclopedia of Ethics*, ed. L. C. Becker (New York: Garland Press, 1992), 350. For a theorist who does not accept even this rather general account of exploitation, see Allen Wood, "Exploitation," *Social Philosophy and Policy* 12 (1995): 135–58.

12. Wertheimer, *supra* note 11, at 17. Also, in the context of research especially, it is important to note that A could be working on behalf of a third party, C, in which case it is sufficient if either C or A benefits from A's transaction with B. On this point, see Wertheimer, *supra* note 11, at 210. For simplicity I restrict myself to talking about transactions between A and B. However, in clinical research multiple parties typically benefit. Researchers benefit in terms of career advancement and prestige. They also work for and represent sponsors who benefit financially, and the general public benefits from the increase in knowledge.

13. *Id.* at 16.

14. *Id.* at 12.

15. Wertheimer claims that procedural flaws are not by themselves sufficient for exploitation. However, it is not entirely clear what he means by this. If he simply means that exploitation must involve as a necessary component A's benefit (which is a feature of the outcome), then we agree and simply represent the material slightly differently. I set up A's benefit as a necessary requirement from the outset and then distinguish between different unfairnesses to B: procedural unfairnesses and outcome unfairnesses. However, if he thinks there must be some form of outcome unfairness to B in addition to any unfairness B suffers as a result of flawed consent, then we do not completely agree in our analysis.

16. How exactly should we describe the unfairness to B in a case where B is harmed? Wertheimer is not completely clear about this. He appears to vacillate between the claim that harming is itself a form of unfairness and the claim that unfairness enters only as a result of the fact that A benefits from the harming. So, for example, he says on page 16, "We may say that the benefit to A is unfair because it is wrong for A to benefit at all from his or her act (e.g. harming B)." The second option seems better to me (on purely linguistic grounds). Wertheimer himself, in e-mail correspondence from March 2005, has admitted to leaning in the second direction as well.

17. For example, some of the subjects in Nicole's trial very likely did not give fully informed consent (revealing that fact appears to have been the primary journalistic motive for the article in note 1). However, I shall set aside those concerns here.

18. Though see note 29 below about coercion.

19. Wertheimer, *supra* note 11, at 216–17.

20. *Id.* at 40, 53. Also see his contribution in chapter 3 of this volume.

21. Wertheimer has also used this case as an example of coercion where the baseline against which threats are distinguished from offers is moralized. *Exploitation*, at 53. On the relationship between my analysis and coercion, see note 29.

22. See, e.g., Participants in the 2001 Conference on Ethical Aspects of Research in Developing Countries, "Moral Standards for Research in Developing Countries: From 'Reasonable Availability' to 'Fair Benefits,'" *Hastings Center Report* 34, no. 3 (2004): 17–27.

23. Some people associate the role of doctor with a duty to rescue. I discuss such duties later at length. While we do often call upon people with medical training in crisis situations ("Is there a doctor in the house?"), I think this is not best viewed as an essential part of the role of doctor. We all have a duty as moral agents to help in crisis situations, and this may include making use of any special skills we have. If someone collapses in a seizure, it may be that, of all the bystanders, the one with medical training is best placed to try to help and may therefore inherit the obligation. But this is not unique to doctors. If a child has fallen down the local well, and the bystanders include someone with extensive experience of climbing and rappelling, then that person may be obligated to let himself be lowered down into the well as part of a rescue attempt.

24. The relationship need not always be formed by explicit agreement, or by some prior personal engagement between doctor and patient, as long as there are institutional norms that make it clear when one person becomes another's patient.

25. See, e.g., Alison McIntyre, "Guilty Bystanders? On the Legitimacy

of Duty to Rescue Statutes," *Philosophy and Public Affairs* 23 (1994): 157– 91; T. M. Scanlon, *What We Owe to Each Other* (Cambridge, MA: Harvard University Press, 1998), 224–28; and Joel Feinberg, *Harm to Others* (Oxford: Oxford University Press, 1984), 126–86.

26. Feinberg notes that although many European countries have instituted laws that penalize people who fail to carry out easy rescues, Anglo-American law has generally not done so. But Anglo-American law does penalize someone in a fiduciary relationship who allows the other party to suffer an easily preventable injury. Hence, Anglo-American law reflects the same distinction I make in the text between two types of positive obligations to help. Feinberg, *supra* note 25, at 127.

27. An illustration: "For example, I am sitting in a lounge chair next to a swimming pool. A child (not mine) is drowning in the pool a few inches from where I am sitting. If I do not save him I violate no rights . . . but would still reveal myself as a piece of moral slime properly to be shunned by all decent people." J. Murphy, "Blackmail: A Preliminary Inquiry," *Monist* 63 (1980): 168, quoted in Feinberg, *supra* note 26, at 130.

28. In this chapter I use "obligation" in the wide sense that carries no implication that if A is morally obligated to do X for B, B has a right against A that A do X.

29. It is worth noting that on a widely accepted account of coercion, placebo cases* would turn out to be not only exploitative but also coercive if, but only if, the critics are right about the type of obligation being flouted. Alan Wertheimer argues that "A coerces B to do X only if A proposes (threatens) to make B worse off with reference to some baseline if B chooses not to do X." The issue of the baseline is tricky, but it is the same one that arises with respect to harm. If we grant both that A has a preexisting moral obligation to aid B and that a failure to fulfill that obligation is harm, then when A offers B a 50 percent chance of receiving treatment, A can be viewed as threatening B with 100 percent chance of harm (non-aid) unless B accepts a 50 percent chance of harm. However, if my argument succeeds, then a failure on the part of researchers to fulfill their obligations is not harm, and so the offer to participate is not a threat of harm and so *not* coercive. For the preceding definition of coercion, see Wertheimer, *supra* note 11, at 26; Alan Wertheimer, *Coercion* (Princeton, NJ: Princeton University Press, 1987).

30. See, e.g., Brennan, "Proposed Revisions to the Declaration of Helsinki— Will They Weaken the Ethical Principles Underlying Human Research?" *New England Journal of Medicine* 341 (1999): 527–31, at 527: "Just as the physician must be committed to protecting the welfare of the patient he or she is treat-

ing, the researcher must be committed to protecting the welfare of the research subject."

31. For a historical overview of the medical model of researcher obligations, see F. Miller and H. Brody, "A Critique of Clinical Equipoise: Therapeutic Misconception in the Ethics of Clinical Trials," *Hastings Center Report* 33, no. 3 (2003): 19–28. Miller and Brody describe the gradual evolution of what they term the "similarity view" (roughly the same as my "medical model"). They argue that this view (a) makes research ethics incoherent, (b) is tacitly accepted by many who nonetheless fail to see the tension between the similarity view and the general aims of research, and (c) ought to be abandoned and an alternative framework for research ethics developed. I am in general agreement with all these claims. However, my aim here is to consider in more depth the philosophical arguments that might be given for and against the medical model.

32. As I use it here, "role overlap" does not refer to the general idea of one person occupying both roles (which remains common), but the more specific idea of occupying both roles in relation to the same person. This is certainly less common than it used to be.

33. I follow Hardimon and Daniels in seeing the role obligations of physicians as contractual: the obligated individual consents to adopt the entire role, even though the specific obligations she acquires form a cluster or group among which she is not free to pick and choose. See M. Hardimon, "Role Obligations," *Journal of Philosophy* 91 (1994): 333–63; Norman Daniels, "Duty to Treat or Right to Refuse?" *Hastings Center Report* 21, no. 2 (1991): 36–47.

34. This ought to be qualified a bit. There is room to disagree about whether, even in resource-rich environments, a researcher's obligations are the same as a physician's or simply similar to them (and constrained by them). But I will not pursue the point here.

35. While there are affluent people even in these destitute countries, the communities selected for such research are generally ones in which no one currently receives the most effective therapy for the condition in question. For example, all the hospitals in Bolivia chosen for the Surfaxin trial served a poor population and had no surfactant for the treatment of respiratory distress syndrome. So there is little danger that someone who would have been able to get effective treatment elsewhere will mistakenly choose research participation out of confusion of the researcher role and the physician role.

36. There is much disagreement about when appeals to personal sacrifice can defeat Good Samaritan obligations. A much stronger view than the one I advocate for here is Peter Singer, "Famine, Affluence, and Morality," *Philosophy and Public Affairs* 1 (1972): 229–43, at 231.

37. Henry Richardson and Leah Belsky also defend the idea that researchers have Good Samaritan obligations—what they call "duties to rescue." H. Richardson and L. Belsky, "The Ancillary Care Responsibilities of Medical Researchers: An Ethical Framework for Thinking about the Clinical Care That Researchers Owe Their Subjects," *Hastings Center Report* 34, no. 1 (2004): 25–33. However, their primary concern is to defend additional positive duties over and above duties to rescue. They neither elaborate on Good Samaritan obligations nor relate them explicitly to placebo-controlled trials.

38. Angell, *supra* note 4, notes that drugs for research are often provided free by drug companies. Of course, drugs are not the only expense of research, and that matters. If offering effective therapy were prohibitively expensive, I might endorse an exception, assuming the first and last of my other conditions (set out later in this chapter) are met. However, the determination of "prohibitively expensive" should not be left to the sponsors of research, but would need independent assessment. I thank Ezekiel Emanuel for pressing me on this point.

39. The phrase "me-too" drug refers to the practice of developing drugs that, at a chemical level, are incredibly similar to existing drugs but just distinct enough to circumvent patent limitations. Although the practice is dubious, not all "me-too" drugs work the same way, and some turn out to be quite valuable (the varieties of SSRIs for depression being an example). For a discussion of this practice, and its negative effects on medicine and drug development, see Marcia Angell, *The Truth about the Drug Companies: How They Deceive Us and What to Do about It* (New York: Random House, 2004), 1.

40. I thank Dan Brock and Dan Wikler for pressing me on this.

41. J. Thomson, "A Defense of Abortion," *Philosophy and Public Affairs 1* (1971): 63.

42. See, e.g., C. Snowden, D. Elbourne, and J. Garcia, "Zelen Randomization: Attitudes of Parents Participating in a Neonatal Clinical Trial," *Controlled Clinical Trials* 20 (1998): 149–71.

43. For more on ancillary care, see Richardson and Belsky, "Ancillary Care Responsibilities."

44. Though see note 38 for a possible second requirement.

45. So, for example, I am explicitly rejecting the kind of stance found in E. M. Meslin and H. T. Shapiro, "Ethical Issues in the Design and Conduct of Clinical Trials in Developing Countries," *New England Journal of Medicine* 345 (2001): 140. They allow for an *exception* to the general presumption against using placebo "in a situation in which the only useful research design, from the host country's perspective, require(s) a less effective intervention in the control group, *if the condition being studied (is) not life threatening*" (emphasis added).

The stipulation that the condition not be life-threatening makes it impossible to distinguish, as I do, between *AZT** and *Surfaxin**, but instead rules out both.

46. This is precisely what happened in *Surfaxin*. After receiving negative publicity about its plans from Ralph Nader's Public Citizen's Health Research Group, the manufacturer abandoned the project and conducted active controlled trials in the United States and Europe instead.

47. This is not mere speculation. Robert Temple of the Food and Drug Administration was quoted as saying, "If they did the trial, half of the people would get surfactant and better perinatal care, and the other half would get better perinatal care. It seems to me that all the people in the trial would have been better off." S. Shah, "Globalizing Clinical Research," *Nation*, July 1, 2002, 28.

48. "'Bizarre as it may seem to most people,' declared the lead editorial in the New York Times on May 6, 1992, 'many black Americans believe that AIDS and the health measures used against it are part of a conspiracy to wipe out the black race.' . . . The consequences of mistrust were nothing short of tragic. As the Times explained, 'At its most destructive, the paranoia causes many blacks to avoid medical treatment.'" J. Jones, *Bad Blood: The Tuskegee Syphilis Experiment*, new and expanded edition (New York: Free Press, 1993), 221.

$$\boxed{9}$$

Addressing Exploitation: Reasonable Availability versus Fair Benefits

EZEKIEL J. EMANUEL AND PARTICIPANTS IN THE 2001
CONFERENCE ON ETHICAL ASPECTS OF RESEARCH IN
DEVELOPING COUNTRIES

(*Names of Participants and Affiliations
Appear at End of Chapter*)

Over the last decade, clinical research conducted by sponsors and researchers from developed countries in developing countries has been the subject of significant controversy.[1] Debate about perinatal HIV transmission studies in Southeast Asia and Africa, sponsored by the National Institutes of Health (NIH) and Centers for Disease Control (CDC), inflamed this controversy and focused it on the standard of care, that is, whether treatments tested in developing countries should be compared with treatments provided locally or the worldwide best interventions.[2] Debate about research in developing countries has expanded to include concerns about informed consent. Less discussed but potentially even more important has been the requirement of "reasonable availability" of tested drugs if proven effective.[3] There seems to be general agreement that reasonable availability is a requirement of research in developing countries in order to avoid exploitation. We reject this consensus. Instead of the reasonable availability requirement, we advocate a fair benefits framework to avoid exploitation, and compare these two approaches in a specific case—the trial of hepatitis A vaccine in Thailand, the Havrix trial.

Current Views on the Reasonable Availability Requirement

Historically, the idea of making interventions reasonably available was emphasized in the Council for International Organizations of Medical Sciences (CIOMS) *International Ethical Guidelines* (1993) and has been reiterated in the 2002 revision in Guideline 10 and its commentary:

> As a general rule, the sponsoring agency should agree in advance of the research that any product developed through such research will be made reasonably available to the inhabitants of the host community or country at the completion of successful testing. Exceptions to this general requirement should be justified and agreed to by all concerned parties before the research begins.

Disagreement has focused on three issues. First, how strong or explicit should the commitment to provide the drug or vaccine be at the initiation of the research trial? (The specifics of various opinions on this question are presented in table 1). CIOMS required an explicit, contractlike mechanism, agreed to before the trial, and assigns this responsibility to the sponsors of research. The Declaration of Helsinki's 2000 revision endorses a less stringent guarantee that does not require availability of interventions to be "ensured" "in advance."[4] Several other ethical guidelines suggest "discussion in advance" but do not require formal, prior agreements.[5] Conversely, some commentators insist that the CIOMS guarantee is "not strong or specific enough."[6] For instance, both the chair and the executive director of the U.S. National Bioethics Advisory Commission (NBAC)[7] contend: "If the intervention being tested is not likely to be affordable in the host country or if the health care infrastructure cannot support its proper distribution and use, it is unethical to ask persons in that country to participate in the research, since they will not enjoy any of its potential benefits."[8] To address these concerns, others advocate that a formal and explicit prior agreement "which includes identified funding" and specifies improvements necessary in the "country's health care delivery capabilities" is ethically required for research in developing countries.[9]

Second, disagreement focuses on who is responsible for ensuring reasonable availability. Are sponsors responsible, as the original CIOMS

TABLE 1
THE RANGE OF RECENT OPINION ON THE
REQUIREMENT OF REASONABLE AVAILABILITY

	Very High	←	Extent of Guarantee
	Annas, Grodin, Glantz, Mariner	Shapiro and Meslin	CIOMS (1993)
Type of Guarantee	A realistic plan, which includes identified funding [and a plan to improve that country's health care delivery capabilities], to provide the newly proven intervention to the population from which the potential pool of research subjects is to be recruited.	If the intervention being tested is not likely to be affordable in the host country or if the health care infrastructure cannot support its proper distribution and use, it is unethical to ask persons in that country to participate in the research, since they will not enjoy any of its potential benefits.	As a general rule, the sponsoring agency should agree in advance of the research that any product developed through such research will be made reasonably available to the inhabitants of the host community or country at the completion of successful testing. Exceptions to this general requirement should be justified and agreed to by all concerned parties before the research begins.
Party Responsible for Reasonable Availability	Sponsors of research, developed countries, and international funders		Sponsors of research
Scope of the Guarantee of Reasonable Availability	Host country	Host country	Inhabitants of the host community or country

TABLE I *(continued)*

of Availability	→	*Limited*
CIOMS (2002)	*Declaration of Helsinki*	*Ugandan Guidelines*
Before undertaking research in a population or community with limited resources, the sponsor and the investigator must make every effort to ensure that . . . any intervention or product developed, or knowledge generated, will be made reasonably available for the benefit of that population or community.	Medical research is only justified if there is a reasonable likelihood that the populations in which the research is carried out stand to benefit from the results of the research.	The investigator shall make a reasonable effort to secure the product's availability to the local community in which the research occurred.
Sponsors of research and investigators	Unspecified; guidance is to "physicians and other participants in medical research"	Researchers
Population or community in which the research is being done	Populations in which research occurred	Local community in which research occurred

guideline called for? Does responsibility rest with host country governments? Or international aid organizations? Does "reasonable" require the drug or vaccine be free, subsidized, or at market prices? Finally, disagreement has focused on to whom interventions should be made reasonably available. Should they be restricted to participants in the research study? Should they include the village or tribe from which individual participants were enrolled? Or the whole country in which the research was conducted?

The Justification of Reasonable Availability

Why is reasonable availability thought to be a requirement for ethical research in developing countries? Research uses participants to develop generalizable knowledge that can improve health and health care for others.[10] The potential for exploitation of individual participants enrolled in research as well as communities that support and bear the burdens of research is inherent in every research trial. Historically, favorable risk-benefit ratios, informed consent, and respecting enrolled participants have been the primary mechanisms used to minimize the potential to exploit individual research participants.[11] Importantly, in developed countries, the potential for exploitation of populations has been a concern, but of less significance since there is a process, albeit imperfect, for ensuring that interventions proven effective through clinical research are introduced into the health care system and benefit the general population.[12] In contrast, the potential for exploitation is particularly acute in research trials in developing countries. It is claimed that target populations typically lack access to regular health care, political power, and an understanding of research. Hence, they may be exposed to the risks of research with few tangible benefits. The benefits of research—access to new effective drugs and vaccines—are predominantly for people in developed countries with profits to the pharmaceutical industry. Many consider this scenario the quintessential case of exploitation.[13]

Supporters deem reasonable availability a requirement of ethical research in developing countries as necessary to prevent exploitation of communities. As one group of commentators put it: "In order for research to be ethically conducted [in a developing country] it must offer the potential of actual benefit to the inhabitants of that developing country. . . . [F]or underdeveloped communities to derive potential benefit from research, they must have access to the fruits of such research."[14] Or as the commentary to the 2002 CIOMS Guideline 10 put it: "If the knowledge gained from the research in such a country [with limited resources] is used primarily for the benefit of populations that can afford the tested product, the research may rightly be characterized as exploitative and, therefore, unethical."

What Is Exploitation?

While initially plausible, there are a number of problems with making reasonable availability a necessary ethical requirement for multinational research in developing countries. The most important problem is that the reasonable availability requirement embodies a mistaken conception of exploitation and, therefore, offers the wrong solution.

There are numerous ways of harming other individuals, only one of which is exploitation. Although oppression, coercion, undue inducement, deception, betrayal, discrimination, and so forth are obviously distinct ways of harming people, they are frequently conflated and confused with exploitation as if they were all the same.[15] It is important to carefully distinguish these different wrongs predominantly because they require very different remedies. Addressing coercion requires removing threats; addressing deception requires full disclosure; yet removing threats and requiring full disclosure alone will not resolve cases of exploitation.[16]

What is exploitation? Party A exploits party B when B receives an unfair level of benefits as a result of B's interactions with A.[17] The fairness of the benefits Party B receives depends upon the burdens that B bears as part of the interaction, and the benefits that A and others receive as a result of B's participation in the interaction. A classic example of exploitation occurs if B runs his car into a snowbank and A offers to tow him out but only at the cost of $200—when the normal and fair price for the tow is $75. In this circumstance, A exploits B.

This Wertheimerian conception of exploitation is distinct from the commonly cited Kantian instrumental conception in which exploitation entails the "use" of someone for one's own benefit. As Allen Buchanan characterizes the Kantian conception: "To exploit a person involves the *harmful, merely instrumental utilization* of him or his capacities, for one's own advantage or for the sake of one's own ends."[18] There are many problems with the Kantian conception. Most important, if the instrumental use of a person alone is the harm, then, as Kantians acknowledge, almost all human interactions are exploitative because we constantly and necessarily use other people.[19] In the snowbank case, not only does A exploit B, but on this Kantian view, B also exploits A because B instrumentally uses A to get his car out of the snowbank. So we have mutual exploitation because we have mutual instrumental use to our own advantage. Sometimes the word "exploit" is merely a neutral version of "use"—he exploited the minerals or his own strength. However, in discussions of research, especially but not exclusively in developing countries, exploitation is never neutral; it is always a moral wrong. Consequently, we do not need to mark out all cases of use but need to identify the cases that are morally problematic. A conception of exploitation is needed to determine which ones are wrong.[20] Consequently, whatever one thinks about the merits of the Kantian conception of exploitation, it seems irrelevant to assessing the adequacy of reasonable availability to prevent exploitation; reasonable availability relies on the idea that sufficient benefits can prevent exploitation.

The Kantian conception of exploitation requires expansion beyond use to include a separate harm. But, in the case of exploitation, what is this "other harm"? For a Kantian to exploit must mean to use in a way that the other person could not consent to, a way that undermines her autonomy.[21] The problem here is that in many cases people do consent to situations—with full knowledge and without threats—and yet we think they are exploited. People in developing countries could give fully informed consent to participating in a research study and yet still be exploited. Similarly, snowbank-bound B does seem exploited even if he consents to being towed out for $200. Mistakenly, the Kantian conception fuses exploitation with inadequate consent. Finally, reasonable availability does not seem to be grounded in a Kantian conception of exploitation as use and violations of autonomy. Rather, reasonable availability is aimed at ensuring that people have access to the interventions that they helped to demonstrate were effective. Reasonable availability is related to the benefits people receive from participating in a research study, not their autonomy in consent.

The Wertheimerian view of exploitation, which locates the core moral issue inherent in exploitation in the fair level of benefits each party of an interaction receives, seems to capture the concern underlying the reasonable availability requirement. There are at least six important observations about this conception of exploitation. First, exploitation is a micro-level not macro-level, concern. Exploitation is about harms from discrete interactions, rather than about the larger social justice of the distribution of background rights and resources. We should not confuse problems of distributive justice with problems of exploitation. Certainly macro-level distributions of resources can influence exploitation, but the actual exploitation is separate. Furthermore, while people may feel exploited and may claim to have been so based upon historical events, the ethical evaluation of exploitation does not depend upon a feeling or past injustices. Exploitation is about the fairness of an individual exchange. Indeed, as we shall note later, exploitation can happen even in a just society and fail to occur when there is gross inequality between the parties:

> While the background conditions shape our existence, the primary experiences occur at the micro level. Exploitation matters to people. People who can accept an unjust set of aggregate resources with considerable equanimity will recoil when they feel exploited in an individual or local transaction. . . . Furthermore, micro-level exploitation is not as closely linked to macro-level injustice as might be thought. Even in a reasonably just society, people will find themselves in situations [which] will give rise to allegations of exploitation.[22]

The reasonable availability requirement recognizes the possibility of exploitation associated with a particular study, asking whether the intervention studied was made available to the host community afterward. Reasonable availability does not require ensuring the just distribution of all rights and resources or a just international social order. This is more than just pragmatic; it also reflects the deep experience that exploitation is transactional.

Second, because exploitation is about interactions at a micro-level, between researcher and community, it can only occur once an interaction is initiated. In this sense, the obligations to avoid exploitation are obligations that coexist with initiating an interaction. When A walks away from a transaction, there is no exploitation of B, even if B remains poorly off. That is, A may bear some responsibility for the poverty of B, but this is based on claims of justice, not of exploitation.

Third, exploitation is about "how much," not "what," each party receives. The key issue is fairness in the level of benefits. Moreover, exploitation depends upon the fairness, not the "equalness," of the level of benefits. An unequal distribution of benefits may be fair if there are differences in the burdens and contributions of each party. The notion of fairness important for exploitation is not Rawlsian. Fairness in the distribution of benefits is common to both Rawls's theory and a theory of exploitation. However, they differ in that the former addresses macro-level and the latter micro-level distributions of benefits. That is, the Rawlsian conception of fairness addresses the distribution of rights, liberties, and resources for the basic structure of society within which individual transactions occur.[23] In other words, Rawlsian fairness is about constitutional arrangements, taxes, and opportunities. Rawls's conception has often but wrongly been applied to micro-level decisions, usually issuing in implausible and indefensible recommendations. Fairness in individual interactions, which is the concern of exploitation, is based on ideal market transactions.[24] Thus, a fair distribution of benefits at the micro-level is based on the level of benefits that would occur in a market transaction devoid of fraud, deception, or force in which the parties have full information. While this is always idealized—in just the way economic theory is idealized—it is the powerful ideal informing the notion of fairness of micro-level transactions. Importantly, this notion of fairness is also relative; it is based on comparisons to the level of benefits for other parties interacting in similar circumstances. Just as the fair price in markets is based on comparability, so too is the determination of fair benefits (to avoid exploitation) based on comparability.

Fourth, that one party is vulnerable may make exploitation more likely, but it does not inherently entail exploitation. Vulnerability is neither necessary nor sufficient for determining whether exploitation has occurred. Exploitation is based upon the level of benefits; examining the status of the parties is irrelevant in determining whether exploitation has occurred. If the exchange is fair to both parties, then there is no exploitation regardless of whether one party is poor, uneducated, or otherwise vulnerable and disadvantaged. In the snowbound case, if A charges B $75 for towing the car out, then B is not exploited even though B is vulnerable. Fairness of the level of benefits, not vulnerability of the parties, is the essential determinant of exploitation.

Fifth, since exploitation is about the fairness of micro-level interactions, the key question is the level of benefits provided to the parties who interact. Determinations of exploitation must focus on the parties to the interaction, not the kind of benefits people unrelated to the interaction receive.

Finally, because fairness depends upon idealized market transactions, determining when exploitation occurs—when the level of benefits is unfair—will require interpretation. But, like the application of legal principles or constitutional provisions, such moral interpretations depend upon notions of fairness and benefits, and reasonable people can disagree. Interpretation and controversy are inevitable, but neither invalidates the practice of judicial adjudication or moral judgment.

Problems with the Reasonable Availability Requirement

The fundamental problem with reasonable availability is that it guarantees a type of benefit—the proven intervention—but not a fair level of benefits and therefore does not necessarily prevent exploitation. For some risky research or research in which the sponsor stands to gain enormously, reasonable availability might be inadequate and unfair. Conversely, for very low-risk or no-risk research in which the population is obtaining other benefits or in which the benefits to the sponsor are minimal, requiring the sponsor to make a product reasonably available could be excessive and unfair. Reasonable availability does not necessarily assure a fair level of benefits.

There are other problems. Reasonable availability embodies a very narrow notion of benefits to the population of developing countries from research participation. Reasonable availability suggests that only one type of benefit—a proven intervention—can justify participation in clinical research. But a population in a developing country could consider a diverse range of other benefits from research, including the training of health care and/or research personnel, the construction of health care facilities and other physical infrastructure, and the provision of public health measures and health services beyond those required as part of the research trial. Reasonable availability ignores such benefits for the purposes of determining a fair level of benefits and, hence, for determining when exploitation has or has not occurred.

Second, the original CIOMS formulation of reasonable availability applied to only a narrow range of clinical research—successful Phase III testing of interventions.[25] It does not apply to Phase I and II drug and vaccine testing, or to genetic, epidemiology, and natural history research that are necessary and common types of research in developing countries but may be conducted years or decades prior to proving an intervention safe and effective. Consequently, either the reasonable availability requirement suggests that such non–Phase III studies conducted in developing countries are unethical, because they provide no possibility of reasonable access to an intervention after a trial (a position articulated in the original CIOMS guidelines but widely repudiated); or there is no ethical requirement to provide benefits to the population when conducting such early-phase research; or reasonable availability is not the only way to provide benefits from a clinical research study.

To address this, CIOMS altered the reasonable availability requirement in 2002: "Before undertaking research in a population or community with limited resources, the sponsor and the investigator must make every effort to ensure that . . . any intervention or product developed, or *knowledge generated*, will be made reasonably available for the benefit of that population or community (italics added)."[26] According to CIOMS, making the knowledge gained reasonably available is acceptable for avoiding exploitation. Knowledge may not constitute a fair level of benefits for many non–Phase III studies, but restricting benefit to the population to the knowledge gained may not match the risks or the benefits to others. Indeed, the requirement could permit pharmaceutically sponsored Phase I and II testing of drugs in developing countries, while shifting Phase III testing and sales to developed countries as long as data from the early studies are provided to the developing countries. This modification to encompass non–Phase III studies might actually invite more exploitation of developing countries.

Third, even in Phase III studies, reasonable availability provides an uncertain benefit to the population depending upon whether the trial is a "successful testing" of a new product. If there is true clinical equipoise at the beginning of Phase III trials conducted in developing countries, then the new intervention will be proven more effective in only about half of the trials.[27] Consequently, reliance on reasonable availability alone to provide benefits implies that the host country will derive benefits from half or fewer of all Phase III studies.

Fourth, reasonable availability does not avert the potential for undue inducement of a deprived population. One worry about research in developing countries is that collateral benefits will be escalated to induce the population to enroll in excessively risky research. If the population lacks access to public health measures, routine vaccines, medications for common ailments, and even trained health care personnel, then providing these services as part of a research study might induce them to consent to the project despite its risks or the fact that it disproportionately benefits people in developed countries.[28] However, guaranteeing reasonable availability to a safe and effective drug or vaccine after a study could also function as an undue inducement to a deprived population that lacks basic health care.

Fifth, it is beyond the authority of researchers and even many sponsors of research to guarantee reasonable availability. Clinical researchers and even some sponsors in developed countries, such as the NIH and the Medical Research Council of the United Kingdom (MRC), do not control drug approval processes in their own countries, much less other countries. Similarly, they do not control budgets for health ministries or foreign aid to implement research results, and may be, by law, precluded from providing assistance with implementation of research results. At best, they can generate data to inform the deliberations of ministers of health, aid officials, international funding organizations, and relevant others, and provide moral suasion to implement effective interventions. Because most Phase III trials take years to conduct, policy makers in developing countries and aid agencies may be resistant to forging prior agreements regarding a specific intervention before knowing the magnitude of its benefits or the logistical requirements for implementation and distribution, and before being able to compare these to other potential interventions. This cautiousness does not seem unreasonable given scarce resources for health delivery.

Sixth, requiring reasonable availability connotes that the population cannot make its own, autonomous decisions about what benefits are worth the risks of a research trial. Inevitably, requiring reasonable availability of a proven drug or vaccine entails cost to sponsors of research. In many cases, these resources could be directed to other benefits instead. Insisting on reasonable availability as an ethical requirement necessitates that these resources be devoted to providing the tested intervention even when the host country might prefer other benefits. Disregarding the host community's view on what constitutes appropriate benefit for them— insisting that a population must benefit in a specific manner—implies a kind of paternalism.

Finally, requiring prior agreement to supply a proven product at the end of a successful trial can become a "golden handcuff"—constraining rather than benefiting the population. If there is a prior agreement to receive a specific drug or vaccine rather than cash or some other transferable commodity, the prior agreement commits the population to using the specific intervention tested in the trial. (Certainly pharmaceutical companies are likely to provide product directly or a specific product at a specific price for a set time and avoid agreements in which they are required to provide the product of a competitor.) Yet if other, more effective or desirable interventions are developed, the population is unlikely to have the resources to obtain those interventions. Hence, prior agreements can actually limit access of the population to appropriate interventions. This suggests that it is not prior agreement to make a proven intervention reasonably available that is valuable, but sufficient benefit for participating in the research trial.

Because of these difficulties, reasonable availability is recognized more in the breech than in its fulfillment; much effort has been devoted to identifying and justifying exceptions.

The Fair Benefits Framework

Ethically, targeted populations in developing countries must benefit from the conduct and/or results of clinical research performed in their communities. While reasonable availability is one way to provide benefits to a population, it is not the only way. Hence, it is not a necessary condition for ethical research in developing countries and should not be imposed without affirmation by the developing countries themselves.

As an alternative to reasonable availability this group proposes the fair benefits framework (table 2, columns 1 and 2).[29]

The fair benefits framework supplements the usual conditions for the ethical conduct of research trials, such as independent review by an institutional review board or research ethics committee and individual informed consent.[30] In particular, it relies on three background principles that are widely accepted as requirements for ethical research. First, the research should have social value by addressing a health problem of the developing country population. Second, fair subject selection ensures that the scientific objectives of the research itself, not poverty or vulnerability, provide a strong justification for conducting the research in a specific population. For instance, the population may have a high incidence of the disease being studied or transmission rates of infection necessary to evaluate a vaccine. Third, the research must have a favorable risk-benefit ratio, in which benefits to participants outweigh the risks, or the net risks are acceptably low.

The fair benefits framework adds three principles that are specified by fourteen benchmarks to these widely accepted principles (table 2, columns 1 and 2).

Principle 1: Fair Benefits

There should be a comprehensive delineation of tangible benefits to the research participants and the population from the conduct and results of the research. These benefits can be of three types: (1) benefits to research participants during the research, (2) benefits to the population during the research, or (3) benefits to the population after completion of the research (table 2, column 2), It is not necessary to provide each of these types of benefits; the ethical imperative based on the conception of exploitation is for a fair level of benefits. Indeed, it would seem fair that as the burdens and risks of the research increase, the benefits should also increase. Similarly, as the benefits to the sponsors, researchers, and others outside the population increase, the benefits to the host population should increase.

Importantly, because the aim of the fair benefits framework is to avoid exploitation, the population at risk for exploitation from the research

TABLE 2
THE FAIR BENEFITS FRAMEWORK

Principles	Benchmarks	Hepatitis A Vaccine Thailand
Fair benefits	• **Benefits to participants during the research**	
	1. **Health improvement:** There are health services essential to the conduct of the research that improve the health of the participants.	Hepatitis A vaccine provided to all participants.
	2. **Collateral health services:** There are health services beyond those essential to the conduct of the research provided to the participants.	Hepatitis B vaccine for all participants; surveillance and triage of illnesses.
	• **Benefits to population during the research**	
	3. **Collateral health services:** There are additional health care services provided to the population.	Hepatitis B vaccine for health care workers and teachers; unlimited disposable syringes and needles.
	4. **Public health measures:** There are additional public health measures provided to the population.	Improved refrigeration at rural health stations; FM wireless network for rural health stations; correction of hygiene deficiencies in schools, report on epidemiology of childhood mortality.
	5. **Employment and economic activity:** There are jobs in the research project for the local population and spending that stimulates the local economy.	Some employment of research personnel.
	• **Benefits to population after the research**	
	6. **Availability of the intervention:** If proven effective, the intervention should be made available to the population.	Registration of hepatitis A vaccine and sales, using tiered pricing, on the private market.
	7. **Capacity development:** There is capacity development through improvements in health care physical infrastructure, training of health care and research personnel, and/or training of health personnel in research ethics.	Limited training and preparation for vaccine trials.

Table 2 *(continued)*

Principles		Benchmarks	Hepatitis A Vaccine Thailand
	8.	**Public health measures:** There are additional public health measures provided to the population.	Identification of possible mechanisms to reduce motor vehicle accidents.
	9.	**Long-term collaboration:** The particular research trial is part of a long-term research collaboration with the population.	Part of a long-term collaboration and may have facilitated securing HIV vaccine trial.
	10.	**Financial rewards:** There is a plan to share fairly with the population the financial rewards and/or intellectual property rights related to the intervention being evaluated.	No sharing of financial rewards.
Collaborative partnership	11.	**Free, uncoerced decision making:** The population is capable of making a free decision, there are no threats, and the population can refuse participation in the research.	Rejecting the trial was possible.
	12.	**Population support:** After receiving an explanation of—and understanding—the nature of the research trial, the risks and benefits to individual subjects, and benefits to the population, the population targeted for the research voluntarily decides it wants the research to proceed.	Consultation with the provincial population, government, and teachers; approval by Ministry of Public Health.
Transparency	13.	**Central repository of benefits agreements:** An independent body creates a publicly accessible repository of all formal and informal benefits agreements.	No repository existed, but the absence of reasonable availability and the provision of benefits were publicly discussed with the government and provincial population.
	14.	**Community consultation:** Forums with populations that may be invited to participate in research, informing them about previous benefits agreements.	

study is the relevant group to receive benefits and determine their fairness. Indeed, determination of whether the distribution of benefits is fair depends on the level of benefits received by those members of the community who actually participate in the research, for it is they who bear the burdens of the interaction. However, each benefit of research does not have to accrue directly to research participants but could benefit the entire community. For instance, capacity development or enhanced training in ethics review could be provided to the community. The important determination is how much the participants will benefit from these measures. In addition, the community will likely bear some burdens and impositions of the research because its health care personnel are recruited to staff the research teams, and its physical facilities and social networks are utilized to conduct the study. Thus, to avoid exploitation, consideration of the benefits for the larger community may also be required. However, analysis of exploitation as inhering in micro-level transactions makes clear that there is no justification for including an entire region or every citizen of a country in the distribution of benefits and decision making, unless the whole region or country is involved in bearing the burdens of the research study.

Principle 2: Collaborative Partnership

The population being asked to enroll determines whether a particular array of benefits is sufficient and fair. Currently, there is no shared international standard of fairness; reasonable people disagree.[31] More important, only the host population can determine the value of the benefits for itself. Outsiders are likely to be poorly informed about the health, social, and economic context in which the research is being conducted, and are unlikely to fully appreciate the importance of the proposed benefits to the population. Furthermore, the population's choice to participate must be free and uncoerced; refusing to participate in the research study must be a realistic option. While there can be controversy about who speaks for the population being asked to enroll, this is a problem that is not unique to the fair benefits framework. Certainly, even—or especially—in democratic processes unanimity of decisions cannot be the standard; disagreement is inherent. But how consensus is determined in the absence of an electoral-type process is a complex question in democratic theory beyond the scope of this chapter.

Principle 3: Transparency

Fairness is relative, determined by comparison with similar interactions. Therefore, transparency—like the full information requirement for ideal market transactions—allows comparisons with similar transactions. A population in a developing country is likely to be at a distinct disadvantage relative to the developed country sponsors in determining whether a proposed level of benefits is fair. To address these concerns, a publicly accessible repository of all benefits agreements should be established and operated by an independent body, such as the World Health Organization. A central repository permits independent assessment of the fairness of benefits agreements by populations, researchers, governments, and others, such as nongovernmental organizations. There could also be a series of community consultations to make populations in developing countries aware of the terms of benefits agreements in other research projects. This will facilitate the development of "case law" standards of fairness that evolve out of a number of agreements.

Together with the three background conditions, these three new principles of the fair benefits framework ensure that (1) the population has been selected for good scientific reasons; (2) the research poses few net risks to the research participants; (3) there are sufficient and long-lasting benefits to the population; (4) the population is not subject to a coercive choice; (5) the population freely determines whether to participate and whether the level of benefits is fair given the risks of the research; and (6) the repository offers the opportunity for comparative assessments of the fairness of the benefit agreements.

Application to the Hepatitis A Vaccine Case

We can compare the reasonable availability requirement with the fair benefits framework in the case of Havrix, an inactivated hepatitis A vaccine.[32] Was the Havrix study ethical? While all the study participants received hepatitis A and B vaccines, the Havrix study did not fulfill the reasonable availability requirement. There was no prior agreement to provide the vaccine to all the people in Kamphaeng Phet province. Since most Thais would not be able to afford the vaccine, committing to registering and selling it on the private market does not seem to fulfill the requirement, making the trial unethical no matter what other benefits were provided to the Thai population.

Conversely the fair benefits framework requires a more multifaceted assessment. First, the study did seem to fulfill the background requirements of social value, fair subject selection, and favorable risk-benefit ratio. Hepatitis A was a significant health problem in northern Thailand and recognized as such by the Thai Ministry of Health. Although the population in Kamphaeng Phet province was poor, the epidemiology of hepatitis A provided an independent scientific rationale for site selection. The preliminary data indicated that the candidate vaccine had an excellent safety profile and probable protective efficacy, suggesting a highly favorable risk-benefit ratio for participants.

What were the benefits of the Havrix trial (table 2, column 3)? By design, all 40,000 children in the trial received both hepatitis A and hepatitis B vaccines. In addition, regional medical services were augmented. The research team contracted with the community public health workers to examine all enrolled children absent from school at their homes, to provide necessary care, and, if appropriate, to arrange transfer to the district or provincial hospital.

There were also benefits for the provincial population. Public health stations throughout Kamphaeng Phet province that lacked adequate refrigeration to store vaccines, medicines, and blood specimens received new refrigerators. Similarly, rural health stations lacking reliable access to the existing FM wireless network link with the provincial hospital's consultants were joined to the network. In the six schools that had hepatitis A outbreaks during the study, the research team arranged for inspection of the schools and identification of deficiencies in toilet facilities, hand-washing facilities, and water storage contributing to the outbreak. At each school, the researchers contracted and paid to have recommended improvements implemented. In addition, public health workers were provided with unlimited stocks of disposable syringes and needles, as well as training on measures to reduce the incidence of blood-borne diseases. Hepatitis B vaccinations were provided to all interested government personnel working on the trial, including approximately 2,500 teachers, public health workers, nurses, technicians, and physicians. Since deaths of enrolled research participants were tracked and investigated, the research team identified motor vehicle accidents, especially pedestrians struck by cars, as a major cause of mortality in the province and recommended corrective measures.[33] Finally, although there was no long-term commitment made by SmithKline Beecham at the initiation of the trial, the training of Thai researchers and experience in conducting the Havrix trial may have facilitated subsequent trials, including the current HIV vaccine trials in Thailand.

Regarding the principle of collaborative partnership, there were extensive consultations in Kamphaeng Phet province prior to initiating and conducting the trial. The provincial governor, medical officer, education secretary, and hospital director provided comment before granting their approval. In each of the 146 participating communities, researchers made public presentations about the study and held briefings for interested parents and teachers. Each school appointed a teacher to maintain liaison with the research team. Parental and community support appeared to be related to the provision of hepatitis B vaccine to all participants, since it was perceived to be a major health problem and the children lacked access to the vaccine. Furthermore, the protocol was reviewed by the Thai Ministry of Public Health's National Ethical Review Committee, as well as two institutional review boards in the United States. The Ministry of Public Health appointed an independent committee composed of thirteen senior physicians and ministry officials to monitor the safety and efficacy of the trial. Importantly, refusing to approve or accept the trial did appear to be an option, since there were serious efforts by some Thai scientists to prevent the conduct of the trial, such as writing to the National Ethics Review Committee to reject it.

At the time of this trial, there was no central repository of benefits agreements to fulfill the transparency principle. However, the measures taken to benefit the population, including provision of the hepatitis A and B vaccines and registering of Havrix in Thailand, were discussed with the Ministry of Public Health and provincial officials and then published.

Did the Havrix study provide fair benefits? Clearly some in Thailand thought not. They argued the trial did not address a pressing health need of the country in a manner appropriate to the country, but did address a health interest of the U.S. Army. Second, some allege there was insufficient technology transfer. In particular, there was no training of Thai researchers to conduct testing for antibody to hepatitis A and other laboratory skills. Third, it was claimed that inadequate respect was accorded to the Thai researchers as none were the study's principal investigators, and none was individually named in the original protocol, but were simply referred to as "Thai researchers." Only after protests were they individually identified. (The American investigators vehemently deny this charge as factually inaccurate.) A prominent vaccine researcher summarized the sentiment against Thai participation:

> Journalists in the country have accused the government and medical community of a national betrayal in allowing Thai children to be exploited. . . . The role of Thailand in rounding up its children for immunization was hardly seen as a meaningful partnership in this research aim. In private, government ministers agreed with this, but the sway of international politics and money was too persuasive.[34]

Conversely, many argued that benefits to the population of Kamphaeng Phet province were sufficient, especially given the minimal risk of the study. Still others are uncertain, arguing that the level of benefits is not clearly inadequate, although more long-term benefits could have been provided to the community depending on the level of benefits to the sponsors, in this case how much SmithKline Beecham profits from vaccine sales. To address the uncertainty of how much a company might benefit from drug or vaccine sales, some propose profit-sharing agreements that provide benefits to the community related to the actual profits.

Importantly, universal agreement is a naïve and unrealistic goal. The goal is consensus among the population to be enrolled in the trial. Consensus on the appropriateness of a research study acknowledges that some disagreement and dissent are not only possible but likely, and even a sign of a healthy partnership.[35] Ultimately, it is the decision of the community—not us—to determine whether the benefits are sufficient to justify research participation. The national ministry, provincial governmental and health officials, and Kamphaeng Phet population seemed to support the trial.

The fair benefits framework makes the considerations of the community much more nuanced and realistic. Rather than having a litmus test of just one type of benefit, the fair benefits framework takes into account all the various ways the community might benefit from the research as relevant in the community's evaluation.

Conclusion

At least since the publication of the CIOMS guidelines, providing reasonable availability of a proven intervention "to the inhabitants of the host community or country at the completion" of a trial has been viewed as necessary to avoid exploitation and, therefore, a requirement for ethical clinical research in developing countries.[36] The precise content of this requirement is not only contentious, but also seriously flawed. It mistakes providing a specific type of benefit with the need to provide a fair share of benefits to avoid exploitation. Furthermore, it applies only to a very narrow range of research, successful Phase III studies, and ignores other substantial benefits to the population that can accrue from the conduct and results of research.

Clearly, it is an ethical imperative that populations receive sufficient benefit from research in which they participate. However, we reject reasonable availability as the only way to fulfill this requirement. Instead, we propose an alternative: the fair benefits framework. Compared with the reasonable availability requirement, the three principles—fair benefits, collaborative partnership, and transparency—are more likely to ensure that populations in developing countries are not exploited, benefit from clinical research, and retain decision-making responsibility.

The Participants in the 2001 Conference on Ethical Aspects of Research in Developing Countries

EGYPT

Maged El Setouhy
Department of Community, Environmental, and Occupational
     Medicine
Ain Shams University

GHANA

Tsiri Agbenyega
Department of Physiology
University of Science and Technology
School of Medical Sciences

Francis Anto
Navrongo Health Research Centre
Ministry of Health

Christine Alexandra Clerk
Navrongo Health Research Centre
Ministry of Health

Kwadow A. Koram
Noguchi Memorial Institute for Medical Research
University of Ghana

KENYA

Michael English
Centre for Geographic Medicine Research-Coast
Kenya Medical Research Institute (KEMRI) & Wellcome Trust
    Research Laboratories

Rashid Juma
Center for Clinical Research
Kenya Medical Research Institute (KEMRI)

Catherine Molyneux
Centre for Geographic Medicine Research-Coast
Kenya Medical Research Institute (KEMRI) & Wellcome Trust
    Research Laboratories

Norbert Peshu
Centre for Geographical Medicine Research-Coast
Kenya Medical Research Institute (KEMRI)

MALAWI

Newton Kumwenda
University of Malawi College of Medicine

Joseph Mfutso-Bengu
Department of Community Health
University of Malawi College of Medicine

Malcolm Molyneux
Director, Malawi-Liverpool-Wellcome Trust Research Programme
University of Malawi College of Medicine

Terrie Taylor
University of Malawi College of Medicine
Department of Internal Medicine
College of Osteopathic Medicine

MALI

Doumbia Aissata Diarra
Department of Pharmacy and Dentistry
University of Mali

Saibou Maiga
Department of Pharmacy and Dentistry
University of Mali

Mamadou Sylla
Department of Pharmacy and Dentistry
University of Mali

Dione Youssouf
Eglise Protestante Bamako Coura

NIGERIA

Catherine Olufunke Falade
Post-Graduate Institute for Medical Research and Training
University of Ibadan College of Medicine

Segun Gbadegesin
Department of Philosophy
Howard University

NORWAY

Reidar Lie
Department of Philosophy
University of Bergen

TANZANIA

Ferdinand Mugusi
Department of Internal Medicine
Muhimbili University College of Health Sciences

David Ngassapa
Department of Anatomy
Muhimbili University College of Health Sciences

UGANDA

Julius Ecuru
Uganda National Council for Science and Technology

Ambrose Talisuna
Resource Centre
Ministry of Health

UNITED STATES

Ezekiel J. Emanuel
Department of Clinical Bioethics
National Institutes of Health

Christine Grady
Department of Clinical Bioethics
National Institutes of Health

Elizabeth Higgs
Parisitology and International Programs
National Institutes of Health, NIAID, DMID

Christopher Plowe
Malaria Section, Center for Vaccine Development
University of Maryland Medical School

Jeremy Sugarman
Center for the Study of Medical Ethics and Humanities
Duke University Medical Center

David Wendler
Department of Clinical Bioethics
National Institutes of Health

Notes

1. Michele Barry, "Ethical Considerations of Human Investigation in Developing Countries: The AIDS Dilemma," *New England Journal of Medicine* 319 (1988): 1083–86; Marcia Angell, "Ethical Imperialism? Ethics in International Collaborative Clinical Research," *New England Journal of Medicine* 319 (1988): 1081–83; and N. A. Christakis "The Ethical Design of an AIDS Vaccine Trial in Africa," *Hastings Center Report* 18, no. 3 (1988): 31–37.

2. Peter Lurie and Sidney Wolfe, "Unethical Trials of Interventions to Reduce Perinatal Transmission of the Human Immunodeficiency Virus in Developing Countries," *New England Journal of Medicine* 337 (1997): 853–56; Marcia Angell, "The Ethics of Clinical Research in the Third World," *New England Journal of Medicine* 337 (1997): 847–49; Harold Varmus and David Satcher, "Ethical Complexities of Conducting Research in Developing Countries," *New England Journal of Medicine* 337 (1997): 1003–5; Robert Crouch and John Arras, "AZT Trials and Tribulations," *Hastings Center Report* 28, no. 6 (1998): 26–34; Christine Grady, "Science in the Service of Healing," *Hastings Center Report* 28, no. 6 (1998): 34–38; Robert Levine, "The 'Best Proven Therapeutic Method' Standard in Clinical Trials in Technologically Developing Countries," *IRB: A Review of Human Subjects Research* 20 (1998): 5–9; and B. R. Bloom, "The Highest Attainable Standard: Ethical Issues in AIDS Vaccines," *Science* 279 (1998): 186–88.

3. World Medical Association, Declaration of Helsinki, 2000, at www.wma .net/e/policy12-c_e.html; Council for International Organizations of Medical Science (CIOMS), *International Ethical Guidelines for Biomedical Research Involving Human Subjects* (Geneva: CIOMS 1993); P. Wilmshurst, "Scientific Imperialism: If They Won't Benefit from the Findings, Poor People in the Developing World Shouldn't Be Used in Research," *British Medical Journal* 314 (1997): 840–44; and P. E. Cleaton-Jones, "An Ethical Dilemma: Availability of Anti-retroviral Therapy after Clinical Trials with HIV Infected Patients Are Ended," *British Medical Journal* 314 (1997): 887-88.

4. World Medical Association, Declaration of Helsinki, *supra* note 3.

5. Medical Research Council of the United Kingdom, *Interim Guidelines— Research Involving Human Participants in Developing Societies: Ethical Guidelines for MRC-Sponsored Studies* (London: MRC, 1999); Joint United Nations Programme on HIV/AIDS (UNAIDS), *Ethical Considerations in HIV Preventive Vaccine Research* (Geneva: UNAIDS, 2000); National Consensus Conference, *Guidelines for the Conduct of Health Research Involving Human Subjects in Uganda* (Kampala, Uganda: National Consensus Conference, 1997); and

Medical Research Council of South Africa, *Guidelines on Ethics for Medical Research*, (1993), www.sahealthinfo.org/ethics.

6. Leonard Glantz et al., "Research in Developing Countries: Taking 'Benefit' Seriously," *Hastings Center Report* 28, no. 6 (1998): 38–42; George Annas and Michael Grodin, "Human Rights and Maternal-Fetal HIV Transmission Prevention Trials in Africa," *American Journal of Public Health* 88 (1998): 560–63.

7. National Bioethics Advisory Commission, *Ethical and Policy Issues in International Research: Clinical Trials in Developing Countries* (Washington, DC: U.S. Government Printing Office, 2001); and Howard Shapiro and Eric Meslin, "Ethical Issues in the Design and Conduct of Clinical Trials in Developing Countries," *New England Journal of Medicine* 345 (2001): 139–42.

8. *Id.* at 142.

9. Annas and Grodin, *supra* note 6.

10. Ezekiel J. Emanuel, David Wendler, and Christine Grady, "What Makes Clinical Research Ethical?" *Journal of the American Medical Association* 283 (2000): 2701–11.

11. *Id.* at 27. See also Robert Levine, *Ethical and Regulatory Aspects of Clinical Research*, 2nd ed. (New Haven, CT: Yale University Press, 1988).

12. Nick Black, "Evidence Based Policy: Proceed with Care," *British Medical Journal* 323 (2001): 275–79.

13. See Wilmshurst, *supra* note 3; and Medical Research Council of South Africa, *supra* note 5.

14. Glantz et al., *supra* note 6.

15. Alan Wertheimer, *Exploitation* (Princeton, NJ: Princeton University Press, 1996), chap. 1; and Ezekiel J. Emanuel, Xolani E. Currie, and Allen Herman, "Undue Inducement in Clinical Research in Developing Countries: Is It a Worry?" *Lancet* 366 (2005): 336–40.

16. Jennifer S. Hawkins and Ezekiel J. Emanuel, "Clarifying Concerns about Coercion," *Hastings Center Report* 35, no. 5 (2005): 16–19.

17. Wertheimer, *supra* note 15.

18. Allen Buchanan, *Ethics, Efficiency and the Market* (Totowa, NJ: Rowman and Allanheld, 1985), 87.

19. Allen Wood, "Exploitation," *Social Philosophy and Policy* 12 (1995): 136–58.

20. Wertheimer, *supra* note 15.

21. Christine Korsgaard, "The Reasons We Can Share: An Attack on the Distinction between Agent-Relative and Agent-Neutral Values," in *Creating the Kingdom of Ends* (New York: Cambridge University Press, 1996).

22. Wertheimer, *supra* note 15.

23. John Rawls, *Theory of Justice*, rev. ed. (Cambridge, MA: Harvard University Press, 1999).

24. Wertheimer, *supra* note 15.

25. Council for International Organizations of Medical Science (CIOMS), *International Ethical Guidelines for Biomedical Research Involving Human Subjects*, (Geneva: CIOMS, 1993).

26. Council for International Organizations of Medical Science (CIOMS), International Ethical Guidelines for Biomedical Research Involving Human Subjects (Geneva: CIOMS, 1993).

27. I. Chalmers, "What Is the Prior Probability of a Proposed New Treatment Being Superior to Established Treatments?" *British Medical Journal* 314 (1997): 74–75; and B. Djulbegovic et al., "The Uncertainty Principle and Industry-Sponsored Research," *Lancet* 356 (2000): 635–38.

28. NBAC, *Ethical and Policy Issues in International Research*, *supra*, note 7.

29. Participants in the 2001 Conference on Ethical Aspects of Research in Developing Countries, "Fair Benefits for Research in Developing Countries," *Science* 298 (2002): 2133–34.

30. Emanuel, Wendler, and Grady, *supra* note 12; and Levine, *supra* note 11.

31. John Rawls, *The Law of Peoples* (Cambridge, MA: Harvard University Press, 1999); and Thomas Pogge, *World Poverty and Human Rights* (Cambridge: Polity Press, 2002), chaps. 1 and 4.

32. See description of case, chapter 2 this volume.

33. B. L. Innis et al., "Protection against Hepatitis A by an Inactivated Vaccine," *Journal of the American Medical Association* 271 (1994): 1328–34; and C. A. Kozik et al., "Causes of Death and Unintentional Injury among School Children in Thailand," *Southeast Asian Journal of Tropical Medicine and Public Health* 30 (1999): 129–35.

34. "Interview with Professor Natth," *Good Clinical Practice Journal* 6, no. 6 (1999): 11.

35. Amy Gutmann and Dennis Thompson, *Democracy and Disagreement* (Cambridge, MA: Harvard University Press, 1996).

36. CIOMS, *supra* note 25.

INDEX

076 regimen: best proven therapy and, 5–6; degree of certainty and, 43; delivery issues and, 2; double standards and, 5; economic issues and, 1–2; placebos and, 3–7; random controlled trials (RCTs) and, 2–3; standard of care and, 3–4; study design and, 4

10/90 gap, 130

active-controlled trials (ACTs), 74, 86–87; community consent and, 93–95; consequentialism and, 154–61; double standards and, 98–99; research ethics and, 30–32, 36; Surfaxin and, 250

acute respiratory distress syndrome (ARDS), 106

Afghanistan, 90

African Americans: American Public Health Service and, 277; HIV/AIDS and, 285n48; Tuskeegee syphilis study and, 3, 18n23, 277

Agbenyega, Tsiri, 308

agency: categorical imperative and, 177–81; degradation and, 184–87; distributive justice theories and, 96, 185–87, 252; humanity and, 179–81; inequality and, 184–87; informed consent and, 177–93; Kantian theory of exploitation and, 181–93; objects of use and, 214–19; subversion of, 182

AIDS. *See* HIV/AIDS

AIDS Clinical Trial Group (ACTG), 1

Alabama, 3

alignment approach, 40–41

American Psychiatric Association, 101n13

American Public Health Service, 277

Androcles, 164–65

Angell, Marcia, 3–4, 12, 18n23, 34, 37, 43

Annas, George, 9–10, 12, 24–26, 103n43, 182–83, 288

Anto, Francis, 308

Arneson, Richard J., 142–74

Arras, John D., 97

avian flu, 132

AZT (zidovudine) trial, 1–2, 21, 246; CIOMS regulations and, 224; clinical equipoise and, 37–38; controlled trials and, 30; cost of, 9–10; cultural issues and, 26–27; Declaration of Helsinki and, 4; degree of certainty and, 39–44; distribution of, 10; dosage and, 40–44; ethics and, 3; Good Samaritan obligation and, 267, 273–75, 278; information from, 249–51; "inseparability of hats argument" and, 266; placebos and, 3–7; standard of care and, 33–35, 224, 238–39; study design ethics and, 3–7

beneficence, 188–90; fair benefits framework and, 298–303 (*see also* fairness); indifference and, 191–93, 204n45; placebo-controlled trials (PCTs) and, 196–201; posttrial benefits and, 194–96; poverty and, 191; reasonable availability and, 225–27, 235–37;